Current Natural Sciences

Carlo ALECI

Visual Rehabilitation of Stroke – A Translational Guide

Science Press | edp sciences

Hemianopia entails the loss of half of one's visual field. The world is halved in hemianopic patients: torn between sight and darkness, just as how the Moon appears to us sometimes divided between light and shadow.

This book seeks to shed light on the obscured aspects of their vision, aiming to restore the fullness of the moon to their sight.

Cover illustration based on image (https://www.pexels.com/photo/half-of-moon-on-black-sky-8795598/) free to use via *Pexels* (https://www.pexels.com/license/). Modification has been applied for adaptation of the book contents.

EDP Sciences – ISBN(print): 978-2-7598-3493-8 – ISBN(ebook): 978-2-7598-3494-5
DOI: 10.1051/978-2-7598-3493-8

Contents

CHAPTER 8
Rehabilitation of Hemianopia: Visual Restitution 91

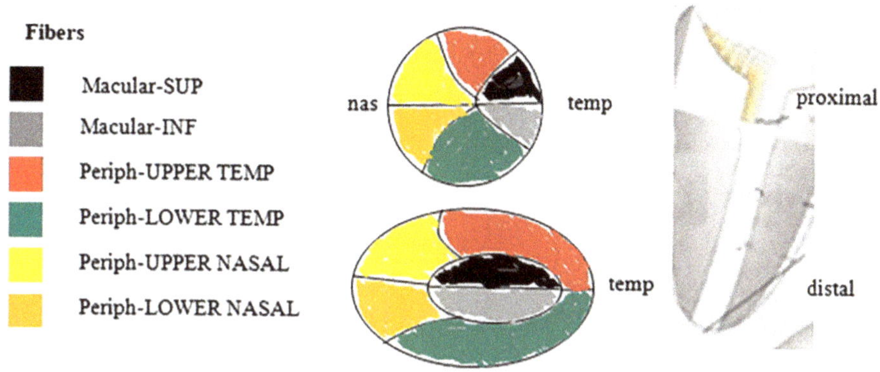

FIG. 1.1 – Topography of the optic nerve. Top: proximal tract (emergence of the optic nerve); bottom: distal intraorbital tract.

In the optic tract, the macular bundle runs in the dorsolateral part, while the lower and upper retinal fibers are localized in the ventrolateral and ventromedial portions, respectively.

The optic tract reaches the lateral geniculate nucleus, a relay station made of six neuronal laminae. Here the signal is transferred to the geniculate ganglion cells that project to the striate cortex *via* the optic radiations.

In the lateral geniculate body, the macular fibers occupy the dorsal (superior) part, and the inferior and superior retinal fibers are localized in the ventrolateral and ventromedial parts, respectively. The projections of the geniculate fibers to the striate cortex emerge from the dorsal part of the lateral geniculate nucleus and form the *optic radiation* (or *geniculocalcarine tract*).

In the optic radiations, the fibers coming from the lower retina loop around the inferior horn of the lateral ventricle (*Meyer's loop or Archambault's loop*) and, *via* the temporal lobe, reach the inferior bank of the striate cortex (lingual gyrus). The geniculocalcarine course of the fibers originating from the superior part of the retina is straight along the parietal lobe and reaches the superior bank of the striate cortex.

Topographically the optic radiations are made up of three bundles:

- the upper (dorsal) bundle that receives projections from the upper portions of the retina of both eyes and reaches the superior bank of the calcarine fissure;
- the central bundle that serves the macular region of both eyes and ends on both lips in the posterior part of the calcarine fissure;
- the lower (ventral) bundle, which receives projections from the lower retina of both eyes, passes through Meyer's loop, and ends in the inferior lip of the calcarine fissure;
- in addition, the uppermost (the most dorsal) and lowermost (the most ventral) part of the optic radiations receives the monocular projection of the inferior and superior peripheral temporal fields, respectively (figure 1.2).

Chapter 1

Recalls of Neuro-Anatomy of the Visual Pathways

It is well known that visual perception begins in the eye but is accomplished by the brain. The visual pathway starts from the cones and the rods, the retinal photoreceptors that transduce light into electric impulses. The electric impulses are transmitted to the bipolar cells then they pass to the retinal ganglion cells. The axons originating from the ganglion cells gather at the posterior pole of the eye forming the first portion of the optic nerve: the optic nerve head or optic disc.[1] The fibers coming from the temporal retina localize in the superior and inferior portion of the optic nerve head, while the nasal bundle forms the nasal and central parts. The macular fibers are in the temporal region. Behind the eye, the intraorbital tract of the optic nerve runs posterior-medially, passes through the optic canal (*intracanalicular tract*), and its intracranial portion reaches the contralateral nerve in the *optic chiasm*, a white matter x-shaped structure located in the forebrain, in front of the hypothalamus. The macular bundle, displaced temporally at the emergence of the nerve, moves centrally in the intracranial portion (figure 1.1).

In the chiasm, the temporal fibers project ipsilaterally to the homolateral optic tract, while the nasal fibers cross the midline (*decussation*) and continue in the contralateral optic tract. The fibers that serve the inferior nasal region of the retina (the upper temporal portion of the visual field) cross the chiasm anteriorly and enter the contralateral optic nerve for about 4 mm, then bend abruptly toward the contralateral optic tract. The knee formed by their course is called the *anterior Wilbrand's knee.* In the posterior part of the optic chiasm, the decussated fibers coming from the superior nasal region of the retina (the lower temporal portion of the visual field) predominate medially and give rise to the *posterior Wilbrand*'s *knee.* The optic tract, therefore, is made up of the ipsilateral temporal fibers and the contralateral nasal fibers (figure 1.2).

The macular fibers form a miniature chiasm, with the decussation of their nasal portion. This explains the occurrence of macular splitting in cases of complete lesions of the optic tract (see section 2.1).

[1]The optic disc is the part of the optic nerve that can be directly inspected at ophthalmoscopy.

DOI: 10.1051/978-2-7598-3493-8.c001

To stimulate interest and prompt the adoption of avant-garde solutions, in this treatise the pathophysiology of hemianopia, its clinical signs and symptoms, and especially the state-of-the-art rehabilitation are described. It is a long translational journey, that sets out from the pioneering studies on the effects of brain lesions in wounded soldiers, passes through the mechanisms of spontaneous compensation of hemianopia, continues with the laboratory results in the psychophysical, electrophysiological, and neuroimaging fields, and comes to describing and discussing the rehabilitative techniques devised in the last decades. Technical details are provided in a series of tables so to make the training procedures replicable step by step. This way, ophthalmologists, orthoptists, and other health rehabilitation personnel can draw inspiration in their daily practice.

This fascinating journey, with its shadows, stops and go, reverses, confirmations, and denials, has not yet come to an end.

But it is firmly determined to re-illuminate the dark side of the Moon in these unfortunate patients.

And you, dear Reader, are going to be the traveler.

Carlo Aleci, March, 2024.

Preface
The Dark Side of the Moon

A consistent amount of patients who suffer from stroke, brain injury, or tumors complain of visual problems. Of these, the most evident is the bilateral loss of light sensitivity in the hemifield contralateral to the damaged hemisphere. This defect, called hemianopia, generates reading and orientation problems and may lead to a profound reduction in the quality of life.

The onset of hemianopia, indeed, is a dramatic event: half of the visual world seems to disappear all of a sudden. And the Moon is always crescent or waning. Never full.

Patients are disoriented, scared by what has just happened, and worried about what will become of their lives. Most of them can no longer drive and independence and sociality are at risk. Add the frustration of not having answers, of not finding solutions. The best neurologists and cardiologists cannot but look for risk factors to reduce to a minimum the probability that a new cerebral accident occurs, and the best ophthalmologists cannot but detect or rule out any concurrent ocular and neuro-ophthalmological disease. In fact, there is nothing they can do to return patients to the wonderful sight of a full Moon.

The Dogma is: "In the brain what is lost is lost". And the Dogma cannot be broken: the vanished part of the visual field is lost forever.

Yet, since the past century research has been challenging the Dogma. Investigations first on animals, then on humans reveal that systematic and repetitive stimulation of the blind region of the visual field helps restore, even if partially, the neuronal function. It is well known that man is a highly adaptive being and specific training may improve the capacity to scan into the lost part of the visual world. Moreover, the intact region of vision can make up for the defective area when appropriate optic devices are developed and applied.

It is weird that despite the high prevalence of stroke and in the face of these experimental efforts visual rehabilitation of hemianopia is not receiving the attention it deserves in the clinical setting.

DOI: 10.1051/978-2-7598-3493-8.c901

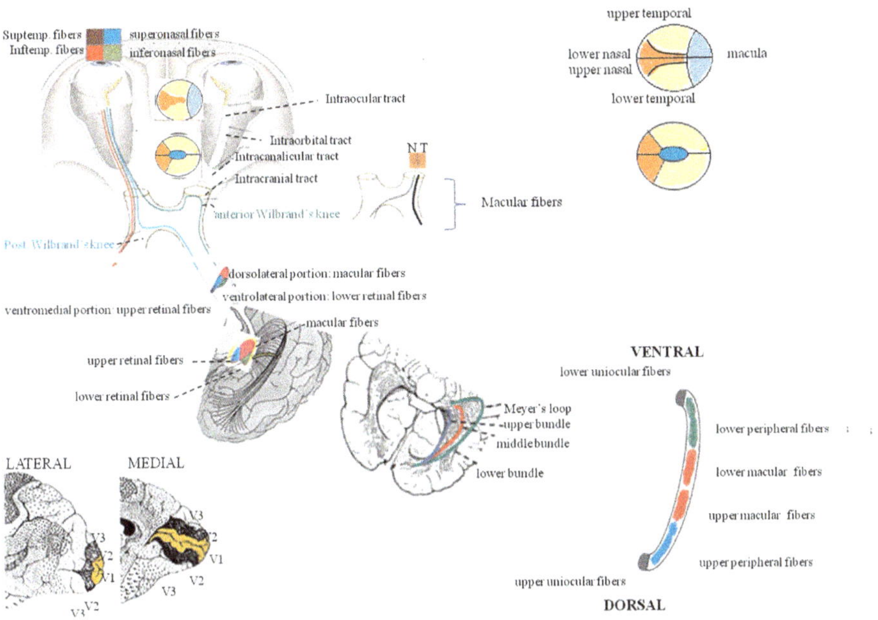

FIG. 1.2 – The visual pathway. See text for explanation.

1.1 Posterior Cerebral Artery

The posterior cerebral artery is the terminal bifurcation of the basilar artery. It passes around the midbrain below the tentorium cerebelli and lies on the medial side of the occipital lobe. Here, it divides into the posterior temporal artery (or *arteries* in 20% of cases), then, more caudally, into two terminal branches: the parieto-occipital artery and the smaller calcarine artery.

The posterior temporal artery, with its branches, anastomoses with the calcarine artery.

The parieto-occipital artery, which terminates in the parieto-occipital fissure, anastomoses with the calcarine artery as well.

The calcarine artery, in turn, heads posteriorly and medially and enters the calcarine fissure (figure 1.3).

Noteworthy, in over 50% of cases, the vascularization of the striate area does not rely solely on the calcarine artery, but it is supplied also by branches of the posterior temporal artery and of the parieto-occipital artery (Kaul *et al.*, 1974). In addition, branches originating from the middle cerebral artery may contribute to feeding the calcarine cortex (McAuley and Russell, 1979), and seem to have a role in the so-called *macular sparing* (see section 2.1).

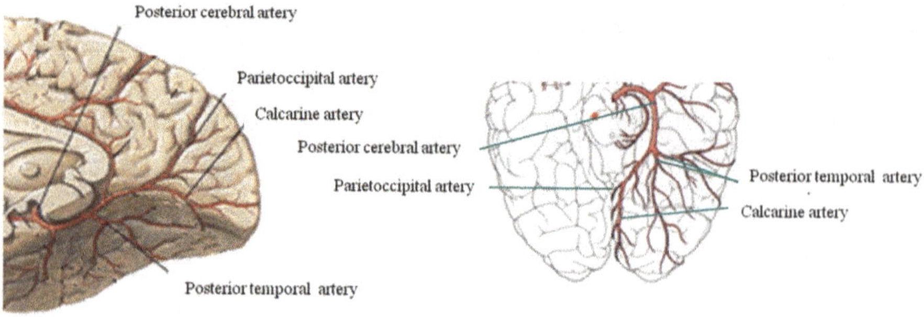

FIG. 1.3 – The vascularization of the occipital region.

1.2 The Visuotopic Mapping of the Visual Cortex

Since the beginning of the last century, a strand of research faced the issue of mapping the visual field on the striate cortex, that is to say evaluating the location and extent of the calcarine area activated by the stimulation of the central (macular), paracentral, and peripheral regions of the visual field. The first contribution to this issue came from a Japanese ophthalmologist, Tatsuji Inouye (1881–1976), who had the occasion, as a medical officer during the Russo-Japanese War (1904–1905), to study the visual defects in head-wounded soldiers. As recalled by Lindegger and Pless (2019), the Russians were using a new rifle (the Moisin Nagant model 91) that fired small-caliber, relatively high-velocity bullets. Since penetration was well-demarcated and did not cause widespread damage, some Japanese soldiers hit by these projectiles survived. By relating the visual field with the injured parts of the occipital cortex of 29 wounded soldiers, Inouye translated the lesions on the scalp into brain spatial coordinates and devised a map that represents the visual field on the striate cortex.[2]

In his map, the upper and lower visual field was represented on the inferior and superior lip of the calcarine fissure, respectively. In addition, the cortical representation of the macular region was located on the occipital pole and was disproportionately large compared to the rest of the visual field.

A confirmation of the findings of Inouye was provided some years later by Holmes, who studied, with the procedure of the Japanese researcher, patients who suffered from penetrating head injuries during wartime (1914–1918). Like Inouye, Holmes elaborated a map representing the visual field on the occipital cortex. Based on his retinotopic (or visuotopic) representation (and in accordance with what was found by Inouye), the occipital lobe serves the central portion of the visual field whereas the peripheral parts are mapped more rostrally on the striate cortex up to the parieto-occipital junction, with the distance from the occipital lobe that depends

[2]Inouye T. (1909). Die Sehstorungen bei Schussverletzungen der Kortikalen Sehsphare nach Beobachtungen an Versundeten der Letzten Japanische Kriege. W. Engelmann. Translated in English in 2000 as: *Inouye T. Visual disturbances following gunshot wounds of the cortical visual area. Oxford; Oftord University Press, Oxford, 2000.*

on the eccentricity from the fixation point. The upper visual hemifield (lower retina) projects to the inferior part of the calcarine fissure, while the lower visual hemifield (upper retina) to the superior striate cortex. The distance from the calcarine fissure is a function of the distance from the horizontal meridian (Holmes, 1945).

The retinotopic map of Holmes has been confirmed by later investigations: in their PET study on seven normal volunteers, Fox and colleagues showed that bilateral visual stimulation of the macular region activated, as revealed by increased cerebral blood flow, the posterior lobe of area V1 (Fox *et al.*, 1987). When the stimulation was directed toward the perimacular region, the anterior and superior portions of the striate cortex were activated, even more so for stimulation of the peripheral retina.[3] Using hemifield stimuli the authors confirmed that the upper and lower retina project, respectively, above and below the calcarine fissure (figure 1.4).

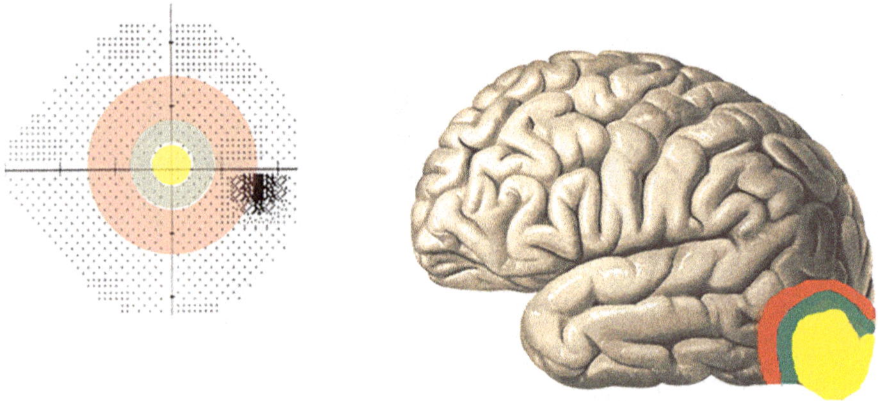

FIG. 1.4 – The pattern of activation of the calcarine cortex during macular, perimacular, and peripheral stimulation. The more eccentric the stimulation, the more rostral the activation on the striate cortex. To be noted is the overrepresentation of the macular region. Adapted from *'Atlas and Textbook of Human Anatomy', 1909, Vol. 3, fig. 626, by Johannes Sobotta and J. Playfair McMurrich. Artist: K. Hajek.*

According to the former estimate of Holmes, up to 25% of the striate area serves the central 15 degrees of the visual field (Holmes, 1945). In revisiting the Holmes'map, Horton, and Hoyt stated with magnetic resonance that the representation of the central 15 degrees of the visual field on V1 is wider, encompassing up to 70% of the total occipital surface[4] (Horton and Hoyt, 1991). Upon this basis, the authors reckoned that testing the central 30 degrees informs about 83% of the

[3]Macular stimulation: anulus 1.5 deg wide made of black and white checks 0.5 deg wide; perimacular stimulation: anulus 5.5 deg wide with checks 1 deg wide; peripheral stimulation: anulus 15.5 deg wide with checks 2 deg wide.

[4]The central 1 deg encompasses 10 mm of striate cortex, and the central 5 deg project to 27.6 mm of striate cortex.

whole visual field. Yet, as pinpointed by Landau and colleagues (1995), a missing temporal crescent (see below section 2.2) generated by a neoplasm can be overlooked in this case.

In substantial accordance with the finding of Horton and Hoyt, McFadzean and colleagues found that the central 10 degrees are represented by 50%–60% of the striate cortex (McFadzean *et al.*, 1994). In turn, Wong and Sharpe (1999) reckoned in a sample of patients with occipital lesions that 37% of the surface of the medial occipital cortex processes the central 15 degrees, and presented a refined visuotopic map of the striate cortex. Their estimate is closer to the measure of Holmes than that of Horton and Hoyt.[5] The same authors provided a correlation between the extent of the stimulated visual field (in terms of eccentricity) and the corresponding extent of the activated striate area (as a percentage). This correlation is linear (figure 1.5).

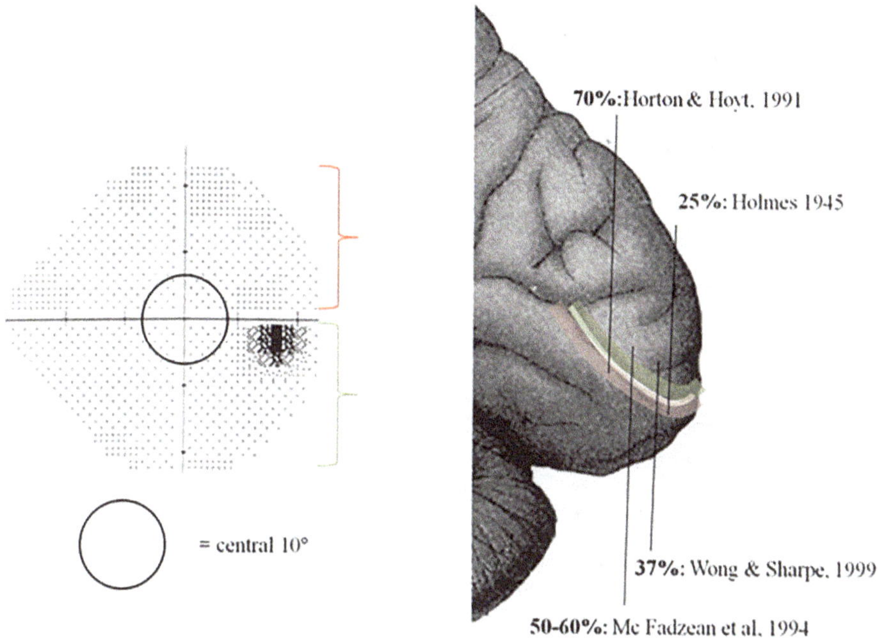

FIG. 1.5 – The visuotopic map on the striate cortex. See text for explanation. The proportions are approximate.

[5]It is worth recalling that not only V1, but also V2, V3, and V4 show a retinotopic representation (Sereno *et al.*, 1995). In this respect, the activation of V1 is accompanied by a significant activation of the peristriate cortex (V2) according to a PET study (Fox *et al.*, 1987). These results were confirmed by a fMRI investigation (Belliveau *et al.*, 1991).

The linear extent of the striate cortex to which each degree of the retina projects, that is to say, the millimeters of cortex per degree of visual angle as a function of eccentricity, is called the *cortical magnification factor*.[6] At 2 degrees of eccentricity, the cortical magnification factor is approximately 4 mm/degree and declines monotonically to 0.5 mm/degree at 25 degrees of eccentricity.[7] The cortical magnification factor emphasizes the central visual field and is directly proportional to visual acuity (Cowey and Rolls, 1974).

[6]The term *Cortical Magnification Factor* (M) was originally coined by Daniel and Wiitteridge in 1961. *Daniel PM, Whitteridge D. (1961). The representation of the visual field on the cerebral cortex in monkeys. Journal of Physiology, 159: 203–221.*

[7]Computed in the lower visual field. Horton and Hoyt (1991) provided a formula to estimate the cortical magnification factor: $M_{linear}(e) = 17.3/(e + 0.75)$, where e is the eccentricity. So, according to this equation, at 2 degrees of eccentricity, 1 degree of the visual field is represented by 6.29 mm of cortex.

Chapter 2

Damage to the Visual Pathways: Perimetric Patterns

Overall, as many as 20%–30% of patients affected by stroke and attending a rehabilitation center have severe visual field defects, including hemianopia (Pambakian and Kennard, 1997; Rossi *et al.*, 1990). In particular, Pambakian reckoned that up to 70% of patients with stroke involving the posterior cerebral artery suffer from hemianopia to a variable extent (Pambakian *et al.*, 2005). The high frequency with which a cerebral injury affects vision should not be surprising given the high proportion of visual fibers in the brain and the size of the cortical visual areas. In the presence of central (*i.e.* cerebral) damage, the visual loss typically manifests itself in terms of visual field defect.

Taking the optic chiasm as a topographical reference, the perimetric patterns due to lesions to the optic pathway can be classified as *prechiasmal*, *chiasmal*, and *retrochiasmal*.

The prechiasmal visual field defects result from an injury to the left/right optic nerve along its course from the posterior pole of the eye to the optic chiasm; the damage produces in the same eye a scotoma localized in the region of the visual field contralateral to the lesion while the visual field of the fellow eye remains intact. If, for example, an orbital tumor exerts compression to the temporal side of the left optic nerve, the nasal portion of the left visual field will be affected to a variable extent, whereas the right visual field will be normal.

When the fibers serving the foveal region are spared, central visual acuity is retained; when all the fibers of the optic nerve are involved, complete loss of vision, *i.e.* amaurosis, takes place.

Chiasmal lesions like pituitary tumors, craniopharyngiomas, sphenoidal meningiomas, and other suprasellar/perisellar tumors may generate bitemporal (heteronymous) hemianopia. The term "heteronymous" indicates that the contralateral hemifields of the two eyes (the left hemifield of the left eye and the right hemifield of the right eye) are affected. The temporal hemifields are lost bilaterally because the decussating nasal projections of each eye are closer to the pituitary/sellar region than the temporal fibers. The characteristics and pattern of progression of the bitemporal defects depend on the position of the lesion and on the

DOI: 10.1051/978-2-7598-3493-8.c002

direction of its extension. For example, hypophyseal tumors may initially give rise to bitemporal superior or inferior quadrantanopia, depending on the anterior or posterior direction of the neoplastic compression. It is worth recalling that, due to the asymmetric extension of the lesion, the temporal hemianopic defect (shape and extent) generally differs to a certain extent in the two eyes (*i.e.* the resulting visual field defects are not completely congruous).

Rarely heteronymous hemianopia can be binasal. This occurs when the compression is exerted laterally toward the chiasm (for instance in the presence of a carotid aneurysm) with its subsequent dislocation. Initially, a homolateral nasal hemianopic defect is expected (the temporal fibers homolateral to the lesion are affected); then, the lateral dislocation of the chiasmatic lamina leads to a contralateral involvement of the temporal fibers, generating a contralateral nasal hemianopic scotoma.

Complete or incomplete homonymous hemianopias are the most represented visual field defects[1] after a lesion of the retrochiasmal visual pathway. The term *homonymous* indicates that the same hemifield (left or right) of the two eyes is affected: after the decussation in the chiasm, the nasal fibers of one eye and the temporal fibers of the fellow eye intermingle so that complete lesions of the postchiasmal left or right pathway generate a loss of the ipsilesional temporal hemifield and of the contralesional nasal hemifield (*homonymous hemianopia*).

In most of the cases (about 70%), homonymous hemianopia follows a posterior cerebral artery infarction (Zhang *et al.*, 2006a, 2006b; Brandt *et al.*, 1995; Trobe *et al.*, 1973) or an occlusion of the middle cerebral artery. Embolism is the most common cause (Pessin *et al.*, 1987; see also The Age-Related Eye Disease Study (AREDS)[2]). Hemorrhages and tumors are other (less frequent) causes.

As recalled by Plow and colleagues (2009), also an infarction of the anterior choroidal artery may determine hemianopia by affecting the optic tract, the lateral geniculate body, or the optic radiation.

When the optic tract is involved, complete or highly incongruous incomplete homonymous hemianopia as well as an afferent pupillary defect (RAPD) and atrophy (pallor) of the optic disc are observed. More rarely Behr's pupil[3] and hemianopic pupillary reaction (Wernicke's sign[4]) is found (Savino *et al.*, 1978). Band or "bow-tie" atrophy of the disc and the nerve fiber layer may occur in the contralateral fundus after some time (Newman and Miller, 1983).

As a rule of thumb, the more caudal the lesion, the more congruous (*i.e.* overlapping) the hemianopic defects. To be considered that the optic radiations fan

[1]In up to 57%–66% of the patients (Rowe *et al.*, 2009; Suchoff *et al.*, 2008; MacIntosh, 2003; Clisby, 1995; Freeman and Rudge, 1988).

[2]Age-Related Eye Disease Study Research Group. The Age-Related Eye Disease Study (AREDS). Natural History Study and Clinical Trial: Design Implications. AREDS Report No 1. Control Clin Trials. 1999; 20: 573–600.

[3]Behr pupil is a condition of a larger pupil (midriasis) controlateral to the side of the damaged hemisphere that occurs in cases of optic tract lesions or cerebral infarction (Herman, 1975).

[4]The Wernicke's sign is the pupillary constriction when light is presented in the normal hemifield associated with failure in constriction when light is presented in the blind hemifield.

out across the parietal and temporal region to reach the occipital cortex: due to the widespread disposition of the fibers, it is unlikely for a lesion to disconnect entirely the occipital cortex from the left or right radiation. As a result, the superior or inferior part is generally preserved so that complete homonymous hemianopia is rarely observed and a quadrantanopia or incomplete hemianopia is more common.

The calcarine lesions can be classified as:

- anterior, when the part adjacent to the parieto-occipital sulcus is involved (10% of the striate cortex). In isolate anterior lesions, the so-called "missing temporal crescent" may occur and the macular function is generally preserved in the affected hemifield ("macular sparing");
- posterior, when the occipital lobe (and the operculum) is interested (50%–60% of the striate cortex). Localized posterior lesions affect the central (10 degrees) contralesional visual field, with loss of the contralesional central visual hemifield corresponding to the macular region ("macular splitting"). In other terms, when the damage is cortical, the visual field around the fixation point is generally spared in the affected hemifield, unless the damage extends to the occipital pole and the operculum;
- intermediate, when the damage is localized between the part adjacent to the parieto-occipital sulcus and the occipital lobe (McFadzean *et al.*, 1994; figure 2.1).

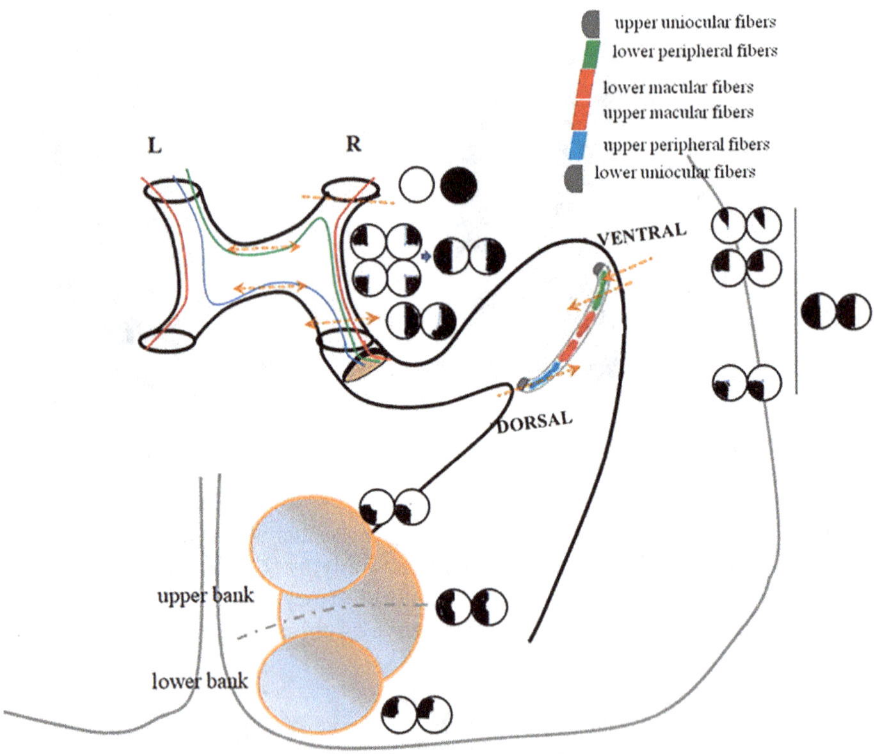

FIG. 2.1 – Damage to the visual pathways and the corresponding perimetric patterns.

2.1 Macular Splitting, Macular Sparing, and Foveal Sparing

As recalled, a prechiasmal damage of the temporal fibers leads to a hemianopic nasal defect and an injury to the nasal fibers produces a hemianopic temporal defect whose severity depends on the extent of the lesion. When the retrochiasmal pathway is affected, a left/right homonymous hemianopia takes place due to the decussation of the nasal fibers. As explained in chapter 1, the projections of the macular ganglion cells located nasally to the foveola are displaced contralaterally, whereas the projection of those located temporally remains ipsilateral in the chiasm.[5] In the presence of a retrochiasmatic lesion, the decussation of the macular fibers sharply splits the macular visual field so that it is abolished in the contralesional region (*macular splitting*).

However, between two-thirds to three-fourths of the surviving patients with left/right-sided occipital infarction show preserved central visual acuity with sparing of the portion of the visual field corresponding to the macular region (Leff, 2004). *Macular sparing* refers, indeed, to retained central visual function in the affected hemifield in the presence of homonymous hemianopia (figure 2.2).

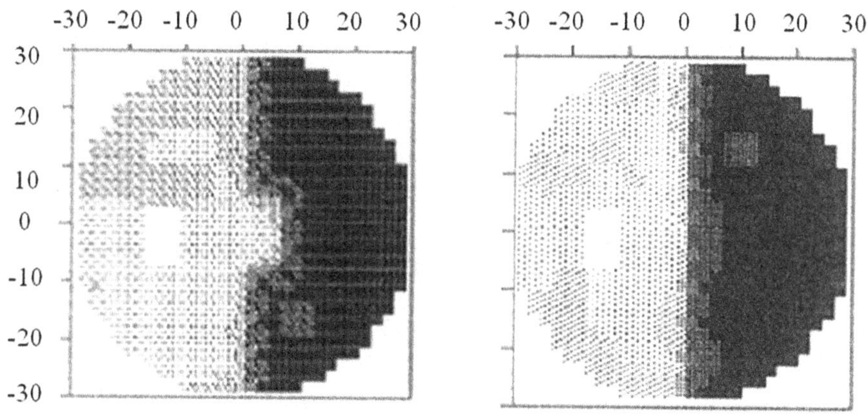

FIG. 2.2 – Macular sparing (left panel) and macular splitting (right panel).

According to McFadzean and colleagues (1994), macular sparing occurs in case the occipital pole and the operculum are fed not only by the calcarine artery but also by an occipital branch of the posterior cerebral artery and of the middle cerebral artery, that, in about half of the subjects, serve as corollary vessels.[6] In these cases,

[5]In the cat and other non-primate mammalians like the grey squirrel and the tree shrew, the projection of the ganglion cells displaced temporally is both ipsi- and contralateral (Stone *et al.*, 1973).

[6]Smith and Richardson (1966).

in fact, the blood supply to the posterior pole and the operculum is preserved despite occlusion of the calcarine artery. On the contrary, when only the calcarine artery vascularizes the whole striate cortex and is occluded, the posterior pole and the operculum will be affected as well, causing macular splitting. In sum, when calcarine infarcts involve the occipital pole (and the operculum), contralateral homonymous hemianopia with macular splitting is expected (figure 2.3).

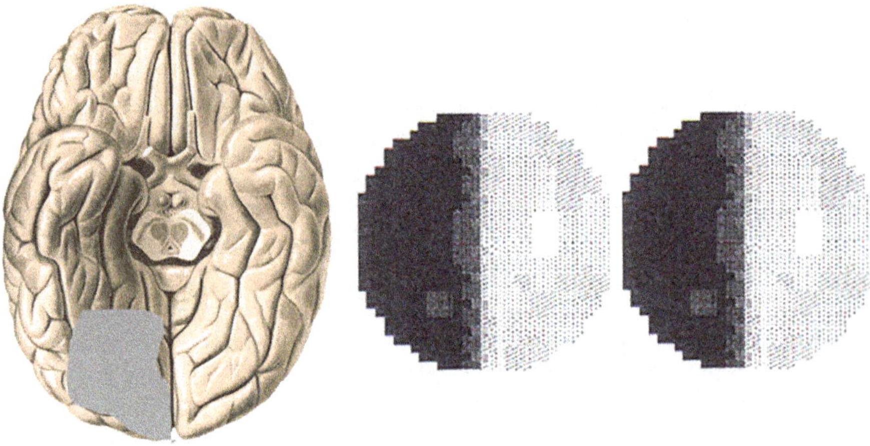

FIG. 2.3 – Lesion of the right occipital lobe including the operculum leads to left homonymous hemianopia with macular splitting.

Macular sparing and foveal sparing are not synonyms. "Foveal sparing" was defined by Huber as a strip of perception in the foveal region of patients with occipital lobectomy detected at perimetry (Huber, 1962). Its extent is consistently smaller than macular sparing (foveal sparing: from 0.5 to 2 deg on either side of the vertical meridian (Reinhard and Trauzettel-Klosinski, 2003; Trauzettel-Klosinski and Reinhard, 1998; Bunt and Minckler, 1977; Bunt *et al.*, 1977; Stone *et al.*, 1973), macular sparing: up to 5 degrees on either side of the vertical meridian). In addition, if the cortical "vascular" theory accounts for macular sparing, foveal sparing is supposed to have a retinal origin.

A strand of research, indeed, supports a bilateral representation of the foveal visual field on the striate cortex (see Lavidor and Walsh, 2004 for references). Stone and colleagues found in monkeys a retinal strip across the fovea formed by ganglion cell fibers that project to the ipsilateral optic tract intermingled with ganglion cell fibers that project to the controlateral optic tract (Stone *et al.*, 1973). The vertical strip of overlap on the retina was about 150 μ wide, corresponding to 1 deg of visual angle (0.5 deg into each hemifield: Stone *et al.*, 1973: figure 2.4).

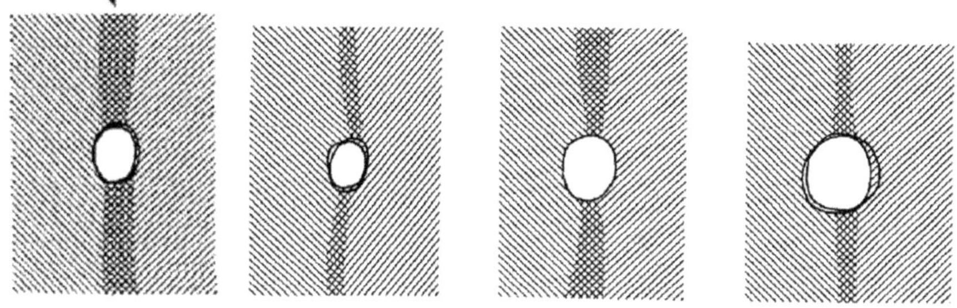

FIG. 2.4 – The vertical strip overlap on the retina of four monkeys ((Macaca irus). From Stone *et al.* (1973). With permission of Wiley Online Library.

According to the authors, the overlap generates a bilateral representation of the central visual field in the primary visual cortex, and this accounts for the residual central vision in post-stroke patients.

Previous and subsequent studies support the finding of the group of Stone (*e.g.* Reinhard and Trauzettel-Klosinski, 2003; Trauzettel-Klosinski and Reinhard, 1998; Huber, 1962, 1992; Terao *et al.*, 1982; Bunt and Minckler, 1977; Bunt *et al.*, 1977[7]; Stone, 1966, but see Lavidor and Walsh, 2004). Since the overlap does not extend beyond 2 deg maximum in the blind hemifield, it is too small to explain the extent of the macular sparing. Macular sparing and foveal sparing, therefore, are likely to rely upon different mechanisms (a double vascular supply for macular sparing *vs.* the peculiar overlapping distribution of the foveal fibers for foveal sparing). Foveal sparing, indeed, can be found even in the absence of macular sparing as in the case of optic tract lesions (Trauzettel-Klosinski and Reinhard, 1998)[8] and of occipital lobectomy with ablation of the whole occipital pole (Huber, 1962). The existence of foveal sparing in hemianopic patients, indeed, has been reported in terms of a vertical strip about 0.5 deg wide in the foveal region. The border of the strip in the hemianopic field can be a straight line or it may show a widening in the upper and lower peripheral region, but it does not expand centrally. Instead, in the foveal region it narrows (Reinhard and Trauzettel-Klosinski, 2003).

The possibility that foveal sparing is an artifact that depends on light scattering of the perimetric stimuli, unstable fixation, scanning eye movements (as hypothesized by Bischoff *et al.* (1995) in their SLO study), or eccentric fixation has been ruled out by Reinhard and Trauzettel-Klosinski (2003).

It remains that, as recalled by Plow and colleagues (2009), homonymous hemianopia is always accompanied by foveal sparing (0.5–1°).

[7]The group of Bunt estimated the overlapping to be about 1.5 deg toward either side of the vertical meridian. Huber computed 1.5–2 deg (1962, 1992).

[8]But see the problems related to the lateral displacement of retinal elements (cones, bipolar, and ganglion cells) in Leff (2004).

2.2 The Monocular Temporal Crescent

The most peripheral temporal portion of the visual field, extending from 60 to 107 degrees lateral to fixation,[9] is called the *temporal crescent* (Lepore, 2001). The temporal crescent projects to the most rostral part of the striate area, *i.e.* adjacent to the parieto-occipital sulcus. This is a peculiar region as it contains only contralateral projections from the outermost nasal retina and lacks ocular dominance columns (Horton *et al.*, 1990).[10] Remarkably, a missing temporal crescent is the only monocular field defect due to retrochiasmal lesions.

The first cases of missing temporal crescent were reported in 1937 by Bender and Strauss. More recently, Landau and colleagues correlated the perimetric finding with MRI imaging of two subjects (Landau *et al.*, 1995). The first patient was a 47-year-old woman with recurrent ophthalmic migraine in the right visual field. Goldmann perimetry revealed on the right eye a peripheral defect on the temporal side, wider in the upper quadrant, whereas the visual field of the left eye was normal. MRI showed a vascular malformation in the left temporo-occipital region, involving mainly the anterior part of the striate cortex. The authors deduced that damage to the most rostral portion of the striate cortex[11] was responsible for the missing temporal crescent (figure 2.5).

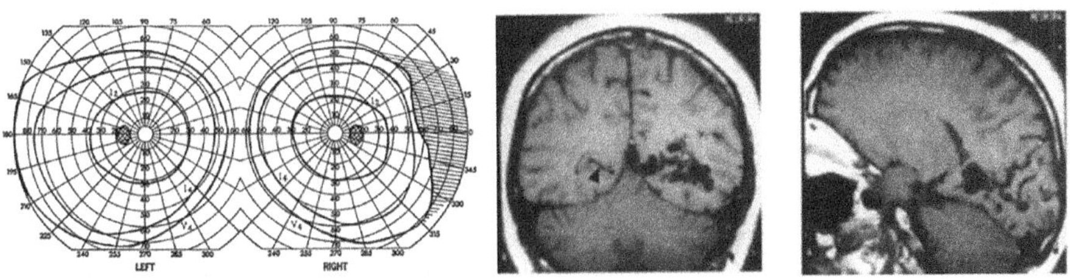

FIG. 2.5 – Missing temporal crescent. The first case was described by Landau and colleagues. In the right panel is shown the T_1 MR imaging showing the vascular malformation in the anterior part of the occipital cortex. From Landau *et al.* (1995). With permission of Elsevier.

The second patient was a 27-year-old woman with recurrent ophthalmic migraine. As in the first case, Goldmann perimetry revealed a peripheral defect on the temporal side in the right eye, wider in the lower quadrant, whereas the visual

[9] The temporal visual field extends up to 107 degrees, and the nasal field does not extend beyond 60 degrees.

[10] The arrangement of the ocular dominance columns in the human primary visual cortex is very similar to that reported in the macaque monkey: a mosaic of irregular parallel stripes oriented at right angles to the boundary of V1. In the rostral part of the striate cortex, the ocular dominance columns of the ipsilateral eye get fragmented until they disappear altogether at the border of the cortical region serving the monocular crescent.

[11] Even if more rarely, a missing temporal crescent can follow a lesion of the posterior part of the optic radiation.

field of the left eye was normal. MRI showed a localized post-stroke lesion in the left anterior striate area, superior bank, of the calcarine fissure.[12]

Rather than being abolished, the temporal crescent can be partially or completely preserved in the blind hemifield of patients with homonymous hemianopia (Lepore, 2001; Benton *et al.*, 1980) or quadrantanopia (McFadzean and colleagues, 1994). Lepore reported sixteen cases (mean age: 62 years) with partial or complete monocular sparing of the temporal crescent. All the subjects suffered from a cerebrovascular event involving the occipital lobe and, in a minority of cases, the optic radiations. In these patients, imaging showed sparing of the most rostral region of the striate cortex, adjacent to the parieto-occipital cortex (Lepore, 2001). McFadzean and colleagues described a case of preserved temporal crescent in left homonymous

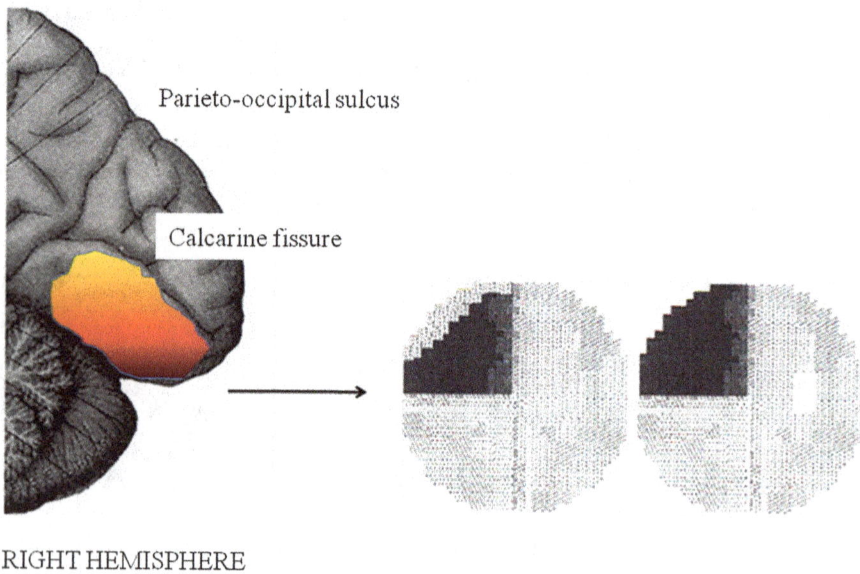

FIG. 2.6 – Simulation of left superior homonymous quadrantanopia with a temporal crescent. A right occipital infarct involves the striate cortex with sparing of the inferior calcarine cortex adjacent to the parieto-occipital sulcus.

[12]Upon considering 215 abnormal (but non-glaucomatous) visual fields, Wellings stated that all the defects due to lesions to the visual pathways can be detected by testing the central 30 degrees; examining the more peripheral regions is unnecessary (Wellings, 1989). In fact, "[...] it is rare for an abnormality to be detected in the peripheral part of the visual field without a defect in the more central visual field." [p. 332]. And yet, cases of missing temporal crescent demonstrate that automated perimetric testing restricted to the 30 central visual fields (as it usually occurs in the clinical practice) informs about as much as 83% of the visual cortex but it is unable to reveal a missing temporal crescent, sign of a rare cerebral lesion in the rostral portion of the striate cortex. For this reason, Goldmann perimetry with the largest stimulus should be included in the clinical protocol (Lepore, 2001; Landau *et al.*, 1995).

quadrantanopia following a right occipital infarction involving the superior bank of the striate cortex with sparing of the calcarine cortex adjacent to the parieto-occipital sulcus. Residual sensitivity of the more peripheral temporal region (temporal crescent) was observed when the 76 degrees of the visual field of the left eye were tested (Humphrey's "crescent program"). An example of a preserved temporal crescent is depicted in figure 2.6.

Interestingly, in the study of Lepore 75% of the patients with a temporal crescent in the right eye developed a reading disability. These were probably cases with involvement of the white matter in the striate cortex; in addition, 44% of the whole sample had release hallucinations (phosphenes, lines, dots, geometric shapes).

2.3 Concluding Remarks

To summarize, a chiasmatic lesion determines heteronymous hemianopia or quadrantanopia (depending on the extent of the damage to the optic fibers); retrochiasmatic lesions to the optic radiations or the striate cortex generate homonymous hemianopias more congruent and more often incomplete compared to a more anterior injury, like damage to the optic tract. Macular sparing is generally a characteristic sign of a cortical lesion, finally, a missing or preserved temporal crescent in one eye can be observed when the most rostral region of the striate cortex is damaged or spared, respectively.

Zhang and colleagues (2006a, 2006b) classified incomplete homonymous hemianopias[13] as follows:

- partial homonymous hemianopias (a portion of the visual field in the scotomatous side is preserved);
- homonymous quadrantanopias (homonymous visual field defects restricted to the superior or inferior quadrant on the left or right side);
- homonymous hemianopias with macular sparing (5 to 25 deg of central visual field preserved in the affected hemifield);
- homonymous central defects (a homonymous loss of sensibility in the central visual field of both eyes enclosed in an area of normal sensitivity);
- homonymous sectoranopias (symmetrical superior and inferior wedge-shaped defects with vertical steps and pointing at the fixation). This pattern can be observed in case of isolated damage to the lateral geniculate nucleus;
- missing temporal crescent.

Light sensibility in the hemianopic region can be depressed (relative hemianopia) or abolished (absolute hemianopia). The hemianopic defect is called "mixed" when

[13]For the sake of clarity, we define "hemianopia" as the binocular condition where the sensitivity in one hemifield of both eyes is reduced or abolished; in turn, "hemianopic defect" is the monocular loss of the nasal or temporal hemifield. So, for instance, a left homonymous hemianopia results from a temporal hemianopic defect in the left eye and a nasal hemianopic defect in the right eye.

in some regions of the affected hemifield the sensibility is depressed and in others it is abolished.

The damage is rarely restricted to the retinocortical pathway and the occipital areas (V1, V2, V3): it generally extends to a variable degree to the white matter connecting occipital, temporal, parietal, and frontal regions (Schuett *et al.*, 2008a). This way, it may produce complex neuro-ophthalmological patterns, accounting, for example, for visual agnosia, diplopia, or cognitive deficits. Indeed, according to a retrospective study, this occurs in 14% of the patients with prevalent occipital damage (Fujino *et al.*, 1986).

After revising a consistent proportion of cases, Zhang and colleagues provided an exhaustive picture, summarized in table 2.1, of the effect a cerebral damage may have on the visual field (Zhang *et al.*, 2006b).

TAB. 2.1 – Data from Zhang *et al.* (2006b).

Laterality	Type of hemianopic defect		Causes of HH
Left HH: 55% Right HH: 45%	Complete HH: 37.6%		Stroke: 69.7% Trauma: 13.6% Tumors: 11.3% Demyelination: 1.4% Other causes: 4%
	Incomplete HH: 62.4%	Homonymous quadrantanopia: 29.2%	
		Homonymous central defects: 12.8%	
		Partial HH: 12.6%	
		HH with macular sparing: 7.3%	
	Associations	Location of the lesion	
	Isolated: 46.5% Associated with diplopia; 14.6% Associated with motor deficits: 34.5% Associated with cognitive deficits: 5.6% Associated with motor and cognitive deficits: 13.5%	Occipital lesions 45% - pure occipital lesions 83.5% - occipitotemporal/ occipitoparietal lesions: 16.5% Optic radiations: 32.2% Optic tract: 10.2% Lateral geniculate nucleus: 1.3% Generalized hemispheric lesions: 11.4%	

Remarkably, damage to the visual field *per se* does not fully account for the perceived vision-related difficulties and consequent degradation of the quality of life of these subjects. Papageorgiou and colleagues examined with a self-questionnaire the ability to perform routinary visual tasks in a group of 33 post-stroke patients (average time from the onset: 2.7 years) with left-sided and right-side homonymous

hemianopic defects and without neglect, aphasia, apraxia, agnosia, physical impairment or cognitive decline. Patients showed a decline in tasks related to near vision (like using hand tools, cooking, and finding objects on crowded shelves) color vision (*e.g.* matching clothes), peripheral vision (*e.g.* avoiding obstacles, vehicles, and people), vision-specific mental health, and driving. Most of the scores actually failed to correlate with the extent of the visual field loss, suggesting that factors other than the perimetric deficit (*e.g.* eye and head movements) play a role in the overall capacity of hemianopic subjects to perform visual tasks in daily living (Papageorgiou *et al.*, 2007).

Reading problems are a main complaint of many patients suffering from brain injury. Indeed, since reading is a complex task that recruits a multi-stage functional activation (from the eye to the higher associative areas), it is not surprising that it is particularly vulnerable to cerebral damage as it occurs in stroke, blood infarction, or tumors. Impaired reading produces a consistent decline in the quality of life, as a great amount of information acquired in the social, educational, and professional fields is conveyed by written documents.

Reading fluently requires correct and fast sequential decoding of words, and successive central integration, and the association of the written sign (grapheme) to the corresponding sound (phoneme).

Brain lesions can affect this complex neural network to varying degrees and with different mechanisms. The reading disability in patients suffering from acquired cerebral lesions, defined as “alexia”,[14] can be associated with aphasic disorders and writing problems (“central alexias”) or may present in isolation (“peripheral alexias”).

In peripheral alexias there is <<[...] a deficit in the processing of visual aspects of the stimulus [Author’s note: the word] that prevents the patient from reliably matching a familiar word to its stored visual form or “visual word form>> (Coslett, 2000, p. 420). From a visual perspective, interest focuses on a particular form of peripheral alexia, namely *hemianopic alexia*, that must be differentiated from *neglect alexia*. In addition, *pure alexia (or alexia without agraphia or letter-by-letter reading)* is worth briefly describing for the close anatomical relationship between the site of the lesion putatively responsible (the so-called VWFA, localized in the left hemisphere between the posterior fusiform gyrus and the inferior temporal gyrus) and the visual occipital areas (see appendix).

2.4 Visual Hallucinations in Hemianopia

Visual hallucinations in the hemianopic field are not a rare occurrence in patients who suffer from occipital lesions. In a retrospective study with 101 patients with homonymous hemianopia, visual hallucinations were reported in about 30% of cases

[14] Even if the terms “alexia” and “dyslexia” are used as synonyms, “alexia” should be reserved for acquired cases of reading disability due to events such as stroke, blood infarction, or tumors, whereas “dyslexia” is a developmental reading disorder diagnosed in childhood.

(Poggel *et al.*, 2007). Since the first report, dating back to 1886,[15] the interest in this topic has grown, and a consistent number of papers have been published: some of them discussed the issue of how to discriminate between epileptic and non-epileptic phenomena (see Kölmel, 1985 for references), others were focused on the phenomenon *per se*. Even if an exhaustive discussion on visual hallucinations in hemianopic patients is tangential to this work, it is worth introducing this topic.

Kölmel interviewed 88 patients with homonymous complete or incomplete hemianopia about visual hallucinations. He found five types of positive phenomena referred by patients in their hemianopic field:

- non-structured (simple) hallucinations in the form of colored or uncolored phosphenes occurring briefly after the onset of the occipital lesion (initial manifestations);
- complex static hallucinations, like rows of small, pale human figures, whose faces were reported to be difficult to recognize;
- complex dynamic hallucinations like marching men or animals or other features (*e.g.* approaching hands) moving from the periphery to the center of the visual field;
- heautoscopia (the patient sees him/herself);
- palinopsia (the identical replication of an object, *e.g.* a gigantic wall of blue tiles stretching from the ground up to the sky). This form of visual delusion differs from monocular diplopia or poliopsia.

Complex hallucinations always occur after the non-structured phenomena, last some days, then decrease in frequency until disappearing as the spontaneous recovery progresses: indeed, hallucinations tend to disappear with the resolution of the hemianopia. This is an important point, as pinpointed by Poggel and associates (see section 8.2.10). During the remission phase, the phenomena tend to reappear in stressful situations.

The frequency of occurrence of visual hallucinations depends on the pre-morbid personality of the patients. However, patients are always aware of the unreality of the phenomenon that they associate with their visual impairment.

According to Kölmel (1985), complex hallucinations are experienced when lesions of the occipital region (that interrupt the flow of visual information to the temporal and parietal lobe) extend rostrally to the subcortical structures so to <<mobilize endogenous visual images>>. However, the strength of neuronal activation (or the loss of inhibition) at the border of the damaged region is more important than the spatial extent of the damage itself (Vaphiades *et al.*, 1996; Anderson and Rizzo, 1994; Kölmel, 1985). Indeed, cortical hyperexcitability at the border of the lesion may be responsible for visual hallucinations (see Eysel *et al.*, 1999), as suggested by their location at the border zone between the seeing and not seeing region (Poggel *et al.*, 2007). An increase in hyperexcitability would determine the switch from simple to complex static hallucinations, then to dynamic hallucinations (in fact, the opposite never occurs). Indeed, according to Lance, the cells of

[15] Seguin EG. A contribution of the pathology of hemianopsis of central origin (cortex-hemianopsia). Journal of Nervous and Mental Disease 1886; 13: 1–38.

the associative cortex are more likely to discharge spontaneously once they are deprived of their normal afferent inflow from the calcarine region, and this would favor the onset of visual delusions (Lance, 1976).

Of interest, hallucinations are reported to disappear with the saccadic movements of the eyes (but not with slow pursuit movements), no matter their direction.[16] Considering that the <<[..] eye movement represents highly ordered volitional activity capable of suppressing the unstable neuronal activity generating complex visual hallucinations>> (Kölmel, 1985, p. 36), multiple possible explanations have been put forward, involving inhibitory impulses from the proprioceptors of the extraocular muscles that reach the cortex *via* the superior colliculi during the saccadic movements (as shown by Donaldson and Long (1980)) and/or the effect of lambda waves, recorded in the occipital lobe during saccadic triggering (Kurtzberg and Vaughan, 1977).

Kölmel found that the involvement of the dominant or non-dominant hemisphere was not relevant to the occurrence of visual delusions, and pinpointed that visual hallucinations in the blind field of hemianopic patients show some features proper of release phenomena (like the latency after the onset of hemianopia, the long duration, and the gradual appearance and disappearance) and other features, namely the frequent stereotyped characteristics, typical of stimulation phenomena like those associated with epileptic seizures.

[16]It is worth reminding for the differential diagnosis that, contrary to complex visual hallucinations associated with hemianopia, epileptic visual hallucinations are not influenced by ocular movements (Kölmel, 1985).

to measure the time required to extract visual information when reading.[5] According to their results, effective foveal and parafoveal processing requires only 50 ms of exposure: now, as the duration of fixations is longer (100–400 ms), the remainder of the fixation time is employed to plan the next saccade (Rayner *et al.*, 1981). Interestingly, the visual space in charge of guiding the saccades during reading goes beyond the fovea and parafovea (the perceptual span) and encompasses a wider and more eccentric region of the visual field (Rayner *et al.*, 1981).[6]

3.2 Saccades

Letters and words must be processed sequentially for the decoding to make sense: so, each fixation has to shift along the string at an even pace. Each repositioning of the fixation is not a smooth movement but it is a sort of leaping and is defined as *saccade* (or FEM, Fast Eye Movement). Saccades are rapid eye movements that move the fixation along the sentence from one letter/syllable to the next one. The direction of the scanning follows the arrangement of the text so that in Western languages the majority of the saccades move from left to right and are referred to as *forward saccades*.

On average, forward saccades are 2 degrees wide so that each one encompasses about 8 characters (McConkie and Zola, 1989). However, as for the fixation time that tends to increase in the presence of difficult texts, forward saccades tend to shorten and their number rises: as a result, the lexical speed is slower when reading demanding passages (Kowler and Anton, 1987).

A small percentage of saccades move in the opposite direction (from right to left): these *regression saccades* bring back the fixation every time the processing of the word has not been satisfactory. Regressions (or *backward saccades*) are shorter than forward saccades and measure about 1 degree, that is 4 letters. Backward saccades are only 15% of the total FEMs (McConkie and Zola, 1989; Rayner, 1978) but their frequency increases with reading difficult or unfamiliar texts (McConkie and Zola, 1989; Rayner and Pollatsek, 1987).

Once the fixation/saccade sequence reaches the end of the line, a wide regression movement, called *return sweep*, repositions the fixation at the beginning of the next line and the process starts again (figure 3.1).

---

[5] Masks 7- and 17-characters wide were superimposed 0–150 ms after the beginning of the fixation to prevent foveal processing. In a second experiment, windows with openings 7- and 17-characters wide were superimposed 0–150 ms after the beginning of the fixation to mask parafoveal processing while allowing foveal processing. The experiment showed that the effective reading rate increased as the mask delay increased, and reached a plateau at a delay of just 50 ms.

[6] Rayner and colleagues used a mask to isolate a window symmetrically centered on the fixation point and extend up to 33 characters (16 characters to the left and 16 to the right of the fixation point: Rayner *et al.*, 1981). The authors measured the size of the forward saccades as a function of the width of the window and found that the saccade length continued to increase up to a window of 29 characters. As the average saccade length encompasses about 7 characters, they came to the conclusion that peripheral regions along the horizontal meridian and distant twice the average saccade length from the landing site play a role in guiding the ocular movement.

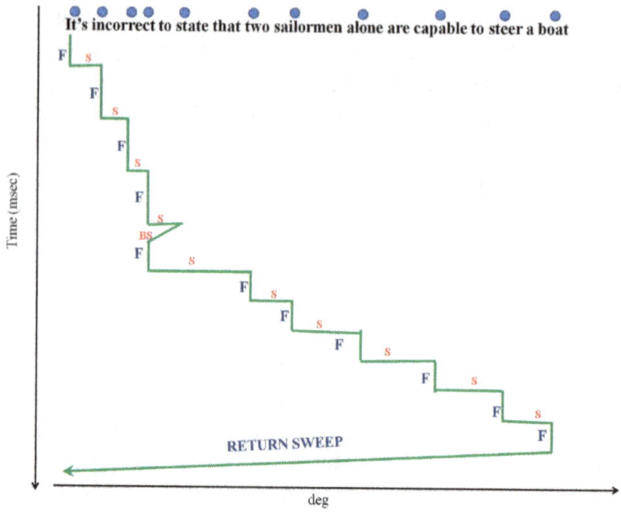

FIG. 3.1 – Schematic representation of the eye movements when reading a line of text ("it is incorrect to state that two sailormen alone are capable to steer a boat"). Abscissa: the amplitude of the saccades that move sequentially along the string; ordinate: (fixation) time. The green line represents the alternation of fixations and saccades. After the first low-frequency (difficult) word, a backward saccade (BS) goes back to the previous fixation. It is to be noted that short, high-frequency words (is, to, that, are, a) are not fixated but foveally pre-processed. In the end, a return sweep moves the gaze back to the beginning of the next line. The dotted spots along the string represent the landing site that matches the preferred viewing location in normal readers (see below).

The position of the fixation depends on the "landing" position of the saccade at the end of its movement. This zone is defined *landing site* and in normal readers is localized between the beginning and the middle of the word (Rayner, 1979) or, according to McConkie, on the third letter of the word (McConkie *et al.*, 1988). This is, indeed, the position that minimizes the fixation time and is therefore called the *preferred viewing location*[7] (*PVL:* Rayner, 1979). The probability of reading correctly a word decreases more and more as the landing site deviates to the left or the right from the PVL. So, the more peripheral the letter fixated (*i.e.* the closer to the beginning or the end of the word is the landing site), the less the information on the word that can be extracted at that fixation, and the higher the probability that a refixation occurs. The relationship is well described by a parabolic function (position of fixation *vs.* frequency of refixation (McConkie *et al.*, 1989: figure 3.2).

[7]The fact that the PVL is not exactly at the center of the word but is slightly shifted to the left allows the recognition of more letters to the right. This is in accordance with the asymmetry of the perceptual span.

Chapter 3

Perceptual and Oculomotor Requirements for Reading

Perceptually, the lexical function relies on the decoding of characters arranged sequentially in the visual space. In the process, the sequential recognition of the symbols as well as of their relative position is crucial. The visual system makes use of fixations and saccades to achieve this goal: fixations are for acquiring information, *i.e.* processing the letters that make up the syllables and the syllables that make up the words; saccades serve to move fixations along the line of text.

3.1 Fixations and the Visual Span

A letter or syllable should fall on the central region of the retina, *i.e.* the fovea, to be identified since the fovea, due to its anatomofunctional structure, has the highest power of resolution. The persistence of a stimulus on the fovea is called *fixation*. When reading, fixations should have an adequate duration: not too short, otherwise the visual system would fail to complete the processing, and not too long, otherwise the reading rate would be too slow.

On average, a fixation lasts 180 ms, but its duration is variable, depending on the difficulty of the text: it may be as short as 30–40 ms and as long as 450 ms (McConkie and Zola, 1989).

Not only foveal processing[1] but also the information provided by the parafoveal region during each fixation, especially on the right side,[2] is critical for fluent reading (Blanchard *et al.*, 1989). In fact, information (shape, length, and

[1]To give an idea of the importance of foveal processing in reading, occluding the fovea with a mask 1 character wide slows down the reading rate from 295 to 160 words per minute (wpm). A mask 3, 5, 7, and 9 characters wide reduces the reading rate to 60 wpm, 50 wpm, 15 wpm, and 10 wpm, respectively (Rayner *et al.*, 1981).

[2]To be noted that the information from the left of the fixation point (the fovea) is not used in ordinary conditions, but when the visual span is restricted (Rayner *et al.*, 1980, 1982; McConkie and Rayner, 1976).

DOI: 10.1051/978-2-7598-3493-8.c003

initial letters) of the word pre-processed by the right parafovea allows faster identification of the same word when it will be foveated at the next fixation. In addition, paracentral processing of short and medium-sized words reduces the probability of their subsequent foveal processing: more precisely, pre-processing a short word (one to three letters) increases the probability that it will be skipped at the next fixation. Preprocessing a medium-sized word (3–5 letters) increases the probability that it will be skipped at the next fixation but if this does not occur it decreases the fixation time of its subsequent (foveal) fixation. Finally, pre-processing a long word (6–10 letters) does not increase the probability it will be skipped at the next fixation, but decreases the duration of its next fixation. This way, parafoveal pre-processing is the main determinant of fixation duration (Blanchard *et al.*, 1989): the (partial) amputation of the right parafoveal region in hemianopic patients (macular splitting or very restricted macular sparing) decreases the probability of skipping short and medium-sized words and prolongs the fixation time of short, medium-sized and long words: as a result reading rate is reduced.

How wide is the visual space (*i.e.* the total number of characters) that can be pre-processed by the parafoveal region during each fixation? First of all, it should be considered that the *visual span*, that is the number of characters readable at each fixation in an extra-lexical context (*i.e.* when the cognitive component is neutralized), is different from the *perceptual span* (or *reading span*), that refers to letters arranged in words (O'Regan, 1990).

Contrary to the visual span, the perceptual span benefits from a cognitive/linguistic anticipatory component that makes it wider compared to the former. This is the reason why in Western readers the perceptual span encompasses up to 11–15 characters (4–5 degrees) to the right of the fixation point[3] and no more than 4 (1–3 degrees) to the left (Rayner and Pollatsek, 1987; Rayner *et al.*, 1980, 1982; McConkie and Rayner, 1975), whereas the visual span is made of 6 letters to the right and 4 letters to the left (Legge *et al.*, 2001).[4]

The parafoveal region not only pre-processes the foveal information extracted at the next fixation, but it helps program the next saccade (Rayner, 1975). Rayner and colleagues used a foveal and parafoveal temporal masking paradigm

[3]Since about 3–4 letters subtend one degree of visual angle in ordinary reading conditions (Leff *et al.*, 2000; Rayner and Bertera, 1979), the perceptual span extends 4–5 deg to the right of the fixation point.

[4]The factors that define the width of the visual/perceptual span are lateral masking (or crowding), the size of the characters, and visual attention. As lateral masking between the characters increases with the eccentricity from the fixation point, beyond a given angular distance the most eccentric characters will be crowded, thereby no more perceivable. Lateral masking is, therefore, a factor that limits the boundary of the visual/perceptual span. In addition, visual acuity decreases with the distance from the fovea so that a letter subtending an angular size that makes it recognizable on the fovea is too small to be recognized beyond a given distance from the fixation point (irrespective of lateral masking). Finally, attentional focus further restricts the span on the left side in Western readers. It is worth recalling that the perceptual span is widely overlapped at each subsequent fixation (Rayner and Bertera, 1979; Ikeda and Saida, 1978).

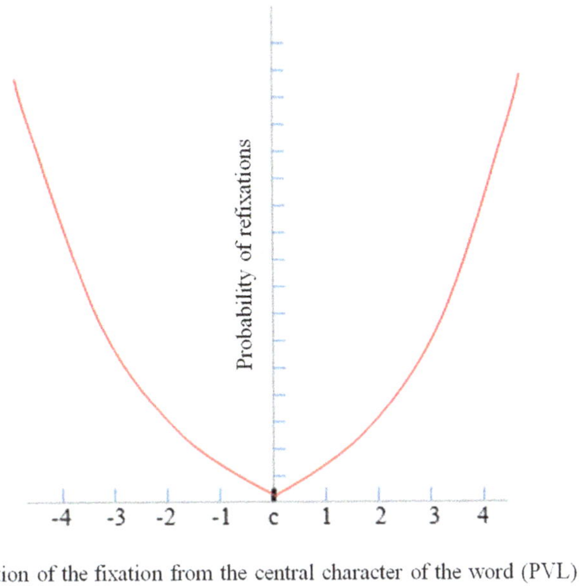

FIG. 3.2 – The parabolic function that relates the distance of the fixated character (the landing site) from the PVL (indicated as "c") with the frequency of refixations.

In sum, the higher the discrepancy between PVL and the actual position of the fixation (the landing site), the lower the information obtained about the word.

Evidently, the correct placement of the fixation depends on adequate saccadic movements: too short or too long saccades drag the fixation to one side or the other side of the preferred viewing location, preventing the correct processing of the word. In this case, additional fixations are required for its recognition (Nazir *et al.*, 1992; McConkie *et al.*, 1989).

3.3 Neuro-Anatomy of the Oculomotor Control

To summarize, from a visual perspective reading fluently requires:

1- normal foveal and parafoveal vision, *i.e.* preserved occipital cortex functioning. This requirement is evident considering the masking effect of a scotomatous hemifield on the left- or right part of the line of text;

2- normal saccadic pattern. A normal saccadic pattern, in turn, refers to:

  i- normal parafoveal (and peripheral) vision, including a visual span wide enough, as seen in the previous section;

  ii- normal functioning of the cortical areas involved in saccadic programming, triggering, and control: of these regions, the Frontal Eye Field paracentral visual loss that prevents text pre-processing (McDonald *et al.*, 2006);

- increased number of backward saccades (thereby more refixations: Schuett *et al.*, 2008a, 2008b; Spitzyna *et al.*, 2007; McDonald *et al.*, 2006; Leff *et al.*, 2000; Trauzettel-Klosinski and Brendler, 1998; Zihl, 1995a; Mackensen, 1962; in simulated hemianopia: Schuett *et al.*, 2009b), especially in RH (Passamonti *et al.*, 2009); in the study of Zihl, left hemianopes showed on average 37% of refixations *vs.*, 44% in right hemianopes: and 15% in controls: (Zihl, 1995a). Of note, there is no dependence of the refixation rate on macular sparing (McDonald *et al.*, 2006);
- reduced width of backward saccades in right-sided hemianopes (McDonald *et al.*, 2006);
- fragmentation of the return sweep into a sequence of small backward saccades in left-sided hemianopia (Trauzettel-Klosinski and Brendler, 1998).

To summarize:
Right hemianopia (RH) is mainly characterized by:

- increased number of forward saccades (and, consequently, fixations);
- reduced size of forward saccades;
- increased duration of fixations;
- increased number of backward saccades thereby of refixations. The higher number of backward saccades depends on the fact that forward saccades on the next word tend to localize more to the left of the preferred viewing location (near the beginning of the word) compared to normal readers[5]: so, refixations are often required to process the words. As pinpointed by McDonald and associates, this finding, which may explain why right-sided hemianopes are less likely to skip short words, is unexpected. In fact, it is not consistent with a compensatory process: a landing site more to the right in right hemianopes would allow more of the word to fall in the intact (left) hemifield, decreasing the number of fixations on the same words and increasing the probability of skipping short words. McDonald and associates explained this lexical behavior: <<fixing to the right of normal runs the risk of placing the initial portion of the word in low acuity left parafoveal vision, and because the beginning of English words is more informative than their endings, this strategy could interfere with word recognition and lead to an excess of regressive saccades>> (McDonald *et al.*, 2006);

[5]Especially for words made of four to seven letters (McDonald *et al.*, 2006).

- reduced width of backward saccades;
- normal return sweep (mean amplitude: 14.7 ± 4.1 deg *vs.* 17.3 ± 3.5 deg in normal subjects: Zihl, 1995a).

In left hemianopia (LH):

- patients have problems finding the beginning of the sentence: the return sweep is fragmented into a sequence of small backward saccades (Passamonti *et al.*, 2009; Schuett *et al.*, 2008a). It follows that on average the return sweep amplitude is smaller than in normal readers (9.4 ± 5.2 deg *vs.* 17.3 ± 3.5 deg in normal readers). It is worth considering that the return sweep needs at least 9 characters (3 degrees with the ordinary print size) of macular sparing to take place (Schuett *et al.*, 2008a). The fragmentation of the return sweep is an inverse function of the distance of the scotomatous border from the fixation point, with a consistent detrimental effect when the distance is lower than 5 deg (Trauzettel-Klosinski and Brendler, 1998).
- the number of backward saccades is higher and their size is reduced (Zihl, 1995a).

Contrary to RH, the size of forward saccades is not decreased (4.1 ± 1.0 *vs.* 4.3 ± 0.7 in normal subjects: Zihl, 1995a).

The main reason for reading slowness in right hemianopia is the increased number of saccades and fixations, as the scotomatous hemifield in the paracentral region hampers the saccadic programming and systematic pre-processing of words on the right side of the fixation point.

In turn, in left hemianopia, the lexical impairment depends mainly on the fragmentation of the return sweep revealing the difficulty in finding the beginning of the new line (Trauzettel-Klosinski and Brendler, 1998). Table 4.1 and figure 4.1 summarize what is reported.

It is evident from table 4.1 and figure 4.1 that the oculomotor pattern is overall less compromised in left-sided hemianopes, and, in fact, reading fluency is better (reading time for a text is almost double and accuracy higher) in LH compared to RH (Zihl, 1995a). In both cases, the proportion of fixations is higher and their duration longer in the affected hemifield, whereas it is normal in the ipsilesional field (Behrmann *et al.*, 1997; Zihl, 1995b; Meienberg *et al.*, 1981).

TAB. 4.1 – Characteristics of the oculomotor pattern in left-sided and right-sided hemianopia during reading.

	Fixations duration	Forward saccades (→ fixations) nb	Forward saccades size	Backward saccades (→ refixations) Nb	Backward saccades size	Return sweep	Dependence fixation-duration-saccade length
RH	↑↑	↑↑	↓	↑↑	↓	~ n	↓↓
LH	↑/n	↑/n	n	↑	↓	Fragmented	↓

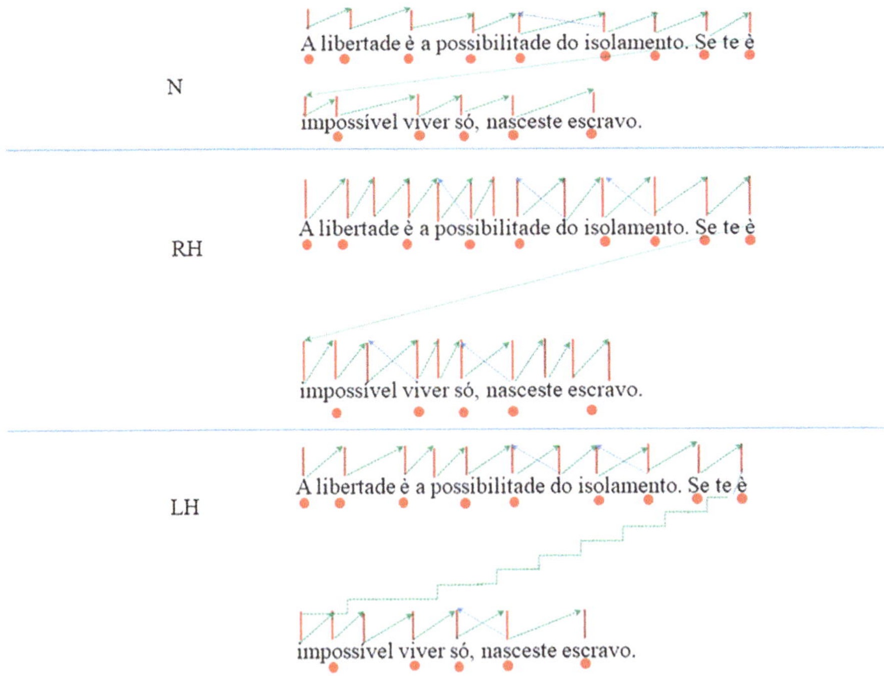

FIG. 4.1 – Characteristics of the oculomotor pattern in left-sided and right-sided hemianopia.

4.3 Visual Field Defect or Cortical Damage: Which is Responsible for the Abnormal Oculomotor Pattern in Hemianopic Dyslexia?

To assess whether the abnormal oculomotor pattern during reading depends on the visual field defect or is mainly related to the cortical damage, Schuett and colleagues studied the oculomotor pattern when reading in a sample of healthy subjects with simulated left- and right-sided hemianopia (with 1 degree of central sparing: Schuett *et al.*, 2009a). The simulation of hemianopia was obtained with the moving-window paradigm (Rayner and Bertera, 1979; McConkie and Rayner, 1975). Subjects with simulated hemianopia read slowly compared to the normal condition, with more fixations, longer fixation durations, more refixations, and shorter forward saccades. These parameters were more compromised in the right-sided simulation. This reading pattern is overall the same as that found in hemianopic patients. This suggests that the reading difficulty in hemianopic patients relies mostly on their visual field deprivation, even if a direct role of the cortical damage cannot be ruled out.

4.4 The Role of Contrast Sensitivity and Visual Attention

Reduced contrast sensitivity (CS) in the presence of normal visual acuity is often associated with cerebral lesions. The loss of CS can be generalized or may be restricted to the medium-high range of spatial frequencies, including 8–10 cycles/deg[6] which is the range most used for decoding words, thereby for reading (Solomon and Pelli, 1994; Bulens *et al.*, 1989; Bodis-Wollner and Diamond, 1976). Actually, Legge and colleagues showed that a reduction in contrast sensitivity may affect reading rate (Legge *et al.*, 1985, 1987) so that, in addition to the disorganized saccadic pattern and the information deprivation due to the hemianopic loss, low contrast sensitivity (when present) may contribute to reducing the lexical fluency. This reduction is related to a prolonged duration of fixations, as longer fixation time is the compensatory mechanism adopted when an elevated contrast threshold hampers the recognition of the letters. So, the reduction of contrast sensitivity to the middle-high spatial frequency, particularly in cases of small macular sparing, may contribute to accounting for the prolonged fixation duration, especially in right-sided hemianopes. Interestingly, the loss at the high spatial frequencies is found to be associated with occipital and temporo-occipital lesions, whereas defects at the low spatial frequencies mainly occur in the presence of temporal or parietal damage (Bulens *et al.*, 1989).

From 16% to 82% of patients with stroke suffer from visuoattentional disorders (Rowe *et al.*, 2011; Rowe and VIS Group UK, 2009): in these cases, top-down visuoattentional modulation, mediated by the frontoparietal areas and physiologically skewed toward the right of the fixation point[7], is disturbed. Visuattentional perturbation, indeed, plays a material role in determining the reading disability in hemianopic alexia: efficient oculomotor adaptation, in fact, is possible only in the presence of efficient visuo-attentional control. When the lesion is restricted to the primary visual cortex, the attentional top-down control of the saccades and their activation at the level of the frontal and parietal cortex is preserved (Schuett *et al.*, 2008a): in these cases, the detrimental effect of the visual field loss on reading is compensated by an efficient, spontaneous oculomotor adaptation. In support of this, Zihl (1995a) found that when the lesion in his

[6]Eight cycles/degree correspond to 3 cycles/letter at a viewing distance of 30 cm and for a character size of 0.2 deg.

[7]The asymmetry is demonstrated psychophysically by the left/right difference in the perceptual span and electrophysiologically by the stronger activation of the left occipital region, of the left posterior parietal cortex, and of the right frontal eye fields compared to the corresponding contralateral regions (Leff *et al.*, 2000). This accounts for the salience of the visual span on the right side over the left side in the Western writing systems, whereas the opposite (visual span wider on the left side) is proper of right-to-left written languages, like Hebrew (Pollatsek *et al.*, 1981).

sample of homonymous patients was limited to the calcarine cortex, without involving the occipital white matter, posterior thalamus, and/or parietal and callosal regions, reading performance was reduced by only 11% and spontaneous recovery of the reading function was observed with no need for rehabilitative intervention.[8] However, if the lesion was larger and extended to part of the ipsilateral occipital white matter, the reduction in reading performance rose to 38%. In the case of more extensive damage to the occipital white matter and the ipsilateral posterior thalamus (structures in charge of the visuo-attentional modulation), the drop in reading performance was up to 68% (Zihl, 1995a).

In substance, despite the severity of the reading problem depends on the entity of the macular sparing (Schuett, 2009; Schuett *et al.*, 2008a), in the presence of lesions of the occipital white matter and/or of the posterior thalamus, a co-existing visu-attentional deficit largely contributes to the problem. Quoting Schuett and colleagues: <<[...] this reading impairment is more than purely visually determined. Hemianopic dyslexia is not caused [*only*: note of the author] by parafoveal visual field loss [..]>> but <<[...] requires widespread damage to the distributed neural network serving the bottom-up and attentional top-down control of visual information processing and saccadic eye-movements in reading. In contrast, patients with sparing of the structures belonging to this neural network usually compensate for their parafoveal visual field loss and show a close to normal reading performance>> (Schuett *et al.*, 2008a, p. 2457).

In conclusion, reading disability of hemianopic patients suffering from stroke (and other cerebral injuries) can be seen as the combined effect of visual hemianopic deprivation, of the oculomotor disorders dependent on the cortical lesion plus the narrowing of the visual span, and of a visuo-attentional disorder (figure 4.2). Hemianopic alexia, indeed, has been defined by Schuett and associates as "*a visual-attentional-oculomotor-network disorder*"[9] (Schuett *et al.*, 2008a, p. 2460).

[8]Interestingly in this case there is evidence that the activation of the posterior parietal cortex is stronger in the hemisphere contralateral to the lesion and that the FEF, PEF, and SEF are bilaterally activated (even if to a lower extent compared to normal subjects). This suggests a re-modulation of the frontal and parietal activation after focal calcarine damage (Nelles *et al.*, 2007).

[9]Within the clinical setting, the demonstration of post-stroke lesions in hemianopic alexics relies on CT and MRI imaging. Yet, there are cases of patients who struggle to read despite low CT/MRI significance or anatomic evidence of the defects. These cases may be explained by functional alterations, as revealed by positron emission tomography (PET), in regions of the brain related to the lexical function and morphologically intact. These "remote effects" (as defined by Zihl), would depend on the interruption of a pre-existing connection between the lesioned subcortical regions and the cortical areas revealed at PET (Bogousslavsky *et al.*, 1988). In support of this, Bosley and colleagues showed that lesions to the optic radiations may lead to changes in glucose metabolism in anatomically intact regions of the brain like the ipsilateral thalamus, and subcortical damage may reduce cortical perfusion (Bosley *et al.*, 1985).

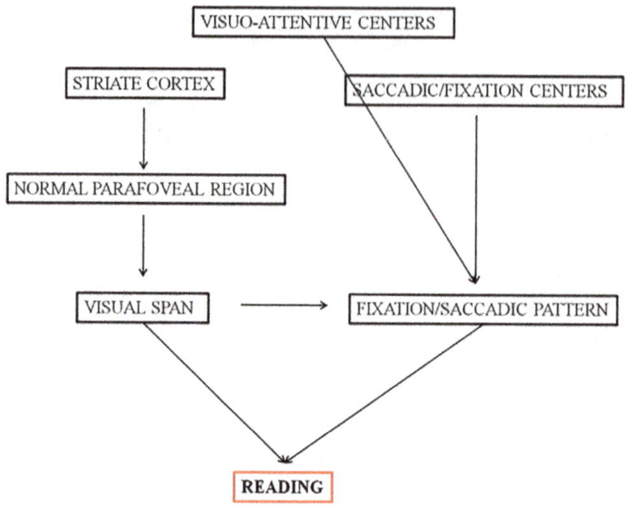

FIG. 4.2 – See text for explanation.

4.5 Quadrantanopia, Paracentral Defects, and Relative Hemianopia

During reading, a preliminary requisite for correct saccade planning is encoding in a coordinate system the visuospatial representation of the boundaries of the text on the page and the visuospatial localization of the words (Kennedy *et al.*, 2003). This process is hampered by hemianopia, whereas a quadrantanopia or (even more) a localized paracentral defect, due to the reduced extent, allows to a various degree the maintenance of such representation. So, the lines above (inferior quadrantanopia) *or* below (superior quadrantanopia), or above *and* below (paracentral scotoma) the string currently fixated can still be used for encoding the boundaries of the text and the relative position of the words, preserving, to a certain extent, the saccadic guidance. This explains why left/right quadrantanopias as well as localized paracentral visual field defects that affect the parafoveal vision degrade the oculomotor pattern, thereby reading, to a lesser extent compared to hemianopia (Schuett *et al.*, 2008a; Zihl, 2000; MacKensen, 1962).

Not only hemianopias and quadrantanopias with absolute visual field loss (light differential sensitivity equal to zero or close to zero) but even relative hemianopias and quadrantanopias (light differential sensitivity partially preserved[10]) affect reading when the parafoveal field is involved (macular sparing less than 4–5 deg: Schuett *et al.*, 2008b). Habekost and Starrfelt (2006) described the case of NS,

[10]The term "cerebral amblyopia" or "hemiamblyopia", used in literature, should be avoided as misleading, and replaced with "relative hemianopia" (where "relative" refers to the depth of the loss of sensitivity, whereas "partial hemianopia" indicates an incomplete hemianopic defect).

a 20-year-old patient who suffered from a cerebral hemorrhage in the left basal occipital lobe and the underlying white matter with sparing of the primary visual cortex. Reading problems were the only complaint of the patient after clinical stabilization. His reading was effortful, slow, and poor in accuracy, with a consistent number of errors, similar to hemianopic alexics. The authors found a relative perimetric defect in the upper right quadrant of the visual field extending 1–2 degrees to the right and 1 degree above the fixation point but failed to relate the presence of this localized loss of sensibility to the reading problem of NS. As a matter of fact, eye movements (saccades mean amplitude, duration of fixations, frequency of regressions) were close to normals.

In a letter to The Lancet (2003), Wang reported the case of a patient with right homonymous hemianopia who was able to read a line almost as before the onset of the cerebral damage by turning her sheet at right angles so that left-to-right turned above-to-below. The author believes that the technique will also work for a patient with left homonymous hemianopia.

Chapter 5

Visual Hemineglect and Neglect Alexia

Strictly speaking, the diagnosis of hemianopic alexia requires the presence of hemianopia and the absence of hemineglect. Patients may suffer from left hemianopia without hemineglect and some patients with left hemineglect have not left hemianopia (Kinsbourne and Warrington, 1962b). Differentiating between left-sided hemianopia and left hemineglect is not easy, especially when they are associated.

Hemineglect or *hemispatial neglect* is a clinical condition following damage of the right inferior parietal cortex or, as stated by Karnath, of the superior temporal gyrus of the right hemisphere (Karnath *et al.*, 2001, 2004; Müller-Oehring *et al.*, 2003).[1] It affects 31%–46% (Allegri, 2000; Dombovy and Aggarwal, 2000) or up to 81%–82% of subjects with right-hemispheric stroke[2] (Stone *et al.*, 1993), and is a negative prognostic factor for functional recovery (Cherney *et al.*, 2001; Sunderland *et al.*, 1987; Denes *et al.*, 1982).

In neglect, the attentional balance between the two hemifields is disrupted so that the attentional focus to the left side is attenuated whereas it is exaggerated to the right side (Kinsbourne, 1987, 1993). In other terms, in hemianopia without neglect, the attentional centers in the left and right hemispheres inhibit reciprocally so that attentional balance is maintained. In neglect, damage to the attentional center in the right hemisphere reduces the right inhibitory input directed toward the left hemisphere: consequently, attention is biased toward the ipsilesional (right) hemifield. Due to the disinhibition of the left hemisphere, the attentional rightward vector is even stronger than in normal subjects (figure 5.1).

[1]There is controversy on the anatomical basis of visual neglect. According to Mort and colleagues, neglect depends on damage to the angular gyrus of the right inferior parietal lobe, whereas lesions to the superior temporal gyrus alone are not sufficient to beget this clinical condition (Mort *et al.*, 2003).

[2]In left brain strokes the prevalence of neglect is 2%–12% (Allegri, 2000).

DOI: 10.1051/978-2-7598-3493-8.c005

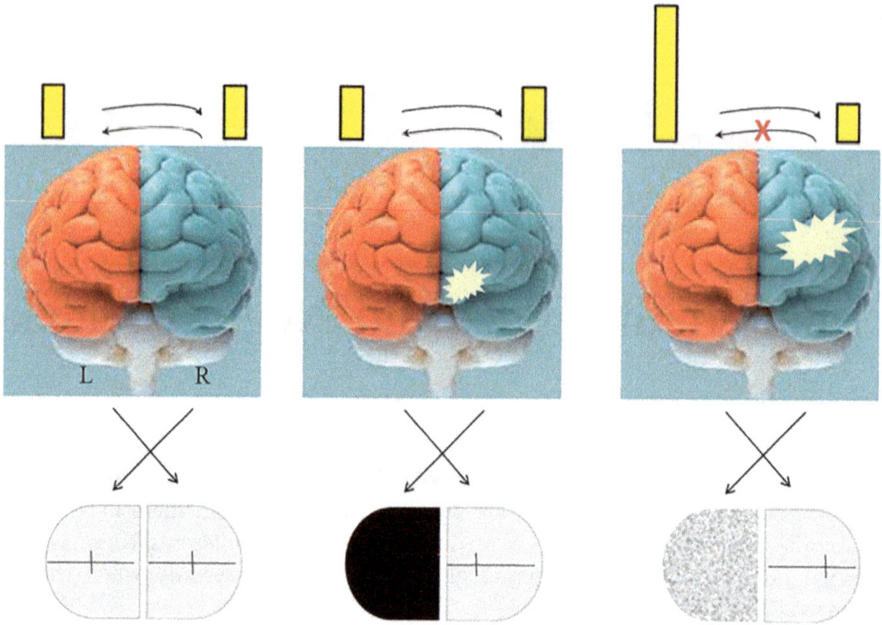

FIG. 5.1 – The model of neglect according to Kinsbourne. Left: normal condition. Middle: hemianopia without neglect: right: left hemineglect. In hemineglect, the attentional balance between the two hemifields is disrupted and the left hemisphere is de-inhibited. It follows that the attentional focus to the left hemifield, driven by the right (damaged) hemisphere, is attenuated, whereas it is exaggerated to the right side. Yellow rectangles: strength of the attentional input in the two hemifields. It is noted that in hemianopia the bisection task is biased toward the blind hemifield whereas in neglect it is biased toward the right (non-neglected) hemifield.

The model of Kinsbourne poses that the difficulty of patients in orienting attention toward the neglected (contralesional) hemifield arises from a difficulty in disengaging visual attention from the ipsilesional space.[3]

[3]The so-called *gap effect* demonstrates that attentional disengagement is crucial: in normal subjects, saccadic latency decreases if a central fixation point is removed before the onset of the target. This suggests that fixation extinction helps disengage visual attention (Walker *et al.*, 1991; Fischer, 1987; Fischer and Bretmayer, 1987; Saslow, 1967). The disappearance of the fixation point before the onset of the stimulus, indeed, decreases the latency of saccades directed toward the target (from 200 ms if the onset of the target and the disappearance of the fixation point are simultaneous to 150 ms if the fixation point is removed 200 ms before the onset of the target: *gap effect*). On the contrary, if the fixation point persists *after* the onset of the target for more than 100 ms, the latency increases to 250 ms (Saslow, 1967).

Likewise, in the *remote distracter effect* a distracter that is presented simultaneously with the target but in the opposite hemifield prolongs the saccadic latency toward the target (Walker *et al.*, 1995, 1997). The *gap effect* and *remote distracter effect* are argued to depend on inhibitory interactions in the superior colliculus (see Ptak *et al.*, 2007 for references).

According to the same author, in subjects with neglect attention decreases progressively from the most eccentric portions of the ipsilesional field to the most eccentric regions of the contralesional space, so that the probability of detecting a target is progressively lower in the more peripheral part of the contralesional hemifield (Kinsbourne, 1970, 1987, 1993).

The group of Behrmann used a visual search task to test this theory (Behrmann *et al.*, 1997): nine neglected patients and nine normal subjects (as well as four hemianopic patients) had to recognize the letter "A" embedded in an array of other letters. Targets were positioned along four pre-established vertical bands. As expected, the performance was worse in the neglect sample, due to a high number of targets omitted on the contralesional side. Patients showed a progressive fall-off of the number of fixations as the target was moved from the ipsilesional to the contralesional hemifield, in agreement with the gradient model of Kinsbourne (figure 5.2).

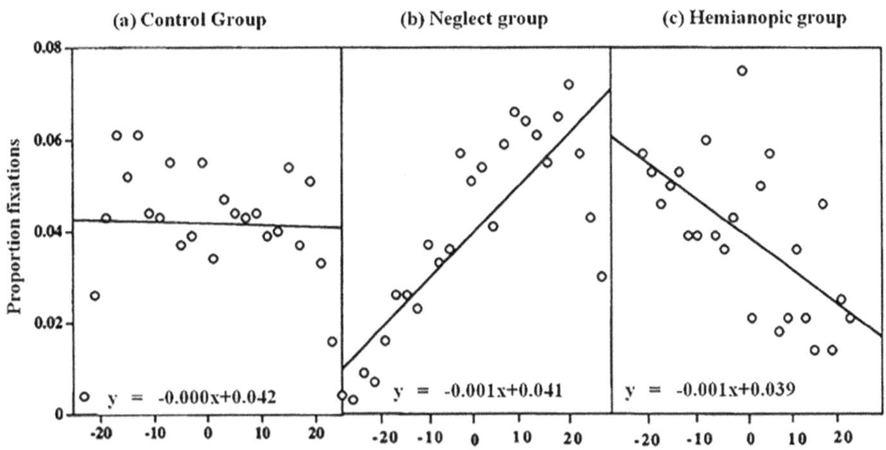

FIG. 5.2 – The proportion of fixations along the horizontal axis for control, neglect, and hemianopic subjects. From Behrmann *et al.* (1997). With permission of Elsevier.

Notably, attention on the ipsilesional side is found to be higher than in normal subjects, as revealed by the longer duration and higher proportion of fixations in the right hemifield compared to non-neglected subjects (Müri *et al.*, 2009; Behrmann *et al.*, 1997).

Since the field of view tested by the group of Behrmann was restricted to ±22.5°, Karnath and colleagues (1998) extended the search area by presenting a stimulus array that surrounded the patients and allowed head movement (*practical field of view*[4]), as it occurs in everyday life. When asked to search for a

[4]It is useful to recall that the *visual field* is the extent of space perceived looking straight ahead, the *field of view* is the extent of space perceived moving the eye, and the *practical field of view* is the extent of space perceived moving both eyes and head.

(non-existent) "A" embedded in an array of other letters, subjects without neglect demonstrated a quasi-flat symmetrical bell distribution of fixations (in terms of exploration time per degree) across the search field, centered to the body axis. On the contrary, patients with neglect showed a bell-shaped distribution displaced to the right (*i.e.* toward the ipsilesional side: figure 5.3). In this study, data obtained within 22.5° were in agreement with the observation of Behrmann (see inset in the rightmost panel), and therefore confirm the model of Kinsbourne. However, the bell-shaped distribution of attention obtained when testing a wider extent of the search field is not consistent with the gradient model. On the contrary, it supports a *deviation model* where patients, like normal subjects, orient their leftward/rightward gaze symmetrically but their egocenter (subjective spatial coordinates) looks deviated ipsilesionally.

In addition, the spatial distribution of fixations across the search field in neglected subjects is narrower compared to normals, and there is a tendency to iterate visual search in previously tested spatial locations.[5] Impairment of the working memory[6] in the ipsilesional hemifield (Husain *et al.*, 2001; Karnath *et al.*, 1998) or a compressed (anisotropic) neural representation along the horizontal axis and toward the ipsilateral side (Halligan and Marshall, 1991) have been invoked to explain this phenomenon.

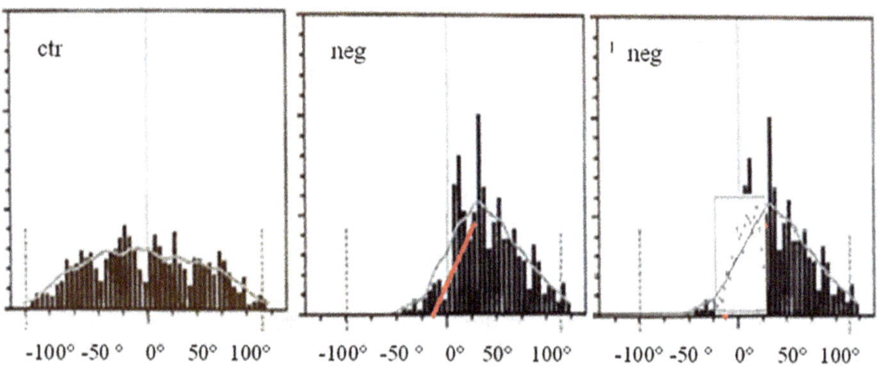

FIG. 5.3 – The flat bell-shaped distribution of fixations across the search field in controls compared to the steep distribution in neglected patients. It is evident the shift of the mode (the subjective egocenter) toward the right. In the right panel, the smooth gradient found by Behrmann, who limited the search field to ±20.5 degrees, is highlighted (compare with figure 5.2, central panel). Modified from Karnath *et al.* (1998). With permission of Oxford University Press.

[5]Neglect patients tend to cancel repeatedly the targets on the ipsilesional side at the cancellation tasks.

[6]The ability to remember which location has already been examined during a visual search depends on the working memory.

5.1 Egocentric and Allocentric Coordinates

As recalled by Hillis and associates (1998), hemineglect may affect the perception of the visual world in different spatial coordinate frames:

i- *Egocentric hemineglect* involves one side of the visual field, of the head, or of the body (Karnath *et al.*, 1997; Chatterjee, 1994; Ladavas, 1987; Bisiach *et al.*, 1985). These three spatial coordinates (retinal-, head-, and body-centered) are defined as *egocentric* or *viewer-centered* and match when, as it commonly occurs, the head and the body are aligned and the eyes are in a primary position.[7] In this form of neglect, the performance worsens when the stimulation is placed farther in the contralesional (left) hemifield or on the contralesional side of the head or the body (Hillis *et al.*, 1998). On the contrary, when the subject looks straight ahead with his trunk rotated 15° to the left relative to the position of the head, the egocenter, actually displaced to the right, shifts to the left, in its ordinary position, and, as a result, left hemineglect improves (Karnath *et al.*, 1997). Chokron and Imbert (1995), indeed, demonstrated in 30 normal subjects with the straight-ahead pointing task (the subject is required to point straight ahead, generally with the eyes closed) a displacement of the egocenter toward the left or to the right when the trunk was rotated 15° respectively to the left or to the right relative to head position. Likewise, the egocenter of the patients with left neglect, that is deviated to the right, shifted to the left by about 17° when the subject turned his body 15° to the left;

ii- *allocentric hemineglect* affects one side of the stimulus, irrespective of its position in the visual field (to the left or to the right) or of the position of the head or the body midline (Tipper and Behrmann, 1996; Hillis and Caramazza, 1995; Chatterjee, 1994; Driver *et al.*, 1994; Driver and Halligan, 1991). This spatial coordinate frame is defined as *allocentric* or *stimulus-centered.* In this form of neglect, performance worsens as a function of the distance of the examined part of the configuration from the center of the stimulus on the side of the contralesional visual space. Instead, the performance does not depend on the position of the stimulus relative to the viewer's visual field, or head/body axis.

In summary, when the boundary between neglected and non-neglected space is the mid-sagittal plane of the patient (his visual field, head, or body), the affected spatial reference is *egocentric*, whereas when the boundary is the center of the object it is *allocentric.*[8]

[7] When the subject looks to the left or to the right with his head and body aligned, the retinotopic-centered coordinate is dissociated from the head- and body-centered coordinate (Ladavas, 1987; Bisiach *et al.*, 1985). Likewise, when the viewer looks straight ahead with his head turned to the left or to the right, the head- and retinal-centered coordinates are dissociated from the body-centered coordinate.

[8] Egocentric and allocentric neglect seem to be related to different anatomical lesions: lesions to the right angular gyrus would be responsible for the former, damage to the right superior temporal gyrus would be associated with the latter (Hillis *et al.*, 2005).

Whether there is a single form of neglect or separate forms of neglect that selectively impair a spatial coordination frame but not the others is a matter of debate (see Hillis *et al.*, 1998 for bibliographic details). Several studies, indeed, provide evidence of subjects suffering from egocentric and patients suffering from allocentric neglect (*e.g.* Hillis *et al.*, 1998; Chatterjee, 1994). In case two separate forms of hemineglect were admitted, in stimulus-centered (allocentric) left hemineglect the initial letters of a word will be neglected even if these letters fall in the intact (ipsilesional) hemifield. On the contrary, in viewer-centered (egocentric) left hemineglect, the initial letters will be recognized if they are presented on the right hemifield: in other terms if they are displayed on the right side of the midplane of the observer (figure 5.4).

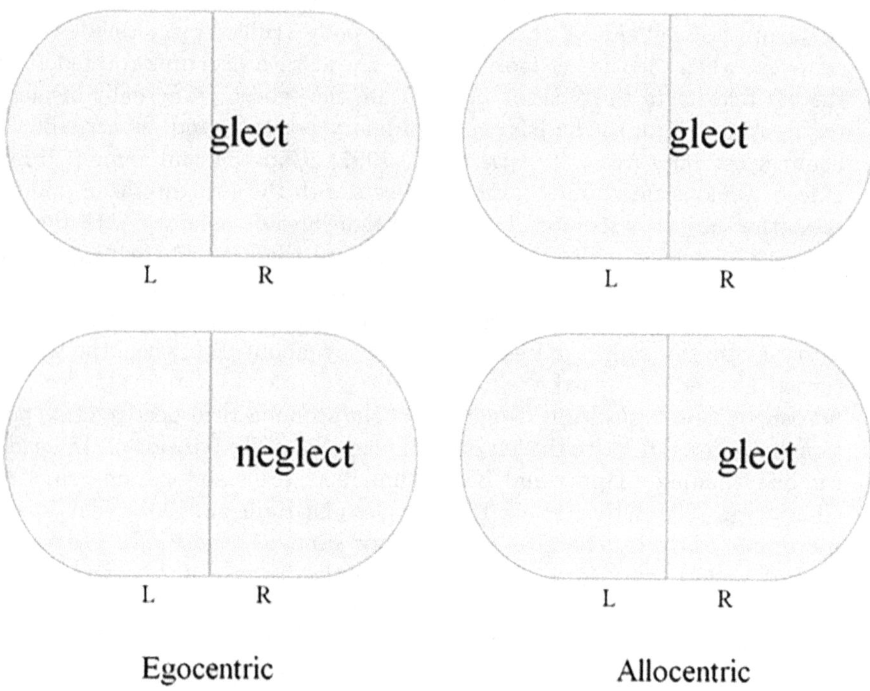

FIG. 5.4 – The perception of a word in egocentric and allocentric neglect. In egocentric hemineglect, the initial letters of a word will be recognized if they are presented on the right hemifield. In allocentric hemineglect, the initial letters of a word will be neglected even if these letters fall in the intact (ipsilesional) hemifield.

5.2 Differentiating Hemineglect from Hemianopia

Even if left hemianopia without left hemineglect and, on the contrary, left hemineglect without left hemianopia may occur (see Halligan *et al.*, 1990), hemineglect and hemianopia are often superimposed. More than 60% of hemianopic patients have reduced or no awareness of their visual field impairment (Kerkhoff, 2000). In this case, hemianopia does not exacerbate the concurrent heminattention

(Halligan *et al.*, 1990); on the contrary, heminattention can mimic hemianopia: even when the lesion is localized and does not involve the primary visual areas, neglect subjects perform poorly at perimetry in the left hemifield, simulating left hemianopia.[9]

The main functional difference between pure hemianopic and neglect patients is clearly explained by Halligan and colleagues: <<The hemianopic patient appears to be able to incorporate the sensory impaired hemifield within his spatial awareness. Patients with neglect, on the other hand, fail to integrate stimuli in contralesional space; they appear unable to conceive therefore to be aware of both the existence of contralesional space and their omission of located stimuli>> (Halligan *et al.*, 1990, p. 490). A differential diagnosis between hemineglect and pure hemianopia is a material point not only from a theoretical perspective but also (and mainly) for practical and rehabilitative purposes.

To summarize, a perimetric hemifield loss can be:

- true hemianopia;
- hemineglect that masks hemianopia: in other words, apparent hemianopia at perimetry may reveal itself as an attentional disorder. This takes place when the lesion involves the parietal area and spares the striate cortex (Müller-Oehring *et al.*, 2003);
- hemineglect superimposed on hemianopia. It occurs when the right parietal or temporal lesion involves also the right optic radiation and/or the striate cortex.

To differentiate hemineglect from pure hemianopia the following aspects may be of avail:

a- Visual extinction

A remarkable sign often (but not always: see Barbieri and De Renzi, 1989) associated with hemineglect is *visual extinction*[10]: patients can detect an isolated target presented in the affected (*i.e.* the left) hemifield, but are unaware of it when both hemifields are stimulated at the same time (Vuilleumier and Rafal, 2000; Rafal, 1994; Bisiach, 1991).[11] The phenomenon is argued to depend on the disruption of the hemispheric rivalry in neglect, which leads to sensory imbalance (Müller-Oehring *et al.*, 2003; Marzi *et al.*, 1996; Farah *et al.*, 1991): the spared (left) hemisphere,

[9]In neglect or suspected neglect patients visual field testing should make use of suprathreshold strategy and be fast, so as to keep the attentive demand at its minimum.

[10]As recalled by Lynch and McLaren, visual extinction is a mild form of visual inattention, Visual inattention, in fact, is divided into two levels of severity. The more severe form, hemineglect, is the complete absence of behavioral response to a stimulus in the visual field contralateral to the damaged hemisphere. The less severe deficit, visual extinction, is the tendency to ignore the contralateral of two visual stimuli when they appear simultaneously and symmetrically with respect to the center of the subject's surroundings (Lynch and McLaren, 1989).

[11]A practical and fast way to assess the presence of visual extinction has been described by Müller-Oehring and colleagues (2003): <<[...] the patients have to indicate the experimenter's movement of one *versus* both hands, positioned in the left and right visual field, respectively, while steadily fixating the experimenter's face [...]. Patients with hemineglect are expected to show a reduced detection rate of the left hand under double (both hands) stimulation (visual extinction), with optimal detection when a single hand is presented in the left visual field>>.

being no more down-modulated by the lesioned (right) hemisphere, becomes hyperactive, therefore induces enhanced inhibition of the affected (left) hemifield *via* the corpus callosum. It follows that if a stimulus can still be detectable when presented in the contralesional (affected) hemifield, it is not detected when a distractor is presented at the same time in the ipsilesional (spared) hemifield: the processing of the distractor, in fact, strongly inhibits the already weak response of the affected hemifield (see Müller-Oehring *et al.*, 2003 for details). Even if also hemianopic patients show a discrepancy between the higher detection rate of single stimuli and the lower detection rate of simultaneous (left/right) stimuli, this discrepancy is three times more marked in neglect patients. In hemianopic subjects, in fact, the detection rate depends on an exquisite loss of sensibility that is not subjected to cortical top-down modulation (Müller-Oehring *et al.*, 2003).

In their study dating back to 2003, Müller-Oehring and associates confirmed this hypothesis. They recruited 11 subjects with pure left homonymous hemianopia due to lesions of the right occipital area and 11 patients with neglect superimposed to hemianopia due to lesions involving also the right parietal region. To test for vision extinction, patients were administered a visual search design (three numbers were presented at three different eccentricities along the horizontal meridian to the left side of the fixation point in the absence or presence of a mirror stimulus displayed at the same time in the right hemifield). The task was to search for the digits, and the parameter under examination was search time. The main findings were:

1- The difference in search time between ipsilesional (right) hemifield (shorter search time) and contralesional (left) hemifield (longer search time) was three times more pronounced in the neglect group compared to the hemianopic sample; the largest difference was at the outermost eccentricity (24 deg).
2- Most importantly, visual extinction evoked by presenting a distractor in the ipsilesional (right, *i.e.* normal) hemifield was more evident in the neglect group, with visual search time in the contralesional (left) hemifield of neglect patients 44% higher than in hemianopes.

Visual extinction, therefore, can help differentiate neglect from true hemianopia.

b- Prolonged search time in the intact hemifield and gap effect

Based on this study, Müller-Oehring and associates stated that if the contralesional hemifield is neglected, a distractor presented within its boundary is processed, even if unconsciously (*i.e.* it is not perceived) and suggested that prolonged search time for stimuli presented in the intact hemifield when a distractor is simultaneously displayed in the contralesional hemifield is a sign of neglect and not of true hemianopia. In turn, a stimulus (like a fixation point) that persists in the normal hemifield tends to worsen the performance of the neglected patient in the contralesional hemifield. Walker and colleagues (1991), indeed, found that removal of the fixation point 100 ms before the appearance of the stimulus in the affected hemifield consistently improved the performance of their neglected patient (B.Q., a 66 years old woman with a right parietal lesion; *gap effect*). This observation revealed that the scotoma affecting her contralesional hemifield actually was not hemianopia. Moreover, the normalized saccadic response in the absence of the fixation point compared to the testing procedure with the fixation point visible during the stimulation confirms that fixation point removal reduces the severity of neglect. Quoting the authors: <<The dramatic effect that fixation point offsets have on B.Q's ability to report contralesional stimuli indicates that standard field plotting techniques, which use a constantly displayed fixation point may be not appropriate for assessing the visual fields of neglect patients. [...]. We believe that testing with a 'gap' procedure may provide a possible means of disentangling neglect and hemianopia>> (Walker *et al.*, 1991, p. 1026). A gap effect with reduced saccadic latency in the contralesional hemifield has been subsequently confirmed by the same authors in four hemineglect patients (Walker and Findlay, 1996).

c- Body axis position

Kooistra and Heilman found that turning leftward the body axis of their patient with apparent hemianopia to direct her eyes toward the spared (right) hemifield led to improvement of the defect, revealing that the patient suffered from hemineglect rather than hemianopia (Kooistra and Heilman, 1989). In this sense, the report by Kooistra and Heilman supports the idea that the visual field differs from the "spatial field".

d- Line bisection task

Line bisection task is one of the most used tests to assess hemineglect (Schenkenberg *et al.*, 1980). The subject is presented with a line with its midpoint aligned to his sagittal midplane and is asked to mark the center of the line. Patients with left hemineglect place the subjective midline mark to the right of the true center of the line, as they subjectively neglect the left side of the visual world. In hemineglect subjects, the average rightward displacement was 8.9% [±12.9] according to previous studies (Halligan, 1999; Barton and Black, 1998; Barton *et al.*, 1997). A criterion for diagnosing hemineglect is a deviation greater than 10% from the true center of the line (Giorgi *et al.*, 2009).

On the contrary, patients with right hemisphere damage and left hemianopia show left displacement, *i.e.* they tend to mark the midpoint of the line toward the affected hemifield (Kerkhoff and Bucher, 2008; Barton *et al.*, 1998).

The displacement in the hemianopic patient is greater in the case of macular splitting (−6.15% ± 4.07), and smaller with macular sparing (−1.90% ± 3.47). This behavioral difference between neglected and hemianopic subjects has been studied by Barton and Black. They posited that the leftward (*i.e.* contralateral to the damaged hemisphere) bisection bias in hemianopes is due to either:

- a non-veridical hemifield representation of space;
- an attentional gradient, adaptively biased toward the affected hemifield. To quote the authors: <<Hemianopic patients show a gradient of fixations with increased search in the contralateral hemisphere [...]. [...] Hemianopic patients tend to search for the end of the line in their blind hemispace. We hypothesize that, because these patients are aware of their deficit, the space on their blind side acquires greater salience, leading to an attentional gradient that is strategically adaptive for their disability. Whether the altered gradient is pathological (in neglect) or adaptive (in hemianopia), the result may be a bias in perceptual judgment in the direction of

the gradient, causing ipsilateral bisection bias in hemineglect and contralateral bisection bias in hemianopia>> (Barton and Black, 1998, p. 662).

e- Cancellation tasks

Subjects with neglect perform poorly at the cancellation tasks: when a page filled with targets embedded in an array of other symbols is presented, the cancellation of the targets is restricted to the ipsilesional side whereas the contralesional targets are neglected (Albert, 1973); on the contrary, it can be completed by hemianopic patients (Mort and Kennard, 2003). The Bell test, a type of cancellation test, can be considered indicative of hemineglect when there is a difference of at least four missed bells between the left and right part of the sheet (Giorgi *et al.*, 2009).

f- Oculography

The different oculographic patterns in neglect and hemianopic patients can be exploited to differentiate the two clinical conditions (Meienberg *et al.*, 1986) (see section 5.3).

Finally, as recalled by Suchoff and Ciuffreda (2004), the differential diagnosis between left-sided hemianopia and hemineglect may be inferred by:

- Medical history: patients with left hemianopia should be asked if one side of the words seems missing. In the case of a positive answer, this is a sign of true hemianopia, whereas a "no" response suggests the presence of neglect as the patient demonstrates to be unaware of his/her defect (anosognosia).
- Behavioral observation: when walking down a corridor, subjects with neglect do not tend to veer toward the left from the midline (since they are unaware of their defect), contrary to left-sided hemianopes who, in addition, make compensatory head turns and scanning movements toward the left.
  Moreover, patients with spatial neglect tend to deviate their head and their gaze to the ipsilesional side (*i.e.* to the right).[12] The deviation appears to be enhanced by the presence of any visual context and its extent is positively correlated with the percentage of omissions at the neglect tests. This postural behavior may serve as a supplementary criterion to diagnose this clinical condition (Fruhmann-Berger and Karnath, 2005).
- Visual acuity examination: during visual acuity testing, neglected patients tend to omit letters on the left side of the chart, even after they are told that letters were being missed on that side. On the contrary, hemianopic patients tend to scan and move their heads toward the left side after they were told they had omitted the left outermost letters.

5.3 Ocular Movements in Neglect

Ishiai and colleagues (Ishiai *et al.*, 1989, 1992) studied the oculomotor pattern of nine severe and moderate/mild neglect patients when performing a line bisection task. By using an eye camera, they found that during the bisection task visual search in the contralesional (left) hemifield never occurred. When asked to mark the left endpoint

[12]This is in agreement with the shift of their egocenter toward the ispilesional field (see section 5.1).

of the line, they started searching slightly to the left of the subjective midpoint. In some cases this point was marked as the subjective left endpoint (*type I leftward search*); in other cases, labeled as *type II leftward search*, the leftward search continued beyond this first mark with stepwise movements or a slow pursuit pattern. Whatever the search strategy, the subjective left endpoint never matched the true left endpoint of the line.

In a subsequent study, Müri and associates (2009) recorded the eye movements of 15 left-sided neglected subjects during a visual search task of naturalistic scenes. They found that:

- The cumulative fixation duration of the neglect group was lower on the left and higher on the right half side of the photographs compared to a control sample (left side: 56.3 ms *vs.* 92.0 ms; right side: 120.2 ms *vs.* 86.4 ms). To be noted that the time spent by neglected patients to explore the left half of the photographs was about half the time spent on the right side. A negative correlation between the severity of visual neglect and the oculomotor exploration time in the contralesional hemifield has been reported by Johnson and Diller (1986). The longer cumulative fixation time compared to controls in the right half field, where visual search is putatively normal, can be accounted for a higher number of re-fixations in a consistent proportion of patients (Mort and Kennard, 2003; Behrmann *et al.*, 1997).
- The number of leftward saccades on the left and on the right side of the photograph was lower in the neglect group compared to the controls (left side, average: 60 *vs.* 139; right side, average: 107 *vs.* 167). The number of rightward saccades on the left side was slightly higher in neglected subjects (average: 212 *vs.* 175), and the number of rightward saccades on the right side was slightly higher in patients (average: 163 *vs.* 120).
- Overall, the saccadic amplitude of neglect patients on the left side of the photographs was smaller compared to controls (leftward saccades: 3.1° *vs.* 4.3°; rightward saccades 4.9° *vs.* 6.4°). On the contrary, the leftward and rightward saccade amplitude of neglect patients did not differ from controls on the right side of the photographs. Indeed, the reduced amplitude of contralesional saccades (but not of ipsilesional saccades) in neglected patients had been previously reported (Ptak *et al.*, 2007; Walker and Findlay, 1996; Heide and Kömpf, 1998).
- On average, the percentage of the first leftward saccades was lower in the neglect group compared to the control sample (22% *vs.* 66%); on the contrary, neglect patients made more first rightward saccades (table 5.1).

TAB. 5.1 – Characteristics of the oculomotor pattern in left-sided hemineglect. Data from Müri and associates (2009).

	Cumulative fixations duration	Rightward saccades nb	Rightward saccades size	Leftward saccades nb	Leftward saccades size
NEGLECT (L) (visual search)	LEFT SIDE ↓ RIGHT SIDE ↑	LEFT SIDE (↑) RIGHT SIDE (↑)	LEFT SIDE ↓ RIGHT SIDE N	LEFT SIDE ↓ RIGT SIDE ↓	LEFT SIDE ↓ RIGHT SIDE N

The activation of reflexive saccades is abnormal as well: neglected patients fail to make saccades in response to a predicted or randomized sequence of stimuli presented in the contralesional field in a consistent number of cases (up to 25% according to Girotti *et al.* (1983)). In addition, reaction time is increased and, when saccades are triggered, they consist of multiple hypometric movements (staircase pattern) aimed to foveate the stimulus in the contralesional field (Walker and Findlay, 1996; Girotti *et al.*, 1983).

According to Walker and Findlay (1996), the defective reflexive saccadic pattern in the contralesional hemifield of neglected patients depends on the fact that unilateral parietal damage unbalances the attention-orienting system at the cullicular level.[13] The parietal cortex projects directly and *via* the substantia nigra to the superior colliculus that is involved in the generation of reflexive saccades toward sudden stimuli (Sparks, 1986). Normally the activity of the right and left colliculus are balanced by reciprocal inhibition mediated by the substantia nigra (Sprague, 1966): damage to the right parietal cortex leads to reduced activation of the ipsilateral colliculus. As a result, the saccadic triggering in the contralesional hemifield is defective.

The oculomotor behavior of neglect patients differs not only from normal subjects but also from hemianopic patients.

Compared to the latter, neglect patients show:

- shorter fixations in the contralesional field and longer fixations in the periphery of their ipsilesional field (Behrmann *et al.*, 1997);
- fewer saccades and fixations in the contralesional field and more fixations in the ipsilateral field (Behrmann *et al.*, 1997; Hornak, 1992; Ladavas *et al.*, 1990), according to a left–right gradient (Behrmann *et al.*, 1997);
- overall smaller saccadic amplitude (Karnath *et al.*, 1998);
- longer saccadic latency (Walker and Findlay, 1996).

During a visual search task, the starting point in normal observers is usually set slightly to the upper left of the visual scene (upper left quadrant). In hemianopes, the starting point does not differ from the normal observers, whereas in neglected patients it is localized to the right of the midline (Behrmann *et al.*, 1997).

The same applies during reading: Behrmann and associates found that the number and duration of fixations in the contralesional (left) hemifield was reduced in patients with neglect alexia compared to normal readers and hemianopic alexics (Behrmann *et al.*, 2002). On the contrary, the number and duration of fixations on the ipsilesional side were markedly increased compared to control subjects and hemianopic alexics, confirming a state of hyperattention in the ipsilesional side in neglect alexics (Behrmann *et al.*, 2002).

[13]To be considered that patients with damage to the parietal region show impairment of automatic (reflexive) gaze orientation, whereas impairment of intentional (voluntary) gaze is predominant in lesions involving the frontal eye fields (FEF: Heide and Kömpf, 1998).

5.4 Altitudinal Neglect

Heminattention along the vertical meridian has been reported after bilateral parietal lesions. Rapcsak and colleagues, for example, described the case of a subject with Balint's syndrome due to parieto-occipital infarction: at the vertical line bisection task, the patient placed the mark well above the true midpoint (Rapcsak *et al.*, 1988). A similar case was described by Adair and associates (1995).

In the presence of bi-parietal damage, altitudinal inattention involves the inferior space, whereas bilateral temporo-occipital injury is associated with superior neglect (Müri *et al.*, 2009).

Noteworthy, altitudinal heminattention can combine with left-sided neglect (Cappelletti *et al.*, 2007).

5.5 Size Distortion in Neglect

An additional sign reported in the contralesional hemifield of neglect patients is illusory spatial overestimation along the horizontal coordinate: a phenomenon that Milner and Harvey defined as *size distortion* and we will call *spatial anisotropy.* Due to contralesional spatial anisotropy, subjects misjudge the horizontal extent of objects like bars or rectangles presented on the left side as longer than normal (Milner and Harvey, 1995; Nichelli *et al.*, 1989). Size distortion can be neutralized by using background moving paradigms. Kerkhoff and associates (1999) asked six patients to adjust the size of a horizontal bar displayed on the contralesional (left) side of a screen to make its length equal to that of a long horizontal bar presented on the right side. Patients demonstrated consistent overestimation of the length of the contralesional bar (left, on average + 35%). The procedure was repeated in the presence of an array of small yellow squares moving coherently and horizontally leftward (speed: 7.5 deg s^{-1}). Leftward motion revealed so efficient in neutralizing the overestimation that in two cases it even reversed the vector of the distortion (underestimation).

5.6 Neglect Alexia

Hemineglect is related to a form of peripheral alexia called *neglect alexia.* Neglect alexia shows different characteristics from hemianopic alexia.

Neglect alexia is a highly heterogeneous condition qualified as a deficit of perceptual awareness, usually following right temporoparietal lesions and associated with left visual hemineglect (Costello and Warrington, 1987; Kinsbourne and Warrington, 1962b): in neglect alexia, the deficit is attentional rather than visual-perceptive and leads to errors in decoding the extreme letters of the word.[14]

[14]As soon as in 1962, Kinsbourne and Warrington (1962b) reported the case of six patients with left hemineglect and left-sided hemianopia due to lesions to the right hemisphere, and suggested that reading errors in the left hemifield depended on their hemineglect rather than on hemianopia.

As recalled by Young and colleagues (1991) and Behrmann *et al.* (2002), typical reading errors of neglect alexia are:

- omissions of the words positioned on the left side of the page and omissions of the initial letters of the words whose beginning is positioned on the left side of the page. On the contrary, words placed on the right side are not omitted. Omissions, according to the authors, reflect an impairment of the saccadic pattern, in particular of the return sweep that does not reach properly the beginning of the next line as a consequence of the neglected left side of the page (Young *et al.*, 1991);
- misreading (substitutions)[15] of the initial letters of words placed on the ipsilesional (right) side of the page.

In other terms, patients make omission errors for words whose beginning is positioned in their neglected hemifield and misread words that fall entirely in their non-neglected hemifield.

Upon this basis, omissions and substitutions derive from the same problem that is heminattention, but at two different spatial scales: whole page and individual words: omissions occur when the target of attention is the whole page and the patient neglects its left side, whereas substitutions take place when the target of attention is restricted to the individual word and the patient neglects its left side (Young *et al.*, 1991).

As recalled, hemineglect may involve two different spatial reference frames: egocentric, when the boundary between neglected and non-neglected space is the mid-sagittal plane of the patient, and allocentric, when the boundary is the center of the object irrespective of its position referred to the mid-sagittal plane of the subject (see Vallar *et al.*, 2010 and Hillis *et al.*, 1998 for references). Based on this difference between egocentric and allocentric neglect discussed in section 5.1, omissions would be the result of the egocentric component while substitutions would depend on the allocentric component of the inattentive defect. By considering the pattern of errors, neglect alexia may be classified as *retinocentric neglect alexia* (Haywood and Coltheart, 2000; Hillis and Caramazza, 1995) (or *viewer-centered* neglect alexia: Hillis *et al.*, 1998) and *stimulus-centered neglect alexia*:

- In viewer-centered (usually left) neglect alexia, errors take place to the left part of the string (*i.e.* on the contralesional side) with respect to the mid-sagittal plane of the body. Since the boundary of the reference frame is the mid-sagittal plane, the error rate decreases by positioning the string from the left toward the right side of the body (Vallar *et al.*, 2010).
- In stimulus-centered neglect alexia, the boundary of the reference frame is the center of the object or, in the case of a word, the optimal viewing position. It is well known that the optimal viewing position of the word is located to the left of the center: so, the majority of the word lies to the right of the fixation point, and, generally, only the first letter is missed (Haywood and Coltheart, 2000).
- Contrary to the previous form, in stimulus-centered neglect alexia reading is not affected by the spatial position of the string relative to the mid-sagittal plane of the

[15] Less frequently: addition errors (di Pellegrino *et al.*, 2001; Behrmann *et al.*, 1990).

body (Vallar *et al.*, 2010): in this case, even when a word is entirely presented in the right hemifield, the first letter(s) will be neglected.

So, omissions and substitutions underlie different impairments in neglect alexia and are not always present in the same patient. The higher frequency of omissions compared to substitutions suggests a more severe attentional component (Vallar *et al.*, 2010). In both types, vertical reading is preserved, and increasing the inter-letter distance is expected to worsen the reading performance (Haywood and Coltheart, 2000; Hillis *et al.*, 1998).

It is worth recalling that not all the subjects with hemineglect suffer from neglect alexia (Lee *et al.*, 2009; Patterson and Wilson, 1990): Lee and colleagues reckoned that only 37.5% of their left hemineglect patients had reading problems (Lee *et al.*, 2009). On the other hand (unexpectedly) not all the patients with neglect alexia show neglect as assessed at the conventional tasks (Bisiach *et al.*, 1986, 1990): in this regard, Bisiach and associates reported that up to 10 of their patients with neglect alexia had a normal distribution of visual attention across the visual field (*i.e.* no neglect: Bisiach *et al.*, 1990). Even patients with neglect dyslexia in the ipsilesional hemifield have been reported (Cubelli *et al.*, 1991; Costello and Warrington, 1987): for example, Costello and Warrington described the case of JOH, a patient with a left parieto-occipital mass associated with right-sided homonymous hemianopia and right-sided neglect (Costello and Warrington, 1987) who, unexpectedly, showed left-sided neglect alexia. JOH tended to omit figures on the right when copying and to bisect lines to the left, following right hemineglect, but he made reading errors on the left side of words, in line with (left) neglect dyslexia.

To explain the dissociation between neglect and neglect alexia, Behrmann and colleagues (2002) suggested that the spatial representation used in the visual tasks adopted for diagnosing neglect differs from the spatial representation of words.

Whether the attentional deficit in neglect alexia hampers reading at an early stage, before word identification, so that the feature of words are filtered in the neglected visual field, or at a late stage, after the word has been identified, is a matter of debate (Ellis *et al.*, 1987; see Behrmann *et al.*, 1990 for a discussion on this topic). According to Behrmann and colleagues, the two effects are not mutually exclusive and depend on the severity of the peripheral attentional disorder. In the first case, physical manipulation of the words is expected to affect the reading performance. The authors examined two subjects, A.H. and H.R., suffering from neglect alexia with different levels of hemiattentional impairment and, in support of the peripheral attentional disruption, they found that the physical variation of words and non-words affects their recognition, even if to a different degree (Behmann *et al.*, 1990). The authors found that A.H. was especially sensitive to physical variations of the words in the left hemifield, namely to their horizontal spatial extent: in this subject, severe peripheral attentional disruption prevents the lexical information from being processed at a higher-level stage. The result is that reading is consistently affected. On the contrary, H.R. showed just a mild peripheral attentional impairment, so late processing remains possible. In this patient, in fact, a word superiority effect (fewer neglect errors at words than at non-words) revealed that the central (top-down) processing may help his residual reading performance provided enough perceptual information from the attentionally defective hemifield reaches the upper-order sites. In other terms, the word superiority effect suggests that high-level ("conceptual") mechanisms may use the attenuated perceptual information "to feed down and enhance the perception of the target item" (Behrmann *et al.*, 1990). The authors postulated that for it to occur the peripheral attentional disruption must be less severe so that some information can get through to allow the high-order lexical processing.

5.6.1 Ocular Movements in Neglect Alexia

Ocular movements of patients with neglect alexia during reading differ substantially from normal subjects and hemianopic patients.

Behrmann and colleagues examined the oculomotor pattern in a sample of patients with neglect alexia when reading words. They found that:

- the number and duration of fixations in the contralesional (left, *i.e.* neglected) hemifield were markedly reduced compared to normal subjects whereas an increase was observed in the ipsilesional side. This reveals inattention on the contralesional side and hyperattention on the ipsilesional side in neglect alexics (Behrmann *et al.*, 2002).

Angeli and colleagues (2004) analyzed the oculomotor pattern in eight patients with neglect when reading words and non-words. The landing site of the first saccade was close to the center of the word (−0.42° on average, where the negative sign refers to the left side from the center), that is about two letter positions rightward compared to the landing site of normal readers that, in fact, was displaced more to the left (−4.7°: between the beginning and the center of the word). Moreover, patients tended to explore more the right side of the words compared to normal subjects, whereas the fixation time spent on the left side was comparable.

The ocular pattern of neglect alexics seems to differ in the presence of words and non-words. Di Pellegrino and associates (2001) recorded the eye movements of a neglect alexic patient when reading words and non-words, and compared his oculomotor pattern with that of a small sample of normal readers. They found that:

- in normal readers the first saccade was localized to the left of the middle of the word, in the neglect alexic subject it was directed to the right side of words and especially non-words,[16] to confirm that the attentional focus is biased to the right.
- normal readers spent more time scanning non-words than words, and on average they spent the same time scanning the left and right side of the words; in contrast, fixation time was longer on the left side of the string when non-words were presented. On the contrary, the alexic subject did not show differences between words and non-words, but fixation times were longer on the left side when words were displayed, and on the right side when non-words were displayed. This means that in neglect alexics the oculomotor scanning depends not only on the spatial position of

[16]The explanation put forward by the authors to explain this difference is that words, being treated as single lexical objects, are less subjected to attention disorder than non-words.

the stimuli in egocentric coordinates but also on their nature (*i.e.* words or non-words). From these findings, the authors infer that "reading of non-words is accompanied by a greater rightward bias in the allocation of attention that reading of words" (di Pellegrino *et al.*, 2001, p. 71). This finding is in agreement with the previous study of Brunn and Farah who showed that lines placed underneath non-words were bisected less symmetrically than those placed underneath words and that neglect patients make more errors reading the contralesional sides of non-words than words (Brunn and Farah, 1981).

As an explanation for this dissociation, words allow the top-down lexical activation to modulate the distribution of attention, enhancing the recognition of the stimuli in the left hemifield: attention drives the eyes toward the left hemifield, accounting therefore for the longer fixation time for words in the left (neglected) hemifield. This top-down lexical enhancement cannot take place with non-words, that, in fact, are associated with longer fixation time on the right side.

Karnath and Huber (1992) studied the oculomotor pattern of a reader with a left-sided hemineglect but without any visual field defect. They found shortened return sweeps that ended in the middle of the next line and were followed by sequences of short backward saccades. According to the authors, the shortened return sweeps could depend on a different body-centered reference system (table 5.2).

TAB. 5.2 – Oculomotor features of neglect alexics compared to normal readers during reading.

Landing site of the first saccade	Cumulative fixation time	Number of fixation	Return sweep
- Closer to the center of the word (*i.e.* rightward compared to normals (Angeli *et al.*, 2004) or to the right side of the center (di Pellegrino *et al.*, 2001) - Rightward bias more pronounced with non-words (di Pellegrino *et al.*, 2001)	- Shorter on the left (neglected) side (Behrmann *et al.*, 2002) - Longer on the right (non-neglected) side (Angeli *et al.*, 2004; Behrmann *et al.*, 2002) - Longer on the left side with words, and on the right side with non-words (di Pellegrino *et al.*, 2001)	- Reduced in the neglected hemifield (Behrmann *et al.*, 2002) - Increased in the non-neglected hemifield (Behrmann *et al.*, 2002)	- Shortened (centered in the middle of the next line) and followed by sequences of short backward saccades (Karnath and Huber, 1992)

5.7 Rehabilitation of Visual Hemineglect and Neglect Alexia

Recovery is fast over the first 10 days and reaches a plateau at 3 months (Stone *et al.*, 1992). According to subsequent studies, most of the improvement occurs by 8–12 weeks after the onset of the stroke (Dombovy and Aggarwal, 2000), or within the first 5–6 months (Katz *et al.*, 1999; Robertson and Halligan, 1999).

Sunderland and colleagues reported that significant neglect is rarely observed 6 months after the stroke, but further recovery may occur between 6 months and 1 year (Sunderland *et al.*, 1987). It remains that residual spatial inattention often persists indefinitely. One year after a cerebrovascular accident, neglect can be observed in one-third of the patients (Allegri, 2000): this makes efforts to investigate rehabilitation procedures mandatory.

A task like grasping a cup of coffee or pressing a button demands the integration of sensory (visual and proprioceptive) mapping and subsequent motor planning: the result of this integration is eye-hand coordination.

Sensory mapping, coded as visuospatial coordinates (VS, centered on the head) and proprioceptive spatial coordinates (PCS, centered on the shoulders), relies on two complementary processes: *spatial alignment* and *spatial calibration* (Redding and Wallace, 2006).

Evidently, for eye-hand coordination to be effective the sensory mapping must be *veridical*, and this goal is obtained only if the VS and PCS reference frames match; this correspondence is provided by a process called *"spatial alignment"* (Redding and Wallace, 2006). Spatial alignment is, indeed, crucial for effective eye-hand coordination as it supplies a veridical spatial map that drives the hand movement toward the target once the target has been visually localized.

Re-alignment occurs when there is a loss of correspondence between the visual and proprioceptive reference frame, as it occurs during the body development when the length of the limb increases, or in case of sensorial neural cell death like in hemianopic patients. In addition, spatial realignment is elicited by *prism exposure that induces a displacement of the visual field.*

In the presence of veridical spatial mapping, eye-hand coordination allows reaching an object of interest by selecting a *local workspace*, *i.e.* a spatial representation that contains the object of interest (the target) surrounded by other objects (obstacles). The selection of the local workspace is an ordinary short-term process called *spatial calibration* (Redding and Wallace, 2006). Calibration takes into consideration the position of the target: if the target is displaced to the right or to the left of the egocentric reference point[17] (straight ahead), the local workspace localizes to the right or to the left, respectively.

Every time relative changes in the coordinate systems are produced by head and shoulder movements, *recalibration,* which is a short-term and iterated spatial remapping, takes place (Redding and Wallace, 2006).

Calibration and alignment are independent, dissociated functions: calibration is a conscious correction that, as such, requires some attention: in fact, calibration

[17]As recalled by Vallar and colleagues (1999), the egocentric reference is the basic coordinate system that defines the mid-sagittal plane. The mid-sagittal plane is the plane that divides the subject's body and extrapersonal space into two halves (left and right). The egocenter, therefore, allows the computation of the spatial position of visual objects with respect to the observer. The egocentric coordinate system is head-centered (visual coordinates) or body-centered (proprioceptive coordinates). One way to test the position of the egocenter is to ask the subject to point straight ahead (*i.e.* to the midpoint) with the eyes closed. As shown by Heilman and colleagues (1983), neglected patients in this condition point to the right of the midpoint.

relies on high-order cortical activation; on the contrary, alignment is a non-conscious, automatic cerebellar-based process (Jeannerod and Rossetti, 1993).

In normal conditions, the visual and proprioceptive reference frame match (VS and PRS references are aligned), and the position of the local workspace (calibration) depends on the position of the object of interest. As a result, eye-hand coordination is effective in reaching and grasping the object (figure 5.5).

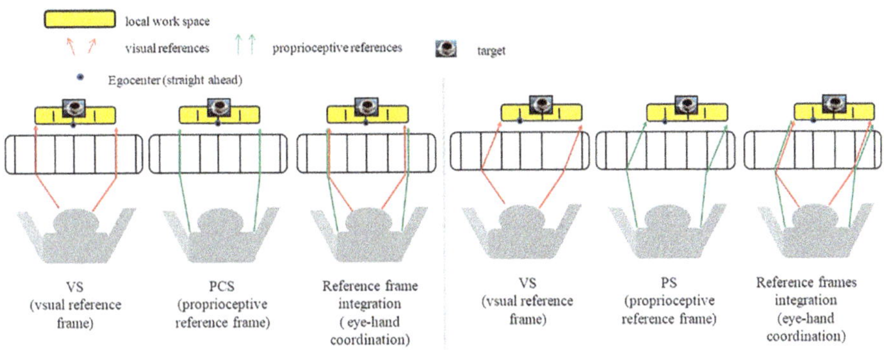

FIG. 5.5 – The visual and proprioceptive reference frame in normal conditions with a straight-ahead target and with a target displaced to the right. With a target displaced to the right, the egocentric straight-ahead is to the left of the target. To be noted the spatial alignment between VS and PCS.

As explained, spatial realignment may be elicited by prism exposure that induces a displacement of the visual field.

Immediately after prism exposure (base to the left) the VS local workspace, including the egocentric straight ahead, is shifted toward the right, The subject misperceives the object to the right of its real position so that the hand fails to grasp the object: the subject who is asked to point toward a target placed straight ahead indicates a region of space to the right because the object appears to him to the right (figure 5.6).

After some practice, VS local workspace shifts to the left (including the egocentric straight ahead). It follows that the eye-hand coordination reference frame restores centering (spatial re-alignment between VS and PCS is achieved) and the hand that points to the object prismatically displaced is again perceived straight ahead (figure 5.7).

In other terms, <<[...] adaptation to prisms may involve a selective shift in the proprioceptive representation of hand position that brings it back into alignment with the prism-distorted visual input>> (Clower *et al.*, 1996, p. 619).

Finally, an after-effect occurs after the prism is removed:

- The VS local workspace is shifted rightward (centering a little to the right of the pre-exposure condition) so that the target placed straight ahead is seen as biased to the right.
- The PCS local workspace is shifted leftward: the hand feels to point straight ahead to the target when it points to the left.

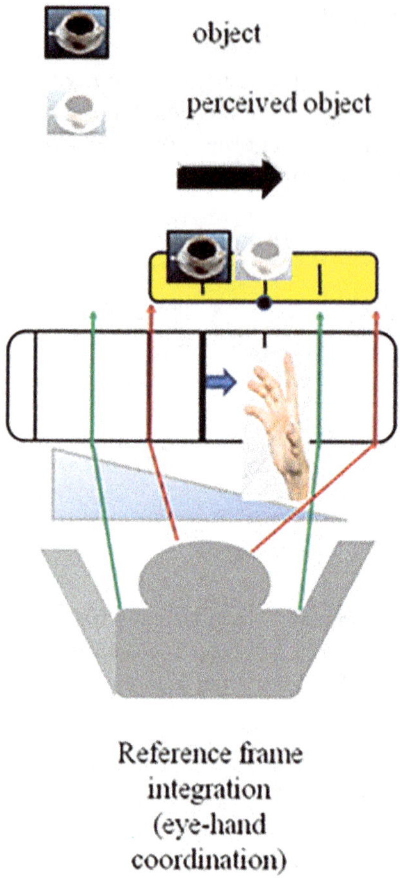

FIG. 5.6 – Displacement of the VS local workspace immediately after prism exposure. The VS workspace is shifted to the right while the PRC workspace is unaffected, thereby there is no realignment. It follows that the subject fails to grasp the object.

As a consequence of the combination of the biased VS and PCS, the eye-hand coordination reference frame shifts leftward (figure 5.8).

5.7.1 Prism Adaptation

When neglect patients are asked to point straight ahead in the dark, they point to the right, demonstrating a rightward displacement of their egocenter reference[18] (Chokron and Imbert, 1995; Heilman *et al.*, 1983).

[18]To rapidly assess the subjective egocenter, the patient is asked to look at a vertical pen moved in front of him from the affected side toward the normal side and *vice versa*. The pen is reported to be centered when it is localized to a various extent to the left or to the right of the midline, depending on the direction and extent of the perceived midline lateralization.

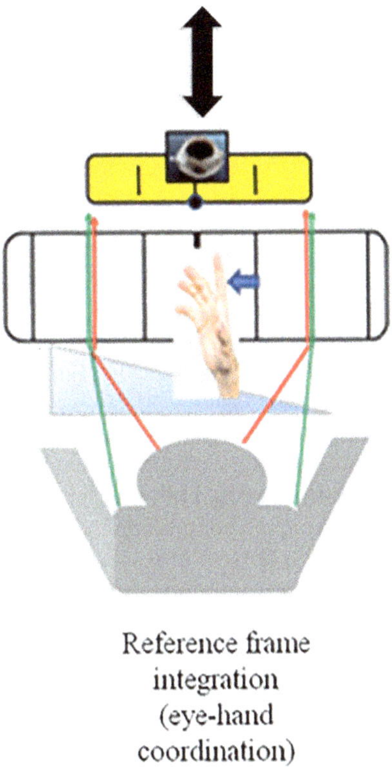

FIG. 5.7 – Realignment during prism exposure. See text for explanation.

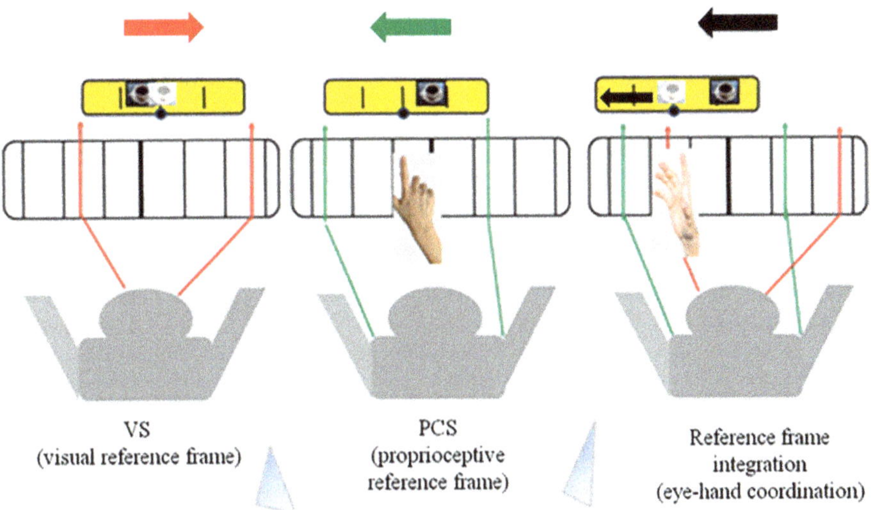

FIG. 5.8 – After-effect after the prismatic displacement is removed. The subject deviates in the direction opposite to the prismatic shift when pointing at an object. See text for explanation.

Prism adaptation has been used to re-align the reference frames of neglect patients, *i.e.* to shift their egocentric reference, biased to the right, toward the left. The shift is induced by the prism after-effect. The after-effect, indeed, restores a centered straight-ahead egocentric reference: this restoration can be verified by measuring the patients' after-effect with their eyes closed. As explained by Angeli and associates, who reported a left after-effect of 4.4° following prism exposure: <<after removal of the prism subjects systematically deviate in the direction opposite to the prismatic shift when manually pointing or reaching for visual objects [...]>> (Angeli *et al.*, 2004, p. 1232). The leftward eye deviation, indeed, helps patients explore the left neglected hemifield.

In the study of Rossetti and colleagues (1998), for example, six neglect patients[19] pointed about 9° to the right before prism exposure and the pointing decreased to 2° to the right after exposure (70% of compensation). The training consisted of fifty repeated fast-pointing movements toward targets randomly placed to the left and the right of the body midline when wearing a couple of prismatic lenses that displaced the visual field 10° to the right. Subjects could not see the trajectory of their hand when pointing ("straight ahead pointing without vision"). The session lasted 3–5 min.

Neglect signs, evaluated with a battery of tests including line bisection task, lines cancellation, and text reading, improved immediately following prism exposure and the ameliorative effect was still observable two hours later. By comparison, the after-effect in normal subjects was smaller (pre-exposure: 0°, post-exposure: about 4° to the left). The authors explained the improvement of neglect after prism adaptation in terms of neural plasticity that normalizes the sensorimotor reference frame and restores the normal function of the right hemisphere. Indeed, the occurrence of cerebral functional reorganization after the reversal of the retinal image induced by prismatic goggles has been demonstrated in monkeys[20] (Sugita, 1996).

Rhode and associates reported similar results in a neglect subject who showed an aftereffect of 9 deg leftward (90% of compensation) at the straight-ahead pointing without vision task (Rode *et al.*, 1998/1999).

Subsequent investigations confirmed the ameliorative effect of prism adaptation on neglect.

McIntosh and colleagues (2002), for example, trained with the procedure of Rossetti *et al.* (1998) a patient with severe chronic neglect by inducing prism adaptation once a week for three weeks. Neglect was assessed before and after

[19] The subjects were examined 3 weeks to 14 months after the onset of the brain damage.

[20] Sugita (1996) studied the plasticity of the visual cortex (V1) in three macaque monkeys using prisms to induce left-right reversed vision. The visually guided behavior was fully disrupted during the first two weeks to the point that the animals could not even move. However, after the third week, they started to recover, and after 6 weeks of adaptation the visuomotor coordination returned to a normal level. In that period, single unit recordings demonstrated that about 36% of the cells isolated in V1 began responsive to stimuli (flash) presented not only in the contralateral visual hemifield, as expected, but also in the ipsilateral region. This took place after completion of visuomotor adaptation, and depended on the formation of ipsilateral receptive fields next to the original contralateral ones. Despite the size of the ipsilateral receptive fields was larger than the size of the contralateral ones, the rate of discharge was higher for the latter. The response to ipsilateral stimulation faded after removal of the prisms.

adaptation by administering two cancellation tests and the line bisection task. Improvement of neglect was observed in terms of reduction of cancellation omissions at the cancellation tasks and of mean directional error at the line bisection task. The effect was greater with the repetition of the training the next week, especially for the cancellation task.

The group of Berberovic *et al.* (2004) used a different approach: instead of administering a battery of tests devised to estimate the degree of spatial hemi-nattention, they evaluated whether the difference in spatial attention between the left and right side is attenuated after prism adaptation using a visual temporal-order-judgment task (VTOJ). Five subjects with left neglect were required to report the order of onset of two subsequent stimuli, one displayed to the left, and the other to the right of the midline. In presence of reduced spatial attention in one hemisphere, as it occurs in neglect patients, perception of the contralesional stimulus should be delayed compared to the ipsilateral one. This way, the amount of attentional asymmetry (rightward bias) could be estimated before and after prism adaptation. Wearing 15° rightward-deviating prisms, subjects had to point repeatedly to a target presented to the left or to the right of the subjective egocentric straight-ahead reference. The adaptation period lasted 10–15 min. The authors reported a reduction of the attentional asymmetry in four of the five patients by more than 50%. Interestingly, no change in spatial distribution was found after prism adaptation in a sample of normal subjects.[21]

The chronicity of the brain accident does not seem to influence the effectiveness of prism treatment (McIntosh *et al.*, 2002).

It is logical to suppose the amelioration of the signs of neglect found by the group of Rossetti depends on the improvement of the egocentric reference bias.

Using the procedure of Rossetti, Pisella and colleagues (2002) obtained a 9° leftward after-effect (95% compensation, measured with straight-ahead pointing without vision) in two neglect subjects immediately after prism exposure. The effect decreased over the first 4 h, but in one patient (PE) it stabilized about the straight-ahead position (0°) and was still observable after four days. On the contrary, in the second patient (SA) it returned to the pre-training value. However, the point of interest is that the line bisection task (adopted as an indicator of neglect) was *not* correlated with the performance of the straight-ahead pointing: contrary to the post-effect, it improved in SA but not in PE. In conclusion, unexpectedly,

[21]And yet, the group of Rousseaux provided a counter-evidence on the effectiveness of prism adaptation in rehabilitating neglect. They tested the effectiveness of prism adaptation on visual neglect signs (bell cancellation, line bisection and drawing) and reading in 10 patients with neglect alexia who suffered a recent right hemisphere stroke. In addition, hemianopia was present in six of them. Subjects were trained with prisms that displaced the visual field 10° toward the right by asking them to point repeatedly with the finger to dots placed 10 degrees to the left or the right of the body midline. The same procedure was repeated with a neutral prism and the results at the neglect tests and reading were compared in the two experimental conditions after 5 min, 3 h, 1 day, and 3 days after exposure. The effect of the prism was not significant in both groups (neglect patients and neglect patients with hemianopia) as for neglect tests and reading, irrespective of the time since prism exposure and of the severity of the hemi-inattention (Rousseaux *et al.*, 2006). The authors attributed the improvement reported in previous studies to a learning effect or an increase of vigilance.

the results of Pisella and associates suggest that the amelioration of the signs of neglect is not causally related to the improvement of the egocentric reference bias. In other terms <<[...] the benefit to prism adaptation on spatial cognition is not mediated by a modification of the egocentric reference>> (Pisella *et al.*, 2002, p. 332).

In the same period, Farnè and associates (2002) investigated the effect of prism exposure in six patients with left neglect. A battery of eight visuospatial tasks, including cancellation tests, line bisection, and two reading tests (made of 50 words, and 50 non-words) was administered before and immediately after prim exposure (according to the method of Rossetti), and 1 day and 1 week later. The training consisted of repeated fast pointing ("without vision") movements toward a target (a red semicircular target) randomly placed centrally (20° to the left and 20° to the right: 25 trials per position) of the body midline when wearing a couple of prismatic lenses that displaced the visual field 10° to the right. The session lasted 5–7 min. The author reported an after-effect of about 3° (33%) that persisted one day after the exposure but disappeared after one week. Neglect symptoms improved by about 25% immediately following exposure; the improvement was maintained after one day but disappeared after one week. The same trend was found in reading (with a reduced rate of omissions of the left portion of the word) up to one day after exposure, but the amelioration was no more evident after one week.

In conclusion, contrary to what was argued by Pisella *et al.*, the findings of Farnè suggest that the after-effect induced by prism exposure *parallels* the improvement of neglect symptoms, and acts as a visual-motor cue.

It is worth considering that a second prism exposure one week after the first led to an improvement of neglect but, since it was not greater than the improvement obtained after the first training session, a cumulative effect is excluded.

Frassinetti and colleagues (2002a) trained six patients with left neglect in the chronic phase (at least three months after the cerebral damage) during prism exposure (10° rightward displacing prisms) twice daily for five days per week (two weeks in total, total number of sessions: 20). The authors used a procedure similar to that described by the group of Rossetti: subjects were seated on a table with a wooden box open on both (patient and operator) sides in front of them. They were asked to point with their finger toward a pen randomly presented by the operator at the center or 21° to the left or to the right of the midline (30 + 30 + 30 presentations during wearing the prisms). The pointing hand was below the top side of the box, so the direction of the arm was not visible ("pointing without vision").

Neglect was assessed with a battery of tests, including line bisection task, a cancellation test, and "ecological" situations (as the description of a room). In addition, a reading test with words and non-words presented at the center of a screen was administered to the sample. The trained group showed a leftward aftereffect of about 2.7°. The effect decreased but persisted over 6–12 h after exposure. In the sample, neglect improved gradually after exposure and over at least 5 weeks after treatment.[22] The same applied to reading errors that decreased up to the next day,

[22]According to the authors, the improvement can last up to 17 weeks after the end of training.

with no further reduction in the subsequent time intervals tested. Two findings are worth to be considered in this study:

i- Contrary to the after-effect, that decays with time, neglect tends to improve after the treatment. The gradual amelioration of neglect would depend on the facilitation of the gaze toward the neglected space induced by the training so that the visual system receives more information than at the pre-training stage. This gain of information is used to explore the left hemifield more and more accurately as time goes by, leading to a progressive and continuous improvement of the inattention parameters.

ii- The difference between the long-lasting effect of prism adaptation on neglect and the short-lasting effect of prism adaptation on the after-effect suggests that the ameliorative effect of prism exposure on neglect involves a high-order level of visuospatial representation (in line with Rode and colleagues, 1998/1999, and Farnè and colleagues, 2002).

So, prism adaptation stimulates high-order processes related to sensorimotor integration and visual-spatial representation. This means the improvement of neglect after prism exposure can be related to the after-effect but is not a mere consequence of it (*e.g.*: McIntosh *et al.*, 2002; Rossetti *et al.*, 1998). Interestingly, the dissociation reported by the group of Pisella *et al.* (2002) and Frassinetti *et al.* (2002a) between the bias revealed by the straight-ahead task and the signs of neglect could be explained by the existence of two different anatomical loci, one in charge of midline computation and activated by the straight-ahead task, the other responsible for the signs of neglect, like bisection task. In an fMRI study, Vallar and colleagues (1999) provided evidence that the main cerebral regions responsible for the subjective setting of the midsagittal plane (the egocenter) are located in the right posterior parietal cortex (including the angular gyrus: Brodmann area 39) and in the right frontal premotor cortex (inferior and frontal gyri).[23] This is overall in agreement with the lesions found in hemiattention syndrome (Robertson and Halligan, 1999; Stein, 1989, 1992), even if a study performed on a sample of patients with severe neglect found that the cerebral lesion responsible for their signs was the frontal-temporal-parietal junction (area 40), a region adjacent to area 39[24] (Vallar and Perani, 1986).

The brain regions stimulated by prism adaptation are the cerebellum (Jeannerod and Rossetti, 1993) and the posterior parietal cortex (more precisely the lateral bank of the intraparietal sulcus), that, in fact, subserve sensorimotor integration (the integration of oculomotor planning and reaching/grasping movements), thereby eye-hand coordination (Clower *et al.*, 1996).

Not only alignment but also calibration is abnormal in neglect subjects: patients suffer from a reduction in the size of the local workspace and difficulty in its selection. More specifically, they have problems in shifting the position of the local

[23]Brain activation was recorded in seven normal subjects who were required to press a button when a horizontal bar shifting across the fronto-paralle plane was perceived straigth ahead, *i.e.* at the egocenter.

[24]See Vallar *et al.* (1999), for a more detailed discussion.

workplace as a function of the localization of the task (Redding and Wallace, 2006), and this may explain the different levels of improvement among patients reported in the previous studies.

5.7.2 *Effect of Prism Adaptation on Reading*

During reading, prism adaptation determines a shift of the landing site toward the left (−1.36°, *i.e.* near the beginning of the word), even if it does not reach the values of normal readers (Angeli *et al.*, 2004), and shorter mean fixation time to the right side of the letters. Due to this reduction, it follows that the difference between fixation time to the left *vs.* the right side of the letters in neglect subjects after exposure approximates the fixation distribution of normal readers (Angeli *et al.*, 2004). Accordingly, improvement in reading performance is obtained, with reading errors reduced by 25% (from 65% to 40%: Angeli *et al.*, 2004).

Surprisingly, the improvement of neglect dyslexia is independent of the recovery from neglect (Cantoni and Piccirilli, 1997).

5.7.3 *Optokinetic Training*

A second line of research uses the optokinetic response to displace leftwards the egocentric reference: a horizontally left-moving serial stimulation that evokes optokinetic nystagmus is used to produce gaze deviation toward the left, thereby to re-orient patient's attention (more precisely the egocentric coordinates) toward the neglected hemifield.

Karnath (1996) obtained a leftward re-orientation of the egocentric reference[25] in three left neglect patients using an optokinetic stimulation made of randomly distributed white dots moving contralesionally (speed: 30 deg/s). With this procedure,[26] Pizzamiglio and colleagues reported a displacement toward the left of the subjective midpoint in normal subjects, right brain-damaged patients, and especially in subjects with left hemineglect, as assessed with the line bisection task. In this group, the extent of the leftward egocenter displacement was positively correlated with the severity of the heminattention (Pizzamiglio *et al.*, 1990). As highlighted by the authors, these findings suggest not only that the optokinetic training can be useful for rehabilitative purposes, but also that the egocentric coordinates of neglect patients are particularly vulnerable to a perturbation of the visual input, like it occurs in the case of moving backgrounds. The procedure, repeated for 8 weeks, confirmed a consistent improvement of neglect in a subsequent study (Antonucci *et al.*, 1992). The generalization of the main outcome of the optokinetic training (normalization of the egocenter) has been subsequently reported in ten patients, where the optokinetic training[27] improved their performance in the cancellation and

---

[25]Assessed with the straight-ahead pointing task.

[26]Viewing distance: 35 cm, speed of the serial stimulation: 50 cm/s.

[27]An array of random small squares moving leftward at a rate of 7.5–50 deg/s, five sessions (each of 40 min) administered.

line bisection tasks, reduced size distortion, and decreased the number of omissions in a reading test (Kerkhoff *et al.*, 2006). These ameliorative effects remained stable after 14 days. Instead, letter/syllables substitutions were unchanged. The same year, similar results were reported by Sturm and associates who administered the training to seven neglect patients for three weeks.

In summary, the therapeutic effect of the optokinetic training generalizes across different domains of neglect but is transitory and seems to last no more than four weeks (Sturm *et al.*, 2006).

5.7.4 Compensatory Prisms

The rehabilitation of hemineglect with compensatory strategies, namely *permanent* yoked full-field prisms, is tangential to this work: we just need to remember that yoked full-field prisms (base to the left) proved to be effective in the visual rehabilitation of neglect patients, since they shift the objective straight ahead (the egocenter), biased to the right, toward the contralesional field. Full-field prisms (base to the left) are more effective than half-field yoked prisms. With full-field prisms the whole visual field is shifted toward the non-neglected side so that the patient is now aware of part of the neglect space; yet, the gain in awareness to the left is accompanied by a correspondent loss of the peripheral right field (see Suchoff and Ciuffreda, 2004 for a review on this topic). To avoid optical distortion and chromatic aberrations related to high-power prismatic lenses, the power of the prism must be the least that improves visual awareness in the affected (*i.e.* left) hemifield (6–8 diopters per eye, and not higher than 10 diopters: Cohen and Wass, 1996).

Chapter 6

Visual Exploration in Hemianopia

Not only reading difficulties (as explained in chapter 4) but also impaired visual exploration[1] affects the quality of life of hemianopic patients (Gall *et al.*, 2009, 2010).

When looking at a visual scene, a wide variety of stimuli is processed by the visual system. Of these, only a small portion, *i.e.* the stimuli of interest, reach our consciousness and influence our actions and behavior. The rest are the surroundings, the background. Visual exploration selects the stimuli of interest but, at the same time, it must keep track of the surroundings. This way, it gets the necessary information for optimal orientation and interaction with the environment.

Key elements for adequate visual exploration are visual acuity high enough to allow perceiving the features of the stimuli, effective saccadic scanning, and preserved visual field (the minimum visual field needed for navigating in normal conditions is 20 deg to the left and 20 deg to the right of the fixation point: Lovie-Kitchin *et al.*, 1990). In addition, visual orientation recruits the attentive function; it is modulated by top-bottom processes like expectations, knowledge, beliefs, and desires.

Based on a standardized anamnesis, Kerkhoff reckoned visual exploration problems in daily life affect up to 70% of subjects with homonymous visual field defects (Kerkhoff, 1999): they lose orientation, collide with obstacles and persons, and miss objects located in the blind hemifield. A main issue is driving: even if the ability to compensate for a visual field loss when driving on a straight road is highly variable among patients (Peli, 2000), most of them have problems with lane keeping, poor steering control, inadequate detection of potential hazards and pedestrians, and difficulties in gap judgment (*e.g.*: Kasneci *et al.*, 2014; Wood *et al.*, 2011; Szlyk *et al.*, 1993). This is attributable to visual field loss and inadequate scanning [see Peli, 2020 for a discussion on this topic].[2] Displacement of the egocenter, size distortion,

[1]Visual exploration is the function responsible for visual scanning, navigation, and location of objects.

[2]Contrary to what was reported, and unexpectedly, Schulte and colleagues found that the extent of the visual field loss is less relevant (Schulte *et al.*, 1999). The authors examined the driving ability of nine hemianopic patients with no further ophthalmological or neuropsychological impairment using a driving simulator. They found that driving errors, driving speed, and reaction time were not different from normal subjects. They went so far as to conclude that patients with homonymous hemianopia can drive a car as safely as normal subjects. However, Sabel, who co-authored the study, in a subsequent paper stressed that patients with complete homonymous hemianopia should refrain from driving (Sabel and Trauzettel-Klosinski, 2005).

DOI: 10.1051/978-2-7598-3493-8.c006

and, in right-sided hemianopic subjects, visual-spatial deficits, play an additional detrimental role (Kasneci *et al.*, 2014).

6.1 Scanning Behavior of Hemianopic Patients in Controlled Experimental Conditions

To address the issue of visual exploration in hemianopes[3] and to find the best rehabilitative program, a strand of research has been devoted to the study of the scanning strategies and compensatory mechanisms put in place by patients.

Hemianopes tend to start exploring their intact hemifield (Zangemeister *et al.*, 1995) and generate irregular, hypometric staircase saccades toward the blind region, with a high number of fixations and re-fixations [*e.g.* Passamonti *et al.*, 2009; Schuett *et al.*, 2009b; Pambakian *et al.*, 2000; Chédru *et al.*, 1973 in simulated hemianopia]. As a result, scanning objects is longer and unsystematic (Passamonti *et al.*, 2009; Zihl, 1995b; Ishiai *et al.*, 1987; Chédru *et al.*, 1973). Fixations of hemianopes during inspection deviate toward the blind hemifield (Roth *et al.*, 2009). This contralesional fixation bias is not a direct effect of the lesion, but, most likely, is a compensatory mechanism to encompass a greater extent of the visual world in the intact hemifield (Machner *et al.*, 2009; Tant *et al.*, 2002; Pambakian *et al.*, 2000; Zihl, 1995b; Ishiai *et al.*, 1987; Chédru *et al.*, 1973).

Zihl (1995b, 2009), who studied in detail this issue, found that fixations, number of saccades required to complete the scan, and search time were very similar[4] to that of normal subjects in almost half (47%) of left-sided and one-third (33%) of right-sided hemianopes.[5] Accordingly, orienting and navigating problems were absent or mild. The author defined this group as "normal hemianopics".

On the contrary, the remaining subjects ("pathologic hemaniopics") showed a disorganized and elaborated pattern, with more repetitions of the scanpath, more saccades, thereby more fixations, more refixations, and longer search time. Instead, fixation duration was within the normal range with no asymmetries between ipsi- and contralateral hemifield (figure 6.1). Unlike "normal hemianopes", "pathologic hemianopes" complain about daily visual difficulties. Zihl hypothesized that additional subcortical damage to the occipital lobe, the posterior thalamus, or the occipito-parietal visual areas prevents efficient spontaneous oculomotor compensatory strategies in this group of patients.

---

[3]To estimate visual exploration in hemianopic subjects, Schuett *et al.* (2008b) adopted a cancellation task with 20 black diamonds randomly embedded in an array of distractors (22 black crosses and dots). The size of the targets and distractors was 0.8 deg, and the size of the sheet of paper (horizontally oriented) was 44.6 deg × 35 deg. Patients were asked to flag all the targets as quickly as possible. The normative performance time, for a sample aged 38 ± 10.7 years, was 13.2 s (±1.3, range 9.1–17.2 s). Left-sided and right-sided hemianopes showed a visual exploration time of about 30–34 s (range: 12–72 s).

[4]At the upper limit of the normal range.

[5]Patients had no neglect, no other ophthalmological diseases, no oculomotor disorders, and normal or quasi-normal visual acuity. The author recorded the saccadic pattern while subjects inspected a cluster of 20 dots scattered over a screen.

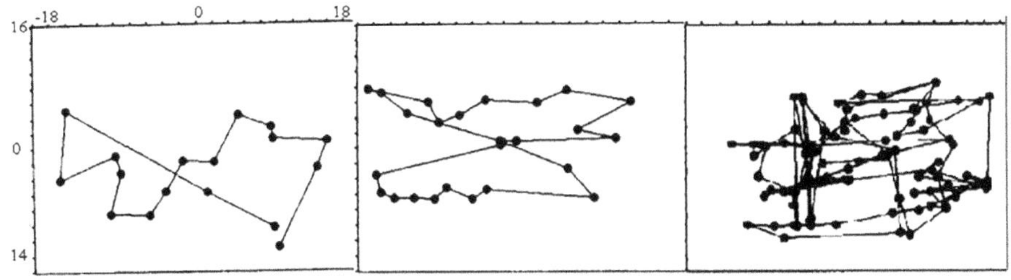

FIG. 6.1 – Example of the scanning pattern of normal subjects (left), *normal hemianopics* (middle), and *pathologic hemianopics* (right panel). From Zihl (1995b). With permission of Elsevier.

Especially the right-sided pathologic hemianopics spent more search time (in line with Barton *et al.*, 1998) and made more saccades in the affected hemifield than in their spared region. Most of them (87%) started to scan in the left (intact hemifield), then transferred a more laborious search to the affected (right) hemifield. Likewise, left-sided pathologic hemianopics started to scan in the right (intact hemifield), and then transferred the search to the affected (left) hemifield.

The group of Machner examined nine acute post-stroke hemianopic patients and overall confirmed the findings of Zihl. Subjects, as expected, showed longer search time, a higher number of fixations and refixations, and smaller saccadic amplitude compared to a control group. This oculomotor pattern, more evident in right-sided hemianopes, is not related to the degree of macular sparing and the overall extent of the visual field defect and takes place immediately after the onset of the cerebral injury (Machner *et al.*, 2009: table 6.1).

TAB. 6.1 – The oculomotor characteristics of hemianopic patients after the onset. See text for explanation.

Start of exploration	Intact hemifield	Zangemeister *et al.*, 1995; Zihl, 1995b
Saccades length	Hypometric staircase saccades toward the blind region	Machner *et al.*, 2009; Passamonti *et al.*, 2009; Schuett *et al.*, 2009b; Pambakian *et al.*, 2000
Saccades nb	↑	Zihl, 1995b
Fixation duration	N	Zihl, 1995b
Fixation/refixation nb	↑, deviated toward the blind hemifield	Machner *et al.*, 2009; Passamonti *et al.*, 2009; Roth *et al.*, 2009; Schuett *et al.*, 2009b; Pambakian *et al.*, 2000; Zihl, 1995b
Scanpath	↑, unsystematic	Machner *et al.*, 2009; Passamonti *et al.*, 2009; Zihl, 1995b; Ishiai *et al.*, 1987; Chédru *et al.*, 1973

Meienberg *et al.* (1981) examined in detail the scanning behavior of three patients: the first with left-sided hemianopia and macular splitting, the second with right-sided hemianopia and macular splitting, and the third with right-sided hemianopia and macular sparing. When a spot of light was presented systematically at 10–20 degrees of eccentricity in the same position in the blind hemifield, the subjects showed a staircase-like saccadic movement to attempt to find the target. Once the target was localized and overshot with a last (hypermetric) saccade, a smooth regressive drift (called "glissade" by the authors) took place. The staircase pattern of the saccades <<…removes the blind hemifield from the target stepwise, the hemifield (which moves with the eye) being pulled back like a curtain>> (Meienberg *et al.*, 1981, p. 540). As soon as the saccadic movement overshoots the stimulus and brings it into the spared hemifield, a backward smooth movement takes place. The first movement of the staircase's saccadic pattern was generally the largest. On the contrary, visual search was normal when the target was presented in the intact hemifield.

Patients were re-examined after 7 months. The authors observed a compensatory strategy: when the position of the spot of light became predictable, the staircase saccades were replaced by an overshoot followed by a quick and wider backward glissade. This way, the stimulus acquisition was faster (figure 6.2).

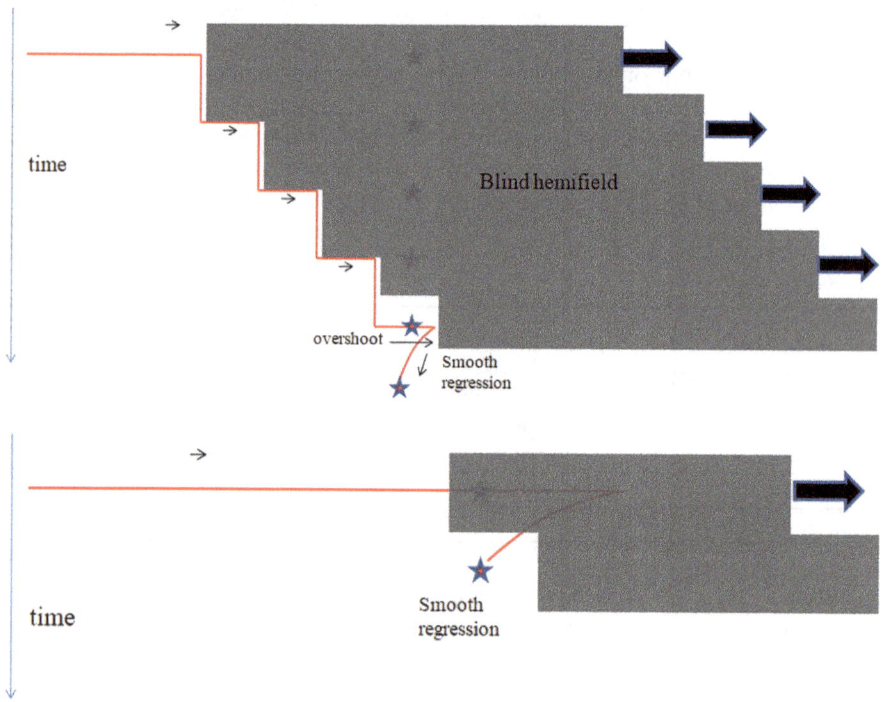

Fig. 6.2 – The staircase pattern during visual search of hemianopic patients when the stimulus is presented systematically at the same position (*i.e.* predictable: upper panel), and after 7 months (lower panel), according to the study of Meienberg and associates. Red line: the ocular movement; stars refer to fixations.

However, when the presentation of the spot of light was unpredictable, the staircase pattern persisted.

Age does not affect the scanning patterns whereas time since the onset of the lesion, as shown, is negatively correlated with search time, number of saccades, and repetitions of the scanpath (Zihl, 1995b).

6.1.1 Visual Field Defect and Cortical Damage: Which is Directly Responsible for the Oculomotor Pattern in Hemianopic Visual Exploration?

The question arises whether the defective visual exploration in patients depends solely on visual deprivation or if it is related also to higher-order dysfunctions.

Tant and colleagues addressed this issue by simulating homonymous hemianopia in normal subjects (Tant *et al.*, 2002). In simulated conditions, the authors found a visual search pattern similar to that reported in hemianopic patients, namely:

- reduced saccadic amplitude in the simulated blind hemifield compared to the controlateral one;
- higher number of fixations and more frequent fixations in the blind hemifield compared to the contralateral side;
- longer scanpath and search time compared to normal conditions;
- poorer visual exploration in left-sided compared to right-sided simulated hemianopia.

Due to the overall correspondence between the visual scanning performed by the simulated hemianopic subjects and real patients, the authors concluded that the abnormal visual scanning behavior is determined by visual deprivation rather than by a concomitant higher-order (*i.e.* cerebral) dysfunction. However, they admit the presence, in hemianopes, of a higher-order dysfunction related to visuospatial organization.

Some years later, the group of Schuett replicated the experiment with a different simulation paradigm: the moving-window paradigm (Rayner and Bertera, 1979; McConkie and Rayner, 1975). Subjects[6] were asked to count some black dots presented in randomized order on a white background. Visual search time was longer, with a higher number of errors in simulated hemianopes compared to normal conditions. Subjects showed longer fixation durations and a higher number of fixations, with reduced accuracy (the saccades toward the blind hemifield tended to be hypometric: Schuett *et al.*, 2009a). Following the study of Tant, the visual exploration pattern in simulated hemianopes was overall the same as found in hemianopic patients (Schuett *et al.*, 2009b): So, the results of Schuett confirmed those reported by Tant, that is visual exploration impairment in hemianopic patients relies mostly on visual field deprivation.

[6]A sample of healthy subjects with simulated left- and right-sided hemianopia (1° of central sparing).

However, it remains to explain why the extent of the visual field defect, quantifiable as the inverse of macular sparing, is not related to the impairment of visual exploration (Zihl, 1995a, 1995b, 2000) and why visual exploration impairment like that of hemianopes is found also in patients with posterior parietal damage but intact visual field (Zihl and Hebel, 1997).[7] Moreover, many hemianopes demonstrate normal visual orientation despite the presence of the scotoma. This suggests that the visual field defect is not the only cause, and orientation and navigation problems do not depend solely on the visual field loss, Additional extrastriate damage, leading to abnormal spatial integration (Zihl, 1995b), is likely to play a substantial role. Spatial integration is provided by the interconnection of receptive fields, and/or by the convergence of neighboring detectors onto higher-order larger receptive fields. Feedback projections help higher-order detectors localize the position of the stimuli across the visual field (spatial orientation). This pyramidal anatomo-functional organization is called *topical convergence* (Zeki and Shipp, 1988). On closer inspection, cerebral lesions involving the topical convergence may contribute to explaining why the compensation of the perimetric loss is more difficult in real compared to simulated patients (Schuett *et al.*, 2009b).

6.2 Displacement of the Egocenter in Hemianopes

An additional problem that may hamper visual exploration of hemianopes is the shift of their subjective "straight ahead" toward the affected side[8] (Ferber and Karnath, 1999; Kerkhoff, 1993, 1999; Barton and Black, 1998; Barton *et al.*, 1998). Due to the mislocalization of the egocenter, shifted toward the blind hemispace, patients (with no neglect) have a contralesional bias to line bisection and tend to localize stimuli as displaced toward the blind region, as shown by errors in pointing tasks (figure 6.3).[9]

Ferber and Karnath (1999) compared the misperception of straight ahead in left-sided hemianopic and neglect patients. As expected, they found an ipsilesional straight-ahead displacement of about 4–5° in neglect patients without hemianopia and a contralesional displacement of about 8° in hemianopic patients without neglect. Interestingly, patients with hemianopia associated with neglect in the same hemifield showed straight-ahead displacement by about 1°, *i.e.* not significantly different from controls.[10] This suggests that the opposite straight-ahead displacement, ipsilesional in neglect and contralesional in hemianopia, counteracts when the two clinical conditions co-exist.

[7]On the contrary, the presence of hemianopia is a constant occurrence in hemianopic alexia and no cases of hemianopic alexia without hemi-visual field defects have been reported (Schuett *et al.*, 2009b).

[8]Contrary to neglect subjects, whose egocenter is displaced toward the spared hemifield.

[9]This phenomenon occurs also in altitudinal hemianopia (Kerkhoff, 1993).

[10]Controls were five patients with right-sided brain damage but no neglect and/or hemianopia.

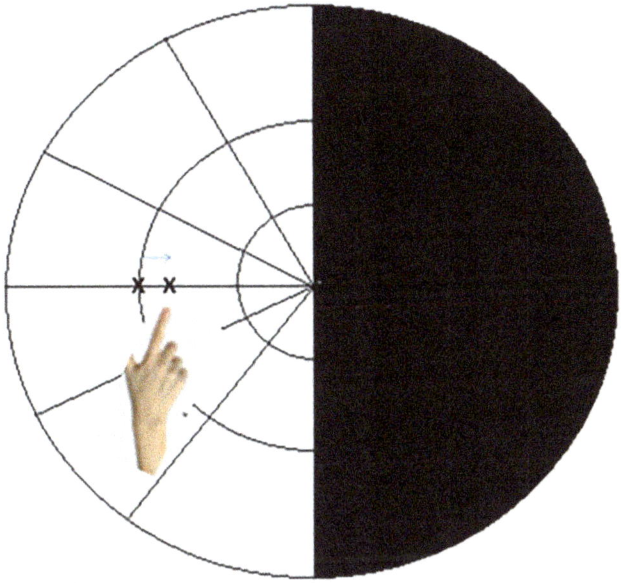

FIG. 6.3 – The mislocalization of the egocenter in hemianopes is shifted toward the blind hemifield.

The parietal cortex (especially the parietoinsular vestibular cortex) is likely to provide a neural representation of space for body orientation (Ferber and Karnath, 1999) so damage to this region could be responsible for the displacement of the subjective egocenter. This may explain the ipsilesional displacement of the subjective straight ahead in patients with neglect, who typically suffer from lesions involving this part of the brain, but fails to account for the contralesional displacement in hemianopic patients with occipital lesions who do not show abnormal parietal function.

6.2.1 Effect of the Displacement of the Egocenter on the Scanning Behavior of Hemianopic Patients

The effect of the displacement of the egocenter on the scanning behavior was studied by the group Barton (Barton *et al.*, 1998). Ocular movements were recorded in seven patients with left- or right hemianopia and no neglect when performing the line bisection task. Subjects were asked to examine the line and to point at its center.

Patients demonstrated a small bisection error toward the contralesional side with median fixation and scanning shifted toward the blind field, as expected. For comparison, nine left-sided hemineglect subjects showed an ipsilesional bisection error with median fixation and scanning shifted ipsilaterally (figure 6.4).

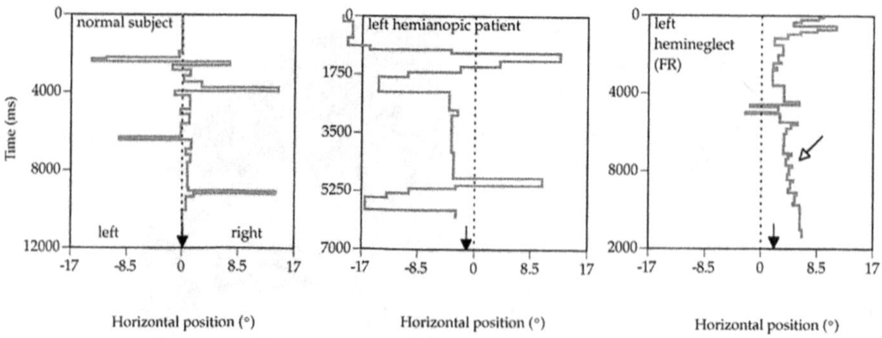

FIG. 6.4 – Oculographic record when performing a line bisection task in a normal subject (left panel), a left hemianopic patient (central panel), and a left hemineglect patient (right panel). The arrow is the subjective straight ahead. From Barton *et al.* (1998). With permission of Oxford University Press.

In addition, fixations along the line showed a bimodal distribution in hemianopes: a peak about the subjective bisection point (*i.e.* shifted 2–4 deg contralesionally), and a smaller one at the end of the line in the contralesional (blind) field. On the contrary, in neglect patients fixations along the line were broadly distributed in the ipsilesional hemifield, without the twin-peak distribution found in hemianopic subjects (figure 6.5). This probably reflects different grades of inattention in the neglect sample (Barton *et al.*, 1998).

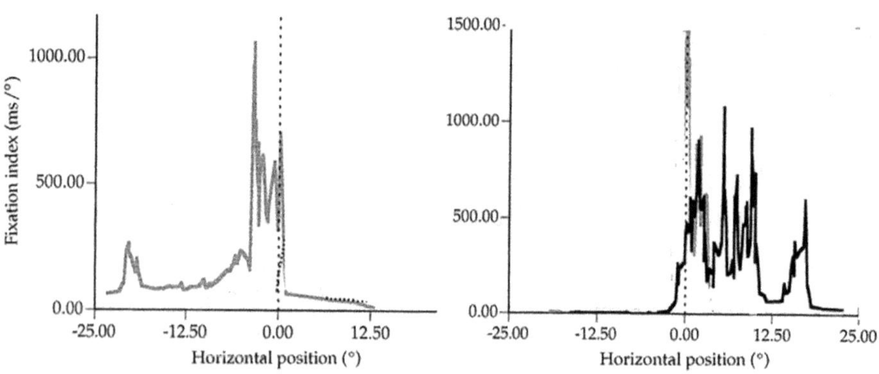

FIG. 6.5 – Fixation density of a left hemianopic patient (left) and a left neglect patient (right) when performing a line bisection task. From Barton *et al.* (1998). With permission of Oxford University Press.

6.3 Size Distortion in Hemianopia

Size distortion is another factor that helps hinder visual orientation. An additional sign in hemianopic patients, indeed, is spatial anisotropy, namely the illusory spatial dilation along the horizontal coordinate (subjects judge spatial distances as longer than normal) in the spared (ipsilesional) hemifield, and spatial compression (spatial distances judged as shorter than normal) in the affected (contralesional) region (*e.g.* Aleci and Pira, 2018; Zihl and von Cramon, 1986).

Chapter 7

Spontaneous Recovery and Compensation of Hemianopia

Overall, hemianopic patients can be classified into two categories: those who show early spontaneous improvement of their visual function (visual field and visual scanning) and those who do not (Zihl, 1995a). What makes the difference is the size of the lesion: patients with lesions restricted to the optic pathways have a better prognosis compared to hemianopic subjects with additional damage to the posterior thalamus and the occipito-parietal cortex (Zihl, 1995a, 1995b).

When present, most of the recovery takes place within the first 48 h,[1] continues during the first 10 days after onset, and is completed some months later. It is evident, especially in right-sided hemianopic patients (*e.g.*: Schuett *et al.*, 2009b; Trauzettel-Klosinski and Brendler, 1998).

Spontaneous improvement of the visual function entails (partial) recovery of light sensibility in the blind region (visual field restoration) and the establishment of adaptive oculomotor strategies.

7.1 Spontaneous Recovery of the Visual Function Due to Visual Field Restoration

Spontaneous restitution of the visual field in the hemianopic region of patients with a cerebral accident has been documented in a series of studies (Tiel and Kolmel, 1991; Gray *et al.*, 1989; Messing and Ganshirt, 1987), but it is limited compared to motor recovery: only 38.4% of the patients with hemianopia benefit from a positive (albeit not satisfactory) prognosis. Among these, complete restitution of the visual field may occur in up to 72% of the patients with incomplete hemianopia, whereas it remains partial in most of the cases of complete hemianopia (72%; Gray *et al.*, 1989).

Functional improvement, which depends on spontaneous healing with reabsorption of perilesional edema and inflammation and reorganization of synaptic

[1]During the first month, according to Cassidy *et al.* (1999).

DOI: 10.1051/978-2-7598-3493-8.c007

connections in the visual cortex (neuroplasticity: Jamara *et al.*, 2003), has been confirmed by neuroimaging. A reduction of the size of the metabolic lesion (improved glucose metabolism) with time has been described with positron emission tomography in hemianopic patients who recovered from the visual field defect, but not in those whose visual field impairment persisted (Suzuki *et al.*, 2016; Bosley *et al.*, 1987). As shown in an fMRI study, spontaneous recovery is associated with a progressive increase of cortical activation next to the lesioned region, with the center of activation displaced toward the occipital lobe (Yoshida *et al.*, 2006).

The improvement of the visual field is not related to the age of the patient and the type of hemianopic defect (Zhang *et al.*, 2006a), but depends on the localization of the cerebral lesion, with the poorest prognosis for damage involving the occipital lobe (Bosley *et al.*, 1987), and on the time since onset. The probability of visual recovery, indeed, decreases with time. Zhang *et al.* (2006a) followed 254 hemianopic patients with complete or incomplete hemianopia and found a spontaneous perimetric improvement in up to 55% of the cases; in these patients, the recovery took place within 1 month with a probability of 50%–60%; after this period, improvement is still possible within 6 months, but with a likelihood of only 20%. After 6 months, the authors found no further reduction of the perimetric loss (figure 7.1).

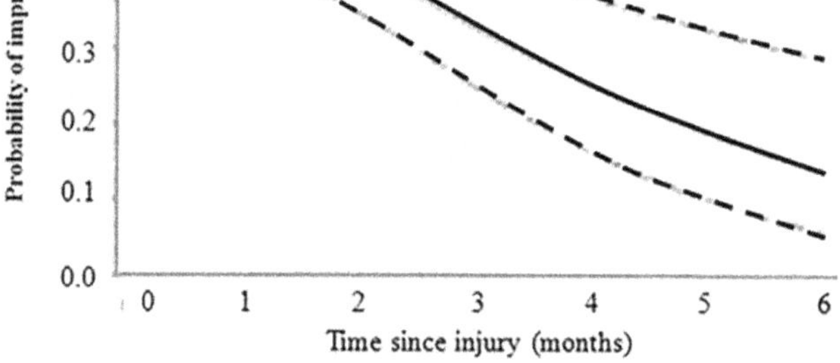

FIG. 7.1 – Probability of recovery as a function of time since injury. From Zhang *et al.* (2006a). With permission of Wolters Kluwer Health publisher.

This finding is overall in line with what was previously found by Gray *et al.* (1989) and by Tiel and Kolmel (1991) (most of the recovery takes place within the first two weeks since onset) and by Messing and Ganshirt (1987) (the improvement reaches its maximum within 6 months).[2] The rate of recovery is higher in the first month after the onset (Ali *et al.*, 2013). Generally, visual field restoration starts from the lower quadrants (Çelebisoy *et al.*, 2011; Tiel and Kolmel, 1991) at the seen/not seen transition zone of the visual field and in the temporal crescent (Tiel and Kölmel, 1991). It involves light detection, then motion, form, color, and finally stereopsis (Gray *et al.*, 1989; Zihl, 1980). Residual vague perception (hand movement) in the affected hemifield is a good prognostic factor (Kaul *et al.*, 1974).

7.2 Spontaneous Recovery of the Visual Function Due to Oculomotor Adaptation

Different visual performances in patients with a comparable visual field loss cannot but depend on more or less effective visual scanning. As an example, the hemianopic drivers who perform better are those who show a higher percentage of glances and compensatory eye, head, and shoulder movements toward the blind field (Kasneci *et al.*, 2014; Wood *et al.*, 2011). So, developing oculomotor strategies suitable to maximize the visual processing in the contralesional hemifield is material to restore the defective visual exploration.

As seen, patients learn to shift their fixation repeatedly toward the blind region, briefly displacing the stimulus of interest to the side of the spared hemifield (Schuett *et al.*, 2008a): in light of the above, it is clear why the prognosis is poor in hemianopic patients with neglect (Schoepf and Zangemeister, 1993).

To a certain extent, the possibility of successful development of an efficient oculomotor strategy in the acquired hemianopic condition has been documented (*e.g.* Machner *et al.*, 2009; Schuett *et al.*, 2009b; Zihl, 1995a, 1995b; Meienberg *et al.*, 1981; Chédru *et al.*, 1973). Immediately after the onset of the brain lesion, eye movements directed toward the blind hemifield are scarce (Chédru *et al.*, 1973) and the oculomotor behavior (*i.e.* the pattern of fixations) is like that of normal subjects; however, with time the scanning behavior adapts to the hemianopic condition (provided neglect is absent).

The findings of Meienberg and colleagues have already been reported. In addition, oculomotor adaptation leading to improvement in visual search was described by Schuett and associates in 24 healthy subjects with simulated hemianopia. After 15 min of visual search practice,[3] search performance and the oculomotor

[2]It is unusual the case described by Poggel *et al.* (2001) of a 29-year-old man with a gunshot lesion in the left occipital lobe extending through the interhemispheric fissure into the right temporal lobe. The subject experienced a complete loss of vision immediately after the injury. After a week, vision had recovered in the upper right quadrant; the improvement continued after the second/third month up to 16 months after the accident: after six months, vision was restored in the contralateral quadrants so that the residual defect was confined to the inferior region of the visual field and best-corrected visual acuity was normal. However, the visuospatial function (form perception, object recognition, spatial relationship perception, visual orientation, speed, and direction estimation) and visual scanning remained impaired.

[3]Practice consisted of counting silently five irregular patterns made up of 19–21 dots as accurately and quickly as possible.

parameters improved with a decreased number of fixations (Schuett *et al.*, 2009b). As a result of spontaneous recovery, patients show fewer refixations (more equally distributed in the blind and spared hemifield), reduced search duration, fewer and wider saccades, and in general a more structured scanpath strategy.

This spontaneous oculomotor compensation takes place in about 40% of the cases (Zihl, 1995b). In 10%–20% of them, the new strategy consolidates within the first two to three months (Kerkhoff, 2000).

In substance, hemianopes adopt two compensatory oculomotor strategies to cope with their field loss:

- i- series of hypometric saccades that approach gradually the stimulus projected onto the blind hemifield (Meienberg *et al.*, 1981). This way, fixation tends to be directed toward the blind region to "push" the visual information to the opposite side. This approach, however, is not efficient and is time-consuming (Schuett *et al.*, 2008a);
- ii- saccadic overshooting toward the blind hemifield (Zangemeister and Utz, 2002; Zangemeister *et al.*, 1995; Meienberg *et al.*, 1981). When subjects are asked to look at a simple stimulus, *e.g.* a white cross presented at 6–30 degrees of eccentricity in the blind field, they perform a series of small saccades. After the presentation of the target is iterated two to four times, its position becomes predictable, and the saccades turn hypermetric. The overshooting is followed by a fast backward glissade toward the target (Zangemeister *et al.*, 1995; Meienberg *et al.*, 1981). This strategy, therefore, can be summarized as a staircase series of saccades, when the position of the target in the blind hemifield is unpredictable, and a large saccade that slightly overshoots the target followed by a backward glissade when it is predictable.

Likewise, when examining complex (natural) scenes, hemianopes replace the global viewing strategy commonly adopted by healthy subjects with a high frequency of local scanning. Quoting the authors: <<Hemianopic patients showed sequences of small amplitude fixational saccades as a local scanpath in both visual hemifields: *i.e.*, they searched for some primarily relevant detail by use of which they could then generate a global scanpath>> (Zangemeister *et al.*, 1995, p. 476). However, practice helps improve visual exploration when inspecting visual scenes: in conditions of simulated hemianopia a sample of normal subjects, who showed a visual scanning similar to that used by hemianopes (with a staircase and overshoot saccadic strategy) improved their oculomotor pattern after 20 min of viewing (*i.e.* practice) with shorter fixation durations and increased saccadic amplitude (Zangemeister and Utz, 2002).

Pambakian and associates (2000) compared the oculomotor pattern of left-sided and right-sided hemianopes with a control group when inspecting natural scenes. The interesting result was that in real-life situations the scanning behavior of the hemianopes with recent lesions (less than six months) did not differ from controls: thereby it was less efficient than controls due to the presence of the visual field impairment. On the contrary, in patients with older lesions the scanning behavior was consistently different, with different positions of fixations, longer scanpaths, and more saccades toward the blind side. Saccades toward the blind side were shorter than those directed toward the intact region, as was observed in the abovementioned experimental studies. This is considered by Pambakian and colleagues as a compensatory oculomotor strategy adopted by patients in real life (Pambakian *et al.*, 2000).

It remains that if the fixation/saccadic pattern of hemianopes differs from controls when performing simple and strictly controlled laboratory experiments, in daily manual tasks it is roughly the same. In a study by Martin and colleagues (2007), the time spent to complete a manual task (namely assembling Wood models), the eye-hand latency as well as fixation and saccade parameters did not show any statistical difference with controls. Patients' gaze was not biased toward the hemianopic field as found in experimental non-naturalistic conditions, the staircase hypometric saccadic pattern was not observed, and the hypermetric/corrective saccadic pattern was found only in one patient. The most relevant difference compared to controls was less predictable sequential gaze patterns, with frequent fixations at intermediate locations, apparently irrelevant. Since fixations in patients were as accurate as in normal subjects, it is concluded that hemianopes compensate for their hemifield loss in daily tasks by relying greatly on visuospatial memory and increasing updating of spatial information in their visual working memory. This is achieved by accurate inspection of different regions of the workspace, not strictly related to the actual task.

In addition, the shift of the head toward the affected hemifield is a form of compensation that should not be discouraged (Kerkhoff *et al.*, 1992a; Zangemeister *et al.*, 1982). Zangemeister and associates (1982) investigated the role of head movement as an additional compensatory strategy. When the target is presented in the blind field, the head movement toward the blind region is reduced or omitted, with a consequent higher frequency of saccades responsible for the staircase search pattern. The authors accounted for the reduction of head movement toward the blind hemifield inasmuch search task in the hemianopic region requires a so complex sensory-motor adaptive strategy that <<[...] brain seemingly responds by simplifying the task: it eliminates the head-movement component of the synkinesis, stabilizing the head in the service of vision>> (Zangemeister *et al.*, 1982). It remains that the head movement could be useful if trained, as it may work in synergy with the oculomotor scanning process in the blind hemifield.

7.3 Spontaneous Recovery of Reading Due to Oculomotor Adaptation

Reading speed of hemianopic patients (without neglect) tends to increase with time since onset, especially in right-sided hemianopia. The improvement depends on a decreased number and increased amplitude of forward saccades, thereby on a decreased number (and duration) of fixations, and fewer backward saccades (Schuett *et al.*, 2009b).

Left hemianopes learn to build the coordinates of the spatial representation of the page starting from the cue provided by the boundaries of the written text: after reading a few lines, the return sweep tends to improve (less fragmented: Schuett *et al.*, 2009b; Trauzettel-Klosinski and Brendler, 1998). The position of the first words of the string of the text, in fact, is always the same, so, with practice, the patient acquires the spatial coordinates of the left boundary of the text and guides the return sweep accordingly (Schuett *et al.*, 2008a).

It is noteworthy that spontaneous compensation of visual exploration in a patient does not help that patient read better, and, *vice versa*, spontaneous improvement of the lexical function has no effect on visual orientation and exploration in the same subject (Schuett *et al.*, 2009b; Zihl, 2000). In other words, spontaneous oculomotor adaptation to the hemianopic loss is task-specific, and there is no transfer of the effect between visual exploration and reading, or reading and visual exploration (Schuett *et al.*, 2009b).

7.3.1 Eccentric Fixation

Compensatory eccentric fixation is often found in hemianopic patients with macular splitting or small sparing of the macular region (about 30% of cases: Trauzettel-Klosinski, 1977). It is an additional compensatory strategy adopted when reading. Trauzettel-Klosinski (1977) demonstrated with a scanning laser ophthalmoscope (SLO) that subjects with homonymous hemianopia or quadrantanopia may develop bilateral parafoveal fixation ("homonymous eccentric fixation"), about 1 deg from the foveola in the spared hemifield, despite normal central visual acuity. This way, the word is shifted toward the healthy retina so that the visual span is enlarged on the side of the blind hemifield. This advantage is achieved at the cost of reduced visual acuity, as visual acuity decreases with eccentricity. However, for stimuli requiring high resolution (*i.e.* high visual acuity), patients (who in most cases have normal foveal visual acuity) can regain central fixation. Trauzettel-Klosinki showed that, compared to a group of patients who did not show eccentric fixation, the reading rate improved in left- and right-sided hemianopic subjects by 26% and by 28%, respectively. According to the same author, eccentric fixation is more frequent in right-sided than in left-sided hemianopia[4] and depends on the distance of the scotoma from the fovea: the closer the hemiscotoma to the center of the visual field, the more probable the development of eccentric fixation in the opposite direction.[5] In the presence of a scotoma closer than 2 deg to the center, fixation is eccentric in the majority of left- and right-sided hemianopes.

Cerebral localization of the lesion (infra/suprageniculate) and age do not affect the development of this function.

Within a rehabilitative framework it should be kept in mind that since the resolution capacity of the paracentral region is lower than the central region, print size should be increased in hemianopic patients who develop eccentric fixation.

[4]Eccentric fixation: 44% of the right-sided hemianopic subjects and 16% of the left-sided hemianopic patients.

[5]Average distance of the border of the scotoma from the fovea: 2.6 deg in RH with eccentric fixation *vs.* 3.9 deg in RH with central fixation, and 2.0 deg in LH with eccentric fixation *vs.* 2.7 deg in LH with central fixation, where 1 degree of retinal eccentricity corresponds to 8.3–9.9 mm in the visual cortex.

7.4 The Effect of the Central Damage on the Development of Spontaneous Oculomotor Adaptation to Visual Search and Reading

Does the central (cerebral) damage affect the development of spontaneous oculomotor adaptation? Schuett and colleagues (2009b) addressed this issue by studying the adaptation of visual exploration and reading in simulated left-sided and right-sided hemianopes.

After 15 min of visual search practice (counting dots), the oculomotor pattern of simulated hemianopes improved with a reduced number of fixations, less fixation duration, shorter visual search time, and fewer errors (omissions of dots: table 7.1). The number of errors decreased to a normal level, whereas search time remained higher compared to the normal, non-simulated condition. Overall, the effect of visual search practice was the same for both left- and right-sided simulated hemianopes.

As for the lexical performance, after 15 min of reading practice, reading time and the oculomotor pattern of simulated hemianopic subjects improved consistently, especially in left-sided hemianopic condition, with a reduced number of fixations, less fixation duration, wider forward saccades, shorter backward saccades, increased amplitude of the return sweep, and shorter reading time (table 7.1).

The right-sided simulated hemianopes needed twice as many reading training sessions to reach the same result.

Regardless of the oculomotor adaptation to a hemianopic scotoma reported in the study of the group of Schuett, the relevant point is that, compared to simulated hemianopes, patients require a much longer systematic rehabilitation (at least 8 h for reading: Zihl, 2000): this strongly suggests, therefore, that central damage does hamper the spontaneous adaptation to visual deprivation.

7.5 Compensation of Hemianopic Patients with Hemineglect

The oculomotor compensation of the hemianopic defect is more difficult in the presence of hemineglect (Halligan *et al.*, 1990; Meienberg, 1988). If "pure" hemianopic patients tend to compensate for their defect by longer inspection on the hemianopic side, patients with additional hemineglect lack this strategy (Ishiai *et al.*, 1987): they tend to fixate and scan a visual scene in the spared hemifield, beginning from the right side. Their saccadic staircase triggering toward the affected hemifield is slower and the compensatory overshoot is missing (di Pellegrino *et al.*, 2001; Behrmann *et al.*, 1997; Meienberg, 1988; Girotti *et al.*, 1983).

So, patients with hemineglect are more handicapped than "pure" hemianopes, as they tend to underestimate or ignore their problem of visual inattention (Meienberg, 1988).

TAB. 7.1 – The effect of practice on the oculomotor pattern in reading and visual search of hemianopes.

		Fixation duration	Forward (rightw.) saccade (→fixation) -number	Forward (rightw.) saccades -size	Backw. (leftw.) saccades (→refixations) number	Leftw. saccades-size	Ret. Sweep	Reading time	
								Visual Search time	Number of errors (omissions of dots)
Reading post-practice	RH	↓	↓	↑	↓	-	↑	↓	-
	LH	↓	↓	↑	↓	-	↑	↓	-
Visual search post-practice	RH	↓	↓	Ns	ns	Ns	-	↓	↓
	LH	↓	↓	Ns	ns	Ns	-	↓	↓

Chapter 8

Rehabilitation of Hemianopia: Visual Restitution

Basically, rehabilitation of hemianopia means rehabilitation of visual exploration and reading. Even if spontaneous oculomotor compensation is more evident in the former than in the latter (Zihl, 2000), in both cases treatment is desirable.

The most straightforward approach to improving both visual exploration and reading is finding a way to

i- restore, at least in part, the blind hemifield;
ii- compensate for the functional loss with oculomotor strategies.

Kerkhoff (2000) categorized the procedures aimed at rehabilitating the blind field as:

- *visual restitution* (also called *restoration*) treatments, when the aim is recovering part of the silent or depressed visual field *via* training with repetitive visual stimulations;
- *visual compensation*, with the aim to help the oculomotor function adapt to the perimetric loss;
- *visual substitution* procedures, when optic devices (*e.g.* prismatic lenses, small mirrors to be mounted over the spectacle frames, o magnification softwares) are developed to supply the loss of function in the hemianopic zone with the spared region of the visual field.

8.1 Rationale of Visual Restitution: Cortical Plasticity

The fact that receptive field (RF) properties and neuronal inter-connections in the adult striate cortex are not fixed but can be modulated by the perceptual context, re-conditioned after cerebral damage, and, last but not least, responsive to repetitive stimulation, is the basic assumption to hypothesize that visual training may restore the visual function of hemianopic patients. In other terms, the precondition is *cortical plasticity.*

DOI: 10.1051/978-2-7598-3493-8.c008

Since the last decades, dogma has been that the properties and anatomical connections of the cortical visual cells are plastic during the age of development but fixed in adulthood. Now, there is wide evidence that a consistent degree of cortical plasticity is retained even after the end of the developmental period.

A clue to the presence of cortical plasticity in adulthood comes from the fact that the functional characteristics of the receptive fields in V1 are modulated by global sensory stimulation, that is to say by contextual stimuli.

For example, the response to a line segment placed within a receptive field is boosted by a line localized outside its boundaries; on the contrary, the response is inhibited by a series of randomly oriented segments surrounding the cortical functional unit. Contextual stimuli can modulate the selective response: lines with a given orientation surrounding the receptive field affect the orientation tuning of a line placed inside it. Another example is perceptual filling-in, which takes place when a permanent or reversible scotoma is filled by the characteristics of the surroundings so that the spatial discontinuity is perceptually removed. These contextual effects operate *via* long-range horizontal connections, with the contribution of higher-order cortical regions like V2 (Gilbert, 1998; Gilbert *et al.*, 1996).

Cortical plasticity is revealed also by perceptual learning: perceptual learning makes use of the practice to improve detection or discrimination tasks of position, motion, line orientation, and so forth. Perceptual learning relies on the enhancement of the subthreshold response consistent with Hebb's rule, and it takes place, probably, on V1: low-level stations along the visual pathway, *e.g.* the lateral geniculate body, seems unlikely, as perceptual learning is specific for the task while the lateral geniculate nucleus is responsive to a broad variety of visual stimulations. In turn, the lack of transfer in terms of the type of task and spatial position in the visual field rules out higher-order cortical regions. Studies using functional magnetic resonance and transcranial magnetic stimulation, indeed, confirm this statement (Karmarka and Dan, 2006).

In the last decades, research shed light on the functional and anatomical mechanisms underlying cortical plasticity. Studies on adult animals (*e.g.* Darian-Smith and Gilbert, 1995; Gilbert and Wiesel, 1992; Kaas *et al.*, 1990) demonstrated that the plastic changes involve the size and position of the receptive fields but not their specific properties, like orientation (reviewed by Das, 1997). The modulation occurs over a wide temporal range: rapid and reversible modifications in neuronal response properties (short-term dynamic reorganization) take place within seconds or minutes; on the contrary, long-term reorganization after surgical manipulations or focal destruction requires weeks to months to consolidate.

8.1.1 Cortical Reorganization After Reversible Cortical Deafferentiation

In the adult cat, Petter and Gilbert (1992) found a consistent enlargement (by a factor of about 5) of the cortical receptive fields after reversible cortical deafferentiation induced by an artificial retinal scotoma. The enlargement took place after 15 min from the deafferentiation; the receptive field size returned to the original dimension as soon as the scotoma was removed. Longer conditioning determines more robust changes and needs prolonged and more vigorous stimulation to bring the receptive field back to the original state (Das, 1997). De-inhibition or enhancement of the horizontal long-range connections between hypercolumns may account for the reversible, short-term variation of the RF size.

8.1.2 Cortical Reorganization After Permanent Retinal Scotoma

As for reversible retinal scotomas, congruous bilateral retinal lesions are shown to induce in animals a two-step cortical reorganization in the deafferentiated region of V1 (Darian-Smith and Gilbert, 1995).

Within 1 h of the lesion, a short-term reorganization takes place with:

- i- no response of the deafferentiated cortical RF to stimulations of the correspondent lesioned retinal region (Darian-Smith and Gilbert, 1995; Gilbert and Wiesel, 1992);
- ii- slight displacement of the receptive fields localized at the periphery of the cortical scotoma, just beyond its boundary (Darian-Smith and Gilbert, 1995; Gilbert and Wiesel, 1992);
- iii- consistent increase (five to tenfold) in receptive field size at the boundary or just inside the scotoma (Eysel and Schweigart, 1999; Gilbert, 1998; Darian-Smith and Gilbert, 1995; Gilbert and Wiesel, 1992).

The response of the re-organized receptive field retained directionality and orientation specificity but was weaker compared with the non-deafferentiated cortex, sluggish, and fatigued after repetitive stimulation (Darian-Smith and Gilbert, 1995).

Two to twelve months later, it can be observed:

- i- response of the deafferentiated cortical RF evoked by perilesional retinal stimulation;
- ii- shift of the receptive fields located inside the scotoma up to 5° outside the border of the scotoma, with a frequent (but not systematic) increase in their size (Darian-Smith and Gilbert, 1995; Gilbert and Wiesel, 1992): this means great expansion of the representation of the perilesional retina.

In sum, cortical reorganization after retinal damage makes the cortical cells close to the deafferentiated region responsive to stimuli directed to the silent region. The cortical receptive fields subserving the scotoma continue to represent the surrounding retinal region: it follows the retinal scotoma is under-represented ("shrinkage").

This way, cortical plasticity accounts for the perceptual filling-in of the scotoma. It remains, however, that it does not restore sight in the damaged retinal region.

8.1.3 Cortical Reorganization After Cortical Damage

In the case of cortical lesions, things are different. Contrary to a retinal scotoma, where the corresponding cortical receptive fields are functionally intact but silenced, in the presence of damage to the striate cortex a neuronal loss takes place, and the cells surrounding the damaged neurons have to take over the topographical representation of the destroyed cortical region. This way, the information from the retinal locus that is no longer represented in the cortex is made accessible by the cells surrounding the damaged tissue. In area 17, 1–5 days after the cortical lesion the activity is suppressed close to the border of the damaged tissue and increases above normal levels in a ring surrounding the lesion, then it decreases further away from the damaged area (Eysel and Schmidt-Kastner, 1991).

After some weeks, excitability normalizes as it increases close to the border of the lesion and decreases along the perilesional ring (Buchkremer-Ratzmann and Witte, 1997). The cortical hyperactivation of the region adjacent to the scotoma, found at magnetoencephalography in nine post-stroke hemianopic patients by Braun and colleagues during stimulation of the perilesional region (the visual field adjacent to the scotoma), reflects the enlargement of the receptive fields surrounding the damaged cortex and may form the basis for the restitution of the visual function (Braun *et al.*, 2001). Enlargement of the cortical retinotopic representation at the border of focal ischemic lesions has been confirmed by Zepeda and colleagues (2003) in a sample of kittens. The enlargement, directed toward the damaged region, occurred within 5 weeks: it follows that the information from the retinal region projecting to the damaged cortex is again effective as it is back to projecting to functionally active, and enlarged, receptive fields surrounding the lesioned cortical area.

In other terms, after cortical injuries the retinal representation of the damaged area on the cortex is displaced toward the neighboring intact regions (Eysel *et al.*, 1999).

8.1.4 Anatomy of Cortical Plasticity

What are the anatomofunctional changes upon which cortical reorganization relies? As seen, brain plasticity in brain-damaged patients makes possible (partial) recovery of the visual function *via* increased size and positional changes of the perilesional receptive fields. This is allowed by functional modulation followed by anatomical reorganization of a complex neuronal network of lateral interactions (Darian-Smith and Gilbert, 1995).

Plastic reversible (short-term) and permanent (long-term) changes on the visual cortex are mediated by horizontal connections between columns with similar receptive field attributes. The excitatory neurons receive excitatory and inhibitory horizontal collaterals that balance each other, producing a subthreshold modulatory effect.

This model assumes that a minimal residual neural substrate, reckoned as 10% of the total neuronal pool, is needed for the reorganization process to take place (the so-called *hypothesis of minimal residual structure*: Sabel, 1997).

Cortical reorganization takes place on V1 and is mediated by structures interacting with the striate cortex, like the superior colliculus (Zihl and von Cramon, 1982) and the suprasylvian gyrus (Baumann and Spear, 1977; Fischman and Meikle, 1965)[1].

Cortical reorganization on V1 includes:

a) potentiation of pre-existing synapses (Hirsch and Gilbert, 1993) according to the Hebbian model: given two or more synapses, when a synapse is coactivated with its target neuron and the other is depolarized, the first strengthens whereas the other remains unaffected (no synaptic competition). If the second synapse is inactive (*i.e.* unable to drive the postsynaptic neuron) when the target neuron is activated, the synapse weakens (synaptic competition: figure 8.1);

b) de-inhibition of pre-existing synapses: about 15%–20% of the population of each cortical layer is made up of inhibitory neurons which exert a high influence on cortical modulation, being more effective than the excitatory counterparts (Reviewed by Das, 1997). So, the process starts with dynamic, short-term de-inhibition of long-range horizontal collaterals at the borders of the nonresponsive regions (reviewed by Das, 1997). De-inhibition leads to the unmasking of subthreshold excitatory inputs (Gilbert, 1998) and allows the incorporation of receptive fields with the same properties. This process accounts for receptive field enlargement, which is initially labile but becomes stable if the deafferentiation continues (Das and Gilbert, 1995);

c) axonal sprouting of long-range horizontal collaterals in the reorganized cortex (Darian-Smith and Gilbert, 1994, reviewed by Das, 1997). The effect of cortical reorganization in animals after bilateral congruous lesions are increased density[2] of axon fibers, 57%–88% greater or even double (Gilbert, 1998; Gilbert *et al.*, 1996; Darian-Smith and Gilbert, 1994) in the reorganized cortex compared to normal conditions. The higher fiber density, taking place over 3–9 months, is associated with increased synapse number but is not accompanied by a topographical extension of fibers beyond the pre-existing fiber plexus. The region involved in long-term cortical reorganization encompassed a cortical area 7–8 mm in size. This extension is in agreement with the lateral extent of the cortical horizontal plexus (Darian-Smith and Gilbert, 1994).

---

[1]The possibility that V1 is the target site of the process is supported by evidence that the post-training improvement of discrimination abilities as orientation discrimination of short-oriented stimuli or bisection or vernier acuity is specific to the trained location. The lack of spatial transfer excludes higher visual areas, like V2 and V3, that show larger receptive fields compared to V1. In effect, due to the larger size of their receptive fields, plastic changes in V2 or V3 are expected to induce improvement not only at the cortical site of the lesion but also in the neighboring areas of the corresponding region of V1: yet, this is not the case (Das, 1997). Likewise, task specificity rules out the role of the LGN in post-lesion plastic changes. In fact, the LGN shows no signs of recovery in the absence of new geniculate-cortical connections (Das, 1997; Darian-Smith and Gilbert, 1995).

[2]Fibre density was defined by the authors as <<the sum of the lengths of all fibre fragments within the sampled volume of cortex>>.

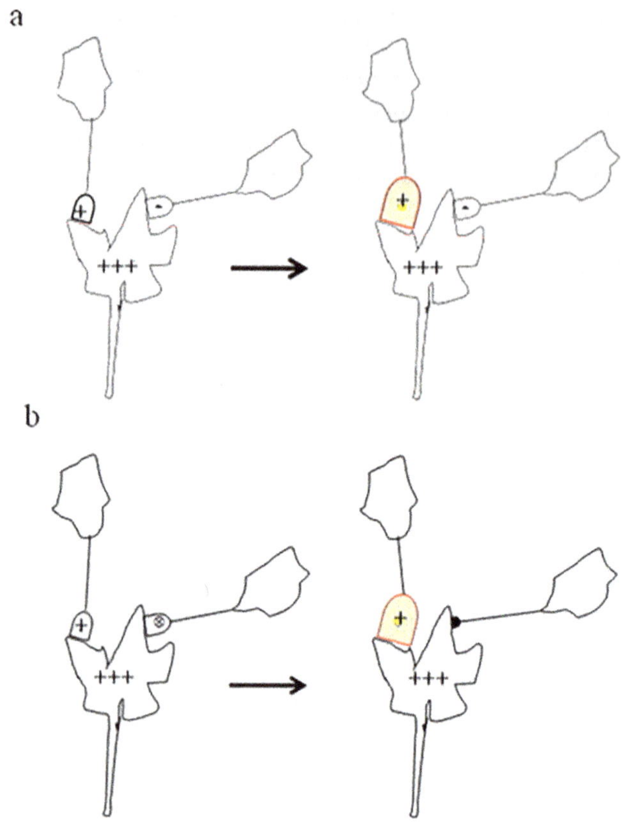

FIG. 8.1 – Hebbian model for synapse strengthening; a: no synaptic competition; b: synaptic competition. See text for explanation. Inspired by Das A. (1997). With permission of Taylor & Francis publisher.

8.1.5 Recovery After Training in Animals

Animal studies support the idea that visual rehabilitation can improve visual function after brain damage. Since the late sixties, Cowey and, subsequently, Mohler and Wurtz, showed that training may improve the visual function after damage to the cortex of monkeys (Mohler and Wurtz, 1977; Cowey, 1967). Likewise, rats without visual cortex regained their ability to perform a visual task after visual training (Spear and Barbas, 1975), and massive training after bilateral removal of the visual cortex led adult cats to recover brightness discrimination (Urbaitis and Meikle, 1968).

In adult cats, the group of Eysel co-stimulated the receptive fields located in layers II and III of areas 17 and 18 with flickering rectangular stimuli (temporal frequency: 1 Hz) aimed at the responsive region of the visual field as well as at an unresponsive region at its border (Eysel *et al.*, 1998). After 10–75 min of co-stimulation, a response was observed also outside the borders of the receptive field, *i.e.* in the previously unresponsive region (figure 8.2). This finding occurred in

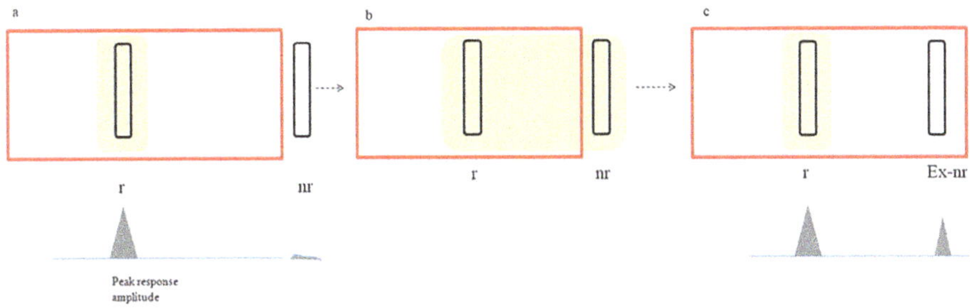

FIG. 8.2 – Effect of co-stimulation on the peak response amplitude of a cortical receptive field. Red rectangle: receptive field; yellow: stimulated region; a: before the training the stimulation of the responsive region (r) generates no response from the nonresponsive region (nr), as expected; b: co-stimulation of both the responsive region within the receptive field and the nonresponsive region at its border; c: after co-stimulation, a response from the previously nonresponsive region is observed. Data from Eysel *et al.* (1998).

57% of the cellular sample and suggested an enlargement of the receptive field toward the non-responsive region that persisted up to 3 h from the end of the co-stimulation. Not only receptive field expansion but also enhanced activation was observed. These results were found for cells in areas 17 and 18, simplex and complex, and were independent of receptive field size or eccentricity.

The observed changes in the size of the receptive field would depend on the activation by suprathreshold inputs of subthreshold synapses within and close to its borders. Intracortical inhibition is likely to be responsible for ineffective co-stimulation as found in 43% of the sample. The next year, the same group confirmed the enlargement of the excitatory area of the targeted receptive field after visual training in one-third of the cases. The enlargement was directed toward the unresponsive co-stimulated area and determined recovery of part of the scotomatous region (Eysel *et al.*, 1999).

As shown in a study on adult rats housed in conditions of light deprivation for 10 days (He *et al.*, 2006, reviewed by Karmarka and Dan, 2006), complete and prolonged visual deprivation brings back the adult visual cortex to a state of cortical plasticity similar to the developmental period, with a decreased ratio of inhibitory/excitatory receptors. This possibility of a cortical reset further confirms the plastic potential of the adult cortex. Taken together, these pieces of evidence legitimate the investigation of rehabilitative solutions based on visual repetitive stimulation in adult human subjects suffering from post-stroke visual deprivation.

8.2 Vision Restitution in Humans: Training at the Transition Zone

Within this framework, since the late sixtieths a strand of research has been investigating the effect of visual training in reactivating the surviving neurons located within the part of the damaged visual cortex representing the *transition zone* between the seeing and non-seeing region. In other terms, the transition zone is the visual space between the intact and the affected hemifield, where light sensibility is depressed but not completely abolished.

After a stroke, neurons in the affected regions can be destroyed, survive with internal damage, or, in small proportion, remain intact. The last two conditions are critical for the recovery: according to Sabel, neurons with partial damage can return to their original state while intact neurons can be potentiated and their activity may be enhanced to compensate for the lost function of the destroyed units (Sabel, 1999). A small amount of surviving cells (say one sixtieth or 10% of cortical neurons: Sabel, 1997; Lashley, 1939), indeed, is enough to allow the recovery of a rudimentary form of discrimination. This quota, more or less damaged but to some extent still responsive, is likely to be localized at the boundaries of the cortical damaged region, corresponding to the transition zone of the visual field. Training strategies have been developed with the scope of enlarging the residual visual field of hemianopic patients by "pushing the curtain" (*i.e.* the transition zone) toward the blind side.

Repetitive stimulation at the transition zone during training would reactivate the cortical neurons in the primary visual cortex that subserve this region (Poggel *et al.*, 2008a, 2008b; Kasten *et al.*, 1998a)[3]. In addition, training is argued to enhance visual attention at the seen/not seen region, increasing the awareness of weak visual signals in this portion of the visual field (Kasten *et al.*, 2000).

Indeed, Bergsma and van der Wildt (2010), in line with Kasten and colleagues, suggested that the effect of visual restoration training (in their case consisting of repeated measurements of detection threshold with a perimetric procedure) relies on a double mechanism: first, the neuronal activity of the spared neurons is increased up to a suprathreshold level. Second, attention directed toward the blind hemifield (and in particular the transition zone) is enhanced.

In this section, the main representative studies on visual restoration training performed on the transition zone of hemianopes are summarized.

8.2.1 Repeated Threshold Measurements across the Transition Zone (Zihl and von Cramon, 1979)

Zihl and von Cramon (1979) stimulated the border of the hemianopic defect by measuring repeatedly light differential threshold[4] at different horizontal eccentricities across the boundary of the scotomatous region (the transition zone) with an automated perimeter. The authors administered 1-h daily sessions, each made of 15–20 measurements, to 12 subjects who suffered from stroke with left- or right-sided hemianopia, quadrantanopia, or central scotoma. The interval between onset since the lesion and training ranged from one month to six years in the absence of other neurological deficits. Stimulation was monocular. After having ruled out

[3]The reactivation would involve a change in the topography of cortical receptive fields, activation of long-term horizontal connections in the visual cortex, and thalamo-cortical feedback loops (Poggel *et al.*, 2008b).

[4]A staircase procedure was used to estimate the threshold, background luminance: 3.2 cd m^{-2}.

spontaneous recovery, the authors reported substantial enlargement of the visual field and increased light sensitivity in their patients (figure 8.3). The characteristics of the recovery can be summarized as follows:

1- the improvement was observable after three to five sessions and ranged from one to several degrees (up to 8–15°);

2- the enlargement of the visual field and the number of sessions required for the improvement depends on the gradient of sensitivity at the transition zone. Shallower gradients (gradual transition) lead to better results. This different behavior may depend on the fact that in the transition zone some cells, intermingled with the non-responsive tissue are intact or quasi-intact. These cells, indeed, would be the recipient of the stimulation: steeper gradients reflect less residual vital cells, thereby poor prognosis;

3- the improvement in terms of spatial extent of the recovered region and increased sensibility was not restricted to the stimulated region at the transition zone, but extended above and below the trained locus: the farther the trained locus from the fixation point along the vertical meridian, the greater the recovered extent and sensibility of the bordering region. In other terms, the effect of the training increased with the eccentricity from the stimulated locus;

4- the improvement showed complete interocular transfer to the occluded (nonstimulated) eye;

5- the improvement was persistent, being still observable after 6 months from the end of the training.

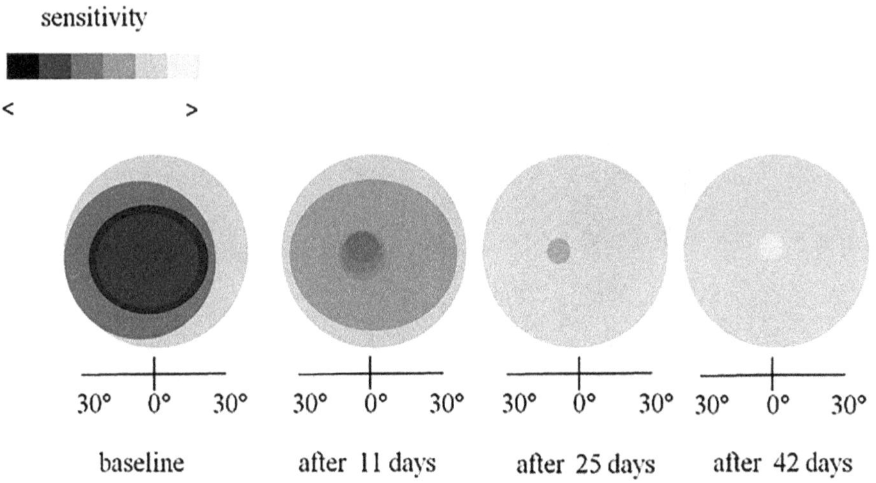

FIG. 8.3 – Restitution of the visual field contrast sensitivity in a case of central scotoma after training. Left eye trained. Data from Zihl J and von Cramon D. (1979).

In a subsequent study, the authors administered the training to 12 patients with post-geniculate lesions and reported an enlargement of the visual field by 10.2° after 9–37 sessions (Zihl and von Cramon, 1982).

8.2.2 Repeated Threshold Measurements across the Transition Zone and Subsequent Saccadic Training (Van der Wildt and Bergsma, 1998)

Van der Wildt and Bergsma (1998) trained two patients[5] with a procedure similar to that adopted by Zihl and von Cramon (1979). By using a Tubinger perimeter, repetitive threshold measurement was obtained in 68 different points of the binocular visual field by using circular stimuli 44 arc min wide (four contrast levels: 3.5%, 10.5%, 31.5%, 94.5%). The trained location was extended from the transition zone to the more peripheral regions of the blind hemifield.

After 28 training sessions (one hour per session), the proportion of detections increased from 61% to 90% (from 0% to 66% for the lowest contrast stimuli). The binocular visual field was enlarged by 5–12 degrees (*i.e.* a shift of the transition zone toward the blind region took place: figure 8.4).

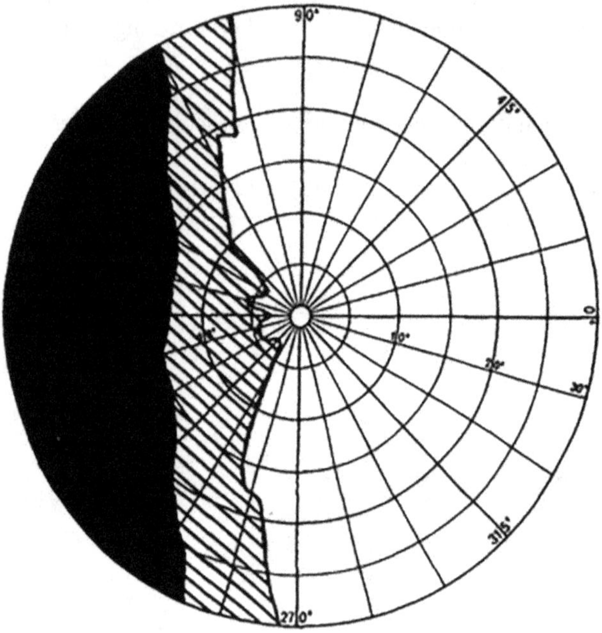

FIG. 8.4 – The enlargement of the visual field after the training of Van der Wildt and Bergsma. From Van der Wildt and Bergsma (1998). With permission of Springer Nature.

[5]A male (58 years old) with left-side hemianopia following surgery for a posterior cerebral artery aneurysm, and a female (58 years old) with upper right quadrantanopia after the remotion of a cerebral tumor.

At the end of this rehabilitation phase, the transition zone now shifted more peripherally, was trained again. Circular stimuli 100 arc min wide were presented on 21 predetermined locations at 10–50 degrees of eccentricity toward the blind hemifield along the horizontal meridian and ±45 degrees from the horizontal (contrast 100%, presentation time 200 ms, binocular conditions).

The subject had to look centrally at a fixation point, and whenever the stimulus was presented he/she had to make a saccade toward it and report its detection and the corresponding meridian. After 33 training sessions (each session lasting one hour), the proportion of stimuli localization increased from 60% to 95%, but the additional visual field enlargement was not significant.

Rehabilitation started 20 months after the onset of the cerebral injury so spontaneous recovery was excluded.

The results persisted after two months and the subjects reported improvement in their daily life.

Fixation was stated to be stable and verified with eye movement recording during one perimetric session (see Van der Wildt and Bergsma, 1998, pp. 288–289 for details).

8.2.3 Visual Training with the Goldmann Perimeter (Bergsma and van der Wildt, 2010)

Bergsma and van der Wildt (2010) trained eleven subjects with hemianopia or quadrantanopia and no neglect (time since onset: 1–8.5 years) with a Goldmann perimeter *via* repetitive static threshold estimation of light sensitivity across the transition zone. The training was administered at different eccentricities from the central vertical axis (background 10 cd m^{-2}, stimulus: Goldmann V, luminance from 4 cd m^{-2} to 318 cd m^{-2}, monocular condition). The duration of rehabilitation was 40 days, one hour per day. In two subjects the location of the stimuli was customized based on the shift of the visual field border, whereas in the remaining patients the presentation of the stimuli was fixed (predetermined). The effect of the training on the visual field was evaluated by kinetic Goldmann perimetry by comparing the exams before and every ten sessions. A visual field enlargement $<2°$ was not considered indicative of the training effect but the unwanted effect of fixation instability.

In addition, the effect of the training on reading was assessed in 7 patients by asking them to silently read two standardized texts. The estimated variables were reading rate (words/min) and reading errors (computed as number of regressions).

An enlargement of the visual field (4–13°) due to a gradual shift of the transition zone was observed in the two patients who received the customized treatment as well as in the sample that received the non-customized treatment. This finding suggests that the visual field enlargement is independent of the customization of the treatment. However, to be effective the stimulation must act on loci close to a region with retained residual function.

The amount of stimulation required to restore detection at a given locus depended on the eccentricity of that locus: the more distant from the midline the trained locus, the more the session required before the stimulus can be finally detected. The authors ruled out that the effect is an artifact due to eye movements.

Of the seven patients tested for reading, four showed an increased reading rate after the training. Those who did not improve were the ones with no visual field enlargement after the training. In the whole sample, the reading rate on average improved by 33 words/min, with fewer regressions compared to the baseline.

8.2.4 The Training Procedure of Poggel and Colleagues (2004, 2008a)

Poggel and colleagues developed a training procedure that made use of stimuli projected onto the transition zone. Stimuli increased in luminance in four steps from 30 to 96 cd m^{-2} over 2000 ms, and the patient had to report detections by pressing a key (Poggel *et al.*, 2004). Nineteen patients (aged between 18 and 75 years) with postgeniculate lesions and no neglect or other neuro-ophthalmological disorders were trained. Two sessions per day were administered (each session lasted about 30–35 min) for about six months. The training was done at home.

After the treatment, the absolute defect within the 30 central degrees of the visual field decreased and the transition zone shifted significantly toward the blind field even if to a small extent (1.31 deg on average). The size of the transition zone increased, the reaction time to stimuli presented across the visual field decreased, and, consequently, visual search became faster. On the contrary, form recognition and color perception remained unchanged. Fifty-eight percent of the patients judged the training useful, reporting more confidence in traffic situations, easier reading, and improved visually-guided navigation (Poggel *et al.*, 2004, 2008a). The authors pinpointed that their results were independent of eye movements and/or eccentric fixation and were not the consequence of enhanced attention.

8.2.5 The Computer-Assisted Training of Julkunen and Colleagues (2003)

Five patients (age 36–59) with chronic stroke and homonymous quadrantanopia without neglect (over 12 months from onset) were trained with the computer program Silmäpeli (University of Turku, dept. of Psychology and Neurology) for 33–47 h (3 sessions a week, each session lasting 1 h; overall duration of the training: three months in average).

The training was carried out on a 17″ PC screen (visual angle: 30°). The transition zone was stimulated by white blinking dots (luminance: 110 cd m^{-2}, duration 490 ms, background: 0.13 cd m^{-2}) randomly presented while the patient was asked to look at a white fixation dot. At each locus, presentations were iterated 3–5 times, and the size of the stimuli was reduced (2°–1°, then 0.5° after correct detection). No active fixation control was provided, but fixation was checked by asking the patient to respond when the fixation point turned red, 200 ms before each presentation. When a stimulus was perceived, the patient had to press a key.

Static and kinetic visual field were performed before and immediately after the training, and after three months from the end of the treatment.

At static perimetry, reduction of the loci with absolute defect was found in three patients, with the recovery that persisted at the end of the follow-up. No improvement was found in the remaining two subjects.

At kinetic perimetry, reduction of the scotoma was observed by 8 up to 15 degrees along the transition zone in three patients; in the remaining two subjects no improvement was found.

Improved VEP parameters in terms of P100 amplitude and/or latency were observed in three patients.

Details are reported in table 8.1.

The authors concluded that homonymous field defects can be reduced with vision restoration therapy even after years from the onset.

To be noted that a control group was not applied.

TAB. 8.1 – The improvement of visual function in the sample recruited by Julkunen and colleagues.

Patient	Static perimetry	Kinetic perimetry	VEP	Daily life improvement
Right upper quadr	–	Unclear	+	+
Right inferior quadr	–	+8°	Unclear	+
Left inferior quadr	+	+15°	+	Unclear
Right upper quadr	+	+5–10°	+	Unclear
Left upper quadr	+	Unclear	Unclear	–

Finally, it should be noted that in this study a clear correspondence between the objective *vs.* psychophysical datum (VEP improvement *vs.* visual field enlargement) took place in three patients over five. The author attributed the lack of agreement in the remaining two patients to problems in collaboration and to the hemifield stimulus used for the VEP recording (Julkunen *et al.*, 2003).

8.2.6 *Training of the Transition Zone with the Lubeck Reaction Perimeter (LRP: Schmielau and Wong, 2007)*

Schmielau and Wong (2007) stimulated the transition zone of 20 hemianopic patients (age 21–81 y) with no neglect with a perimeter developed on purpose, the Lubeck Reaction Perimeter (LRP). The LRP is made of a bowl (background: 0.014 cd m^{-2}) whose inner surface is covered by small green LEDs with luminance that can be modified in steps of 0.2 log units (maximum luminance: 3200 cd m^{-2}). Patients had to respond whenever they perceived the stimuli (randomly presented) by pressing a key, and the reaction time was recorded and taken as the indicator of performance level (see Wall *et al.*, 2002 for the relationship between visual threshold and reaction time). With their perimeter, the authors trained their patients with repetitive stimulations that started in the intact field and moved to the defective region. After two missed responses, the next stimulus was presented 12 deg toward the intact region: this way, the stimulations were constantly focused on the transition zone. The procedure was reiterated at each eccentricity across the vertical meridian. The training was administered binocularly in 13 subjects, monocularly in 7 patients, two sessions per week (from 34 to 169 sessions in total), each session lasting on average 45 min (about 500 stimulations per session). The overall training period ranged from 2 to 27 months.

Static and kinetic perimetry was repeated at the end of the treatment and after at least six months, and the difference between the proportion of correct response before and after the treatment was evaluated at the LRP static perimetry.

The time lapse between the onset of hemianopia and the beginning of the training was no less than six months in the majority of the patients.

At the end of the treatment, the visual field was wider by $11.3 \pm 8.1°$ with an improvement of detection rate in the stimulated region of $18.6 \pm 13.5\%$. The improvement was still observable in 86% of the patients after six months and was independent of the nature (ischemic/hemorrhagic) of the lesion. In 70% of the sample the quality of daily living, investigated with a semi-structured interview, was better after the rehabilitation.

Interestingly, the binocular training turned out to be three to four times more effective than the monocular administration, and interocular transfer was observed (the visual field of the non-treated eye after the training showed roughly the same improvement as the treated one) in 70% of the sample. Taken together, the binocular superiority effect and interocular transfer confirm that visual restoration acts at a cortical level.

8.2.7 The Vision Restoration Therapy of Kasten and Sabel (VRT: Kasten et al., 1998a)

The group of Kasten has provided a main contribution to the subject of vision restoration, developing a specific computer-based training called *vision restoration therapy* (*VRT*: Kasten *et al.*, 1998a). The rehabilitative program of the authors includes a series of training sessions to be done at home on a 17-inch PC for one hour (divided into two 30-min sessions) per day, 6 days a week for 6 months. The program projected suprathreshold stimuli onto the seen/not seen zone (the *transition zone*) while the subject looked binocularly at a central target. The difficulty of the training parameters was adjusted and customized once or twice a month based on the improvement of the patient.

The transition zone between the intact and the blind hemifield was assessed with the suprathreshold binocular "High Resolution Perimeter" (see Sabel *et al.*, 2004; Kasten *et al.*, 1997, 1998b for technical details). The authors defined the transition zone as the region between the intact and the blind hemifield where the probability of detecting suprathreshold stimuli (size 0.15°, luminance 95 cd m^{-2} presented for 150 ms on a <1 cd m^{-2} dark background) is between 20% and 80%. In this region, therefore, the response probability (computed on 5 presentations per locus) to respond to suprathreshold stimuli is highly variable and the authors hypothesized it corresponds to the transition region of relative defect at conventional automated perimetry (even if this correlation was found to be not significant). The transition zone has been classified into three types: type I with a very steep gradient ("sharp border": size <1 SD below mean), type II with a medium gradient (borders about 1 SD), and type III, a wide "fuzzy" region of defect and a large fluctuation of detection with a shallow gradient (borders >1 SD above mean) (figure 8.5).

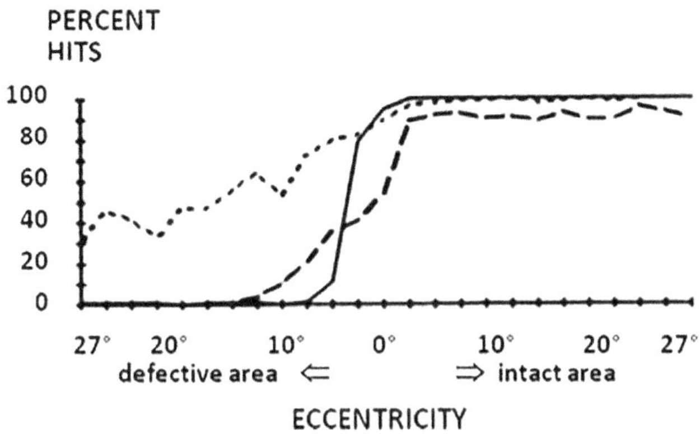

FIG. 8.5 – The three types of transition zone According to Kasten and colleagues. Continuous line: type I, dashed line: type II, dotted line: type III. From Kasten *et al.* (1998b). With permission of Taylor and Francis Publisher.

The authors stressed that the transition zone is not the result of saccades or eccentric fixation, as the number of losses of fixation was not correlated with its size, it does not show an indentation around the fixation point, and it does not change in size as a function of the distance from the fixation point (Kasten *et al.*, 1998b).

In brief, VRT is made up of two training procedures, named *Visure* and *SeeTrain* to be administered binocularly. In *Visure*, the program stimulates systematically the transition zone with a white square (2 deg wide) that rhythmically changes in size and shifts across the boundary from the seen-toward the blind region. The patient is asked to press a key as long as the moving stimulus is perceivable. When the observer releases the key, indicating that he is no longer able to detect the square, its direction is reversed. The procedure is repeated at different horizontal meridians so to stimulate the entire border of the hemianopic scotoma. Whenever a pre-defined level of performance is reached, the size and contrast of the square are decreased, making the task more difficult. *SeeTrain* is the second step of the training strategy, administered after the performance at Visure has reached 90 percent of detections. In *SeeTrain*, suprathreshold stationary small stimuli (white dots: 15 pixels [0.15°] in diameter) are presented with increasing luminance in random locations across the transition zone on a monitor (42° × 32° wide) at a viewing distance of about 30 cm. The patient has to press a key as soon as the target is perceived, according to the method of adjustment [see Aleci, 2021 for a review of the psychophysical methods]. On a monthly basis, parameters are adjusted according to the level of performance achieved by the trainee. Adjustment includes the location of the stimuli in the transition zone and their luminance that is decreased (or increased) according to the reaction time of the subject. The treatment is contraindicated in cases of epilepsy, cognitive deficits, and binocular visual acuity <20/100[6].

Compared to a placebo group, the authors reported a higher frequency of perceived stimuli after the training and enlargement of the visual field (shift of the border of the scotoma) in the stimulated region of 0.4 deg[7] when measured at conventional automated perimetry; on the contrary, no enlargement was found in the non-stimulated regions. The authors pinpointed that 72% of the trained sample reported a subjective improvement in vision (Kasten *et al.*, 1998a). The results of the training were observed after 50–100 h of practice.

In a subsequent analysis performed on a subset of these data, a transfer effect of the trained function (light sensibility) in the site of stimulation on functions not specifically trained, namely color and form recognition[8] was observed (Kasten *et al.*, 2000). However, changes in color and form perception after the training were not significant, and a subsequent study with a more rigorous control of the two parameters concluded that higher-order visual functions like form and color require specific training (Poggel *et al.*, 2008a).

Subsequently, Mueller, Mast, and Sabel collected the VRT data from 302 patients treated in eight clinical centers in Germany, Austria, and Switzerland between 1998 and 2004 (Mueller *et al.*, 2007). They analyzed the perimetric results gathered with suprathreshold high-resolution perimetry (HRP) and threshold conventional perimetry before and after vision restoration therapy (carried out according to the paradigm of Kasten and colleagues: 1997, 2000). After the training, the percentage of detected stimuli was increased by 17.2%, and the visual field was 4.9° larger at HRP. Unfortunately, no data on the expansion of the visual field at conventional perimetry is reported.

In another study (Sabel *et al.*, 2004), Sabel trained 16 patients with homonymous hemianopia due to cerebral injuries that occurred at least one year before. At the baseline and after the six months of vision restoration therapy, patients underwent high-resolution perimetry and conventional Tübinger automated perimetry. Visual field data were compared with the results from scanning LASER ophthalmoscopy (SLO)[9] obtained in a previous investigation. After the training, the proportion of stimuli detected at the high-resolution perimetry was increased by 6.59%. The absolute defect at conventional perimetry disappeared, on average, in 8 tested loci. In addition, the border of the absolute defect at

[6]See Kasten *et al.* (1997, 2000) for details.

[7]As measured at standard automated perimetry (Tübinger automated perimetry, TAP).

[8]Color and form perception was estimated by presenting tachistoscopically three colored squares (blue, green, and red) and lines of different orientations or letters (namely "A", "B", "C", "D") across the transition zone of the visual field. The patient had to differentiate the stimuli.

[9]SLO is a procedure that rules out the biasing effect of light scattering and avoids artifacts like unstable and/or eccentric fixation.

conventional perimetry was localized more peripherally (by 1.94° in the right eye and 0.98° in the left eye).

Changes induced by training are more evident in the peripheral regions of the transition zone than in the central area. This is explainable as an effect of cortical magnification: a large amount of cortex subserves small portions of the visual field in the central region, so more training is required to achieve results comparable to the periphery (Kasten *et al.*, 1999).

Relying upon the answers of the patients who filled in a standardized questionnaire at the end of the rehabilitation program, visual confidence and mobility improved in 75.4% of cases, reading improved in 43.5% of cases and bumping into objects was less frequent in 31.9% of the trained patients (Sabel *et al.*, 2004; Mueller *et al.*, 2003). No correlation was found between improvement of the activity of daily life and the type of lesion or age of the patient. Time since the lesion was found to correlate with reading improvement (older lesions were associated with greater reading improvement: Mueller *et al.*, 2003).

Unexpectedly, the visual field enlargement did not correlate with better visual confidence, mobility, ability to avoid obstacles, and the general activity of daily life (Mueller *et al.*, 2003). Indeed, single-case analysis revealed that in some patients the improvement of the activity of daily life correlated with visual sensitivity after the training, while in others this was not the case (Mueller *et al.*, 2003). In other terms, the correlation between objective and subjective improvement after rehabilitation was weak, albeit significant. This finding suggests that factors other than field improvement contribute to improving daily life activity after training: for example, increased reaction time and/or the fact that visual training could make patients more aware of their defects. In other terms, they pay more attention to their visual function (Mueller *et al.*, 2003).

It should be noted that those with less severe visual field defects before the training have a greater chance to experience greater subjective improvement in daily life activity (Mueller *et al.*, 2003).

The improvement after vision restoration therapy (in terms of number of detected suprathreshold stimuli) persisted up to 23 months from the end of the 6-month training (Kasten *et al.*, 2001) and even up to 3.5 years according to Gall and colleagues (2006). The stability of regained vision was not conditioned by the type of lesion (hemianopia or quadrantanopia), by age, and by the duration of the treatment (6 *vs.*12 months). More specifically, the authors identified three main clusters: patients who showed a further increase after the end of the training, patients whose performance remained stable, and subjects who showed a decline in performance.

8.2.8 The Vision Restoration Training of Schreiber et al. (2006) and Romano et al. (2008)

Schreiber and associates further investigated the effect of VRT on 16 patients (age 18–75) with stable homonymous hemianopia occurring more than 1 year before.

Binocular stimulation of the transition zone with the procedure of Kasten and Sabel (VRT) was administered 1 h daily 6 days a week for 6 months, and the results were evaluated at static automated perimetry (TAP, central 30°) performed monocularly and binocularly.

In each eye, the extent of the hemianopic defect (number of loci with absolute defect[10] over the total number of tested loci) was computed. The *training effect (E)* was defined as the difference in the proportion of absolute loci before and after the training. So, the higher E, the stronger the training effect. A training effect >0.12 was considered relevant.

Monocular visual field examination revealed, on average, improvement of eight loci with an absolute defect with a mean training effect in each eye of 0.05. E was relevant in only 2 patients.

At the binocular examination E, computed on the total 30°, was 0.04 which rose to 0.08 in the treated region (the transition zone). The average shift of the border of the scotoma was 1.62°, with two patients who showed a shift of more than 2 degrees in the central region.

It is worth pinpointing once more the difficulty in obtaining a visual field enlargement in the central region compared to the periphery. This may depend on the fact that the central retina is made up of a higher number of (small) receptive fields compared to the peripheral region: so, the latter requires a greater rehabilitative effort to achieve the same outcome (Poggel *et al.*, 2008b).

Finally, the group of Romano used VRT to treat 161 patients, of whom 84% suffered from occipital stroke. Subjects underwent training 30 min twice daily, 6 days a week for about 6 months. Time since onset ranged from 1 to 451 months. After rehabilitation, the proportion of detected stimuli increased by 13%, and the visual field enlarged by about 5 degrees. The extent was estimated with the suprathreshold high-resolution perimetry, not with conventional perimetry (Romano *et al.*, 2008).

8.2.9 Counterevidence and Controversies About Visual Restitution

The results obtained with visual restitution, and particularly with the visual restoration training developed by the group of Sabel and Kasten (VRT) are controversial and have been questioned by Horton in two editorials (2005a, 2005b). The arguments against VRT can be summarized as follows:

1- the perimetric software developed by the authors to estimate the results after visual restoration (named high-resolution perimetry) is the same used for the training. Now, visual field enlargement at conventional

[10]Loci with an absolute defect were defined as those not responsive to stimuli of luminance 1000 cd m^{-2}.

automated perimetry should be demonstrated as well to clinically validate the procedure. In fact, standard automated perimetry does not seem to confirm the positive results recorded by high-resolution perimetry (Kasten *et al.*, 1998a, 1998b).

2- Eye movements are not accurately controlled during VRT so subjects may learn with VRT practice to shift fixation and direct saccades toward their blind hemifield: this could generate an artifactual visual field enlargement. This is suggested by the increased number of saccades into the blind hemifield after the training (Pambakian *et al.*, 2000), with latency so short to remain undetected during the training and post-training visual field testing (Plant, 2005).

Sabel (2006) replied in his letter that the rate of stable fixations remained unchanged after the treatment (stability of fixation: >90% before and after the training). In addition, the position of the blind spot was unchanged after the training, and this argues against eccentric fixation and saccadic movements during the examination. Finally, the shift of the transition zone cannot be an artifact of eye movements as in this case the entire visual field border (and not only a portion of it) should be displaced toward the spared region. Indeed, Kasten, Bunzenthal, and Sabel studied the eye movements of 15 patients with homonymous visual field defects with an eye tracker and reported that patients did not show changes in fixation or trend for eccentric fixation[11] after the training. In addition, they did not tend to make more saccades toward the blind hemifield after vision restoration therapy. The authors concluded that "VRT has no effect on either the direction or the amplitude of horizontal eye movements during visual field testing" and "these results argue against the theory that the visual field enlargements are artifact induced by eye movements" (Kasten *et al.*, 2006, p. 18).

It remains that when the stability of fixation is accurately controlled, no significant effect of visual restitution training is found, as demonstrated by the SLO (*Scanning Laser Ophthalmoscopy*) study of Reinhard and colleagues (2005, see below). Sabel replied that the absence of perimetric improvement at SLO may depend on the more demanding task (recognizing triplets of dots rather than simple dot detection) and on the different parameter settings at SLO compared to the conventional perimetry. A limited number of residual neurons in the transition zone may still be effective in processing simple tasks like stimulus detection but fails in the more complex tasks required by SLO (Sabel, 2006; Sabel *et al.*, 2004). This would explain also the mismatch between the position of the hemianopic border measured at SLO, closer to the fixation point, and its more eccentric position measured at conventional perimetry.

The author recalled, indeed, that the extent of the visual field is sensitive to the type and size of the stimulus, and stimuli presented at SLO differ from those used at

[11]Eccentric fixation was indirectly checked by analyzing the position of the blind spot before and after the treatment.

standard automated perimetry (SAP)[12]. Finally, he asserted that relative defects are misinterpreted as absolute at SLO, making the latter less effective than standard perimetry in recording subtle improvements in sensitivity.

In sum, according to Horton (2005a, 2005b) and Plant (2005), visual field improvement after VRT is an artifact and depends on the biasing effect of:

- fixation instability;
- eccentric fixation;
- eye movements.

Balliet and colleagues (1985) trained with a procedure similar to that used by Zihl and von Cramon (1979, 1982) 12 patients with stabilized homonymous hemianopia or quadrantanopia following occipital lesions in order to verify the effective improvement of the visual field in hemianopic subjects after removing potentially biasing experimental variables. Two up to eleven months of training (consisting of repeated determinations of the light threshold at the transition zone with static Goldmann perimetry) provided no clinically significant visual field enlargement (as measured at Goldmann perimetry) in their hemianopic subjects (less than 1 degree of improvement toward the blind region).

Likewise, Pommerenke and Markowitsch on the one hand obtained improvement in visual exploration after specific training in patients with stable visual field defects following postgeniculate lesions, on the other they did not observe any visual field enlargement (Pommerenke and Markowitsch, 1989).

Nelles *et al.* trained twenty-one subjects with homonymous hemianopia for four weeks with single stimuli presented on a wide board placed 1.5 t away (Nelles *et al.*, 2001). Patients were asked to look at the center of the board and respond as soon as they could detect the stimulus[13]. Visual field was performed before, after the training, and after 8 months from the end of the training. In addition, changes in stimuli detection and reaction time were assessed.

No difference was found in the number of detected stimuli and reaction time between pre- and post-training. The authors concluded that visual restitution therapy is ineffective in enlarging the visual field of hemianopic patients.

Some years later, in a study dating back to 2005 (Reinhard *et al.*, 2005), visual restitution training was administered to 15 patients with homonymous visual field defects following ischemic, hemorrhagic, or traumatic brain lesions occurring at least one year before. The procedure aimed to stimulate the border of the scotoma with

[12]The differences between SLO and conventional perimetry are the following: three black dots presented on a red background at SLO ("inverse stimuli") *vs.* single white dots on a clear background ("positive stimuli") at conventional perimetry, binocular viewing *vs.* monocular viewing, and discrimination task of the three dots *vs.* detection task of a single dot (see Reinhard *et al.*, 2005 for details). After having examined the visual field of a patient with post-stroke quadrantanopia (previously trained with VRT) after replacing the conventional "positive" single stimuli with black-on-red "inverse" targets, Kasten and colleagues concluded that the worse visual field performance at SLO compared to conventional automated perimetry depended on the "inverse stimuli" presented in the former, and was not an artifact related to eye movements, as posited by Horton.

[13]Presentation time: 205 ms; two daily sessions, each lasting 30 min.

home sessions to be performed binocularly on a PC screen. Repetitive stimulation in the seen/not seen transition zone of the scotoma was carried out daily, six days a week for six months, according to the procedure developed by Kasten *et al.* (1998a). Each session lasted 1 h. With a scanning laser ophthalmoscope (SLO), the absolute border of the hemianopic defect was determined before and after the training period. No significant enlargement was found after the training period in terms of reduction of absolute defects. However, the authors admit a possible reduction of the relative defect in the transition zone of the scotoma that, in fact, is not detectable at SLO.

The improvement after visual restoration is therefore controversial and, if present, is argued to depend on a resetting of the oculomotor pattern and on adaptive strategies learned during the training rather than on a true increase of sensitivity (Reinhard *et al.*, 2005; Zihl and von Cramon, 1985).

In sum, quoting Horton and Plant: "Regrettably, it still remains true that no therapeutic intervention [...] can correct effectively the underlying visual field deficit" (Horton, 2005a, p. 1), and "[...] there is no expansion of the seeing field as a result of VRT [...]" (Plant, 2005, p. 2). In fact, Bach-y-Rita (1983) observed that when the head is kept perfectly still by replacing the chin rest with a bite bar and ocular movements are strictly controlled, the post-training apparent enlargement of the visual field vanishes.

Despite these considerations, the question is not closed. The final word and definitive solution to this issue cannot but be provided by the study of functional objective changes in the cerebral activity of the trained cortical region.

8.2.10 The Functional Studies and the Clue of Hallucinations

In the opinion of the writer, a decisive contribution to the controversy is provided by a series of investigations that made use of VEP, PET, and fMRI to assess functional changes in cortical activation after rehabilitation. If the effect of training, namely the improvement in visual sensitivity in the transition zone, is real, VEP, PET, and BOLD activity should increase after the treatment compared to the baseline.

In a study dating back to 2006, the group of Julkunen studied a patient with stable right superior quadrantanopia due to a left occipitotemporal stroke that occurred 18 months earlier. The authors correlated pre/post training visual field data and subjective light perception with pre/post training visual evoked potential (VEP) and regional blood flow change as measured by positron emission tomography (PET: Julkunen *et al.*, 2006).

Rehabilitation consisted of repetitive stimulation along the transition zone (see Julkunen *et al.*, 2003). Three sessions (each lasting one hour) a week for 37 h in total were administered. The visual function before, immediately after the training, and after three months, was assessed with static automated perimetry (Octopus 101, central 30°), kinetic manual perimetry, and pattern shift VEP. In addition, subjective light perception was estimated according to a subjective-scale judgment of the visibility of white blinking dots used as visual stimuli during PET acquisition. For this purpose, the stimulation was directed toward the intact visual field, the blind visual field, and the transition zone.

The main results of this study were:

- the hemianopic scotoma was reduced after the training at both static and kinetic perimetry, with an increase of the responsive region by 5–10° from the vertical meridian. The improvement in light sensitivity took place in the transition zone, not in the blind or the intact regions of the right (*i.e.* affected) hemifield;
- subjective improvement of light perception in the transition zone was observed after the training;
- VEP P100, not recordable before the training, became evident after the training (amplitude 1.94 μV) and was still present, even if with reduced amplitude (1.50 μV), at the end of the follow-up (figure 8.6);
- cerebral blood flow increased after the training in the left and right occipito-parietal and occipito-temporal cortices as well as in the frontal cortex, cerebellum, thalamus, basal ganglia, and insula. After three months, increased cerebral blood flow was recorded in the left occipital cortex close to the perilesional area and in the right occipital cortex;
- a positive correlation was found between cerebral blood flow in the right lingual gyrus and improvement of perimetric sensitivity in the transition zone. The same was reported with cerebral blood flow and subjective light perception in the transition zone.

The authors concluded that "[...] visual training can cause plastic changes in the brain in chronic stroke, and these changes can be detected with different methods" (Julkunen *et al.*, 2006).

At functional MRI, increased visual perilesional cortical activation after a training program was demonstrated by the group of Pleger in three patients[14] (Pleger *et al.*, 2003). Based on previous results on animals (*e.g.* Eysel *et al.*, 1998, 1999), the authors interpreted the enhanced BOLD signal following repetitive stimulation in terms of activation of the perilesional neurons (Pleger *et al.*, 2003). Supposedly, the activation state may persist indefinitely as a result of long-term axonal sprouting, as shown in the striate cortex of visually lesioned cats (Darian-Smith and Gilbert, 1994).

Likewise, cerebral BOLD activity was assessed before and after 1 month of rehabilitation with functional fMRI by Marshall and associates. The BOLD activity was examined during stimulation of the transition zone (within 4° of the edge of the affected hemifield) with a checkerboard stimulus (width: 4°) before and after one month of training in six patients with stroke and right homonymous hemianopia (Marshall *et al.*, 2008). Rehabilitation followed the paradigm of Kasten and colleagues (training procedure: *Visure*, Kasten *et al.*, 1997, 2000) and was done at home, one hour per day, six days a week. At the end of the month, the patients,

[14]The training (eight-week period, 1–2 h per day) involved three subjects, started two years after the onset of the cerebral lesions, and consisted of a detection task of white flashes followed by a discrimination task with big/small circles, a shape discrimination task with circles, triangles, and squares as targets, a pattern discrimination task (*e.g.* diagonal *vs.* horizontal or vertical bars), and, finally, a color discrimination task.

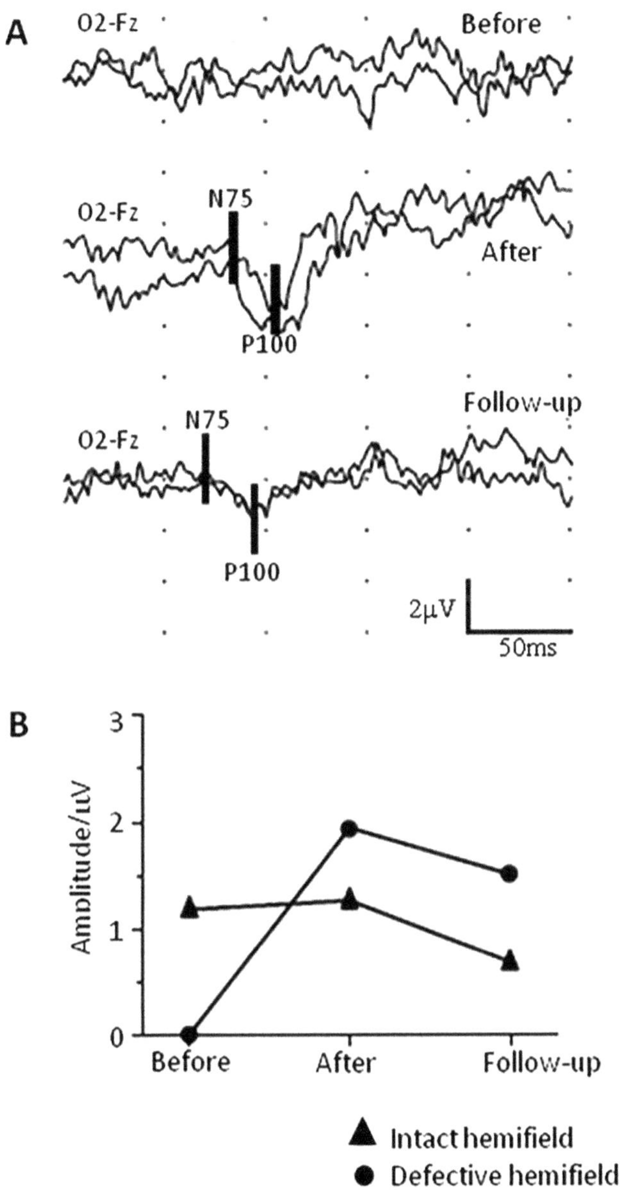

FIG. 8.6 – VEP in the affected hemifield before, after the training, and after the follow-up. Reprinted from Restorative Neurology and Neuroscience. Vol. 24, Julkunen, L, Tenovuo O, Vorobyev V, Hiltunen J, Teräs M, Jääskeläinen SK, Hämäläinen H. (2006). "Functional brain imaging, clinical and neurophysiological outcome of visual rehabilitation in a chronic stroke patient", pages 123–132, 2006, with permission of IOS Press.

who had reached a level of accuracy >90% in the transition zone, showed increased BOLD activity in the medial frontal region, bilaterally, and in the right dorsolateral prefrontal cortex. These regions, indeed, would enhance visual processing in the transition zone, mediating the attentional shift from the seeing region toward the border zone. Despite these results, the authors failed to find a positive correlation between the improvement of visual perception in the transition zone and BOLD activity. In addition, no enlargement of the visual field was reported at the end of the one-month treatment (Marshall *et al.*, 2008).

A phenomenon that seems to confirm an effective neuronal activation in the striate area is the onset of simple hallucinations (phosphenes or flashes) occurring exclusively during VRT sessions. Poggel and associates, indeed, found that the improvement after VRT was greater in those patients who experienced simple hallucinations during rehabilitation. They explained this finding as higher responsiveness of these patients to VRT, thereby as neuronal hyperactivation. It is revealing that most of the hallucinations were experienced in the early phases of the training period, when the visual field improvement was faster and more marked, and this trend would be a sign of striate cortex activation. In the late phases of rehabilitation, when visual field improvement was less evident, hallucinations gradually disappeared, indicating, presumably, normalization of the previous neuronal hyperactivation. Of note, these hemianopes had experienced similar visual delusions at a pre-training phase, during spontaneous recovery, and were those who reported greater subjective spontaneous improvement of the visual field compared to the patients without hallucinations (Poggel *et al.*, 2007).

In conclusion, the potential of training paradigms that make use of light stimuli repeatedly presented at the borders of the hemianopic scotoma to foster the restoration of the visual field in hemianopic patients remains unclear. The rationale behind visual restoration therapy is that if the seen/not seen transition region of the hemianopic visual field is repeatedly stimulated, the visual cells subserving that region (that are not completely silent) can be reactivated to a suprathreshold level. Even if this strategy may be effective in reducing the size of the scotoma or its depth, the enlargement of the parafoveal visual field is limited to a few degrees, and the ameliorative effect, if any, occurs only in case the gradient of sensibility between the normal and scotomatous hemifield is shallow. Last but not least, visual restoration therapy is costly and time-consuming (90–180 h: Schuett, 2009).

8.2.11 Predictors of the Outcome of Vision Restoration Therapy

Poggel and colleagues (2008a) examined the independent variables that may affect the outcome of VRT. They made use of the high-resolution perimeter (HRP) devised on purpose[15] for their evaluations.

[15]HRP, Nova Vision, Magndeburg, Germany. See Poggel *et al.* (2004) for details.

Etiology, sex, laterality (left/right hemianopia) and time since onset do not affect the outcome of vision restoration therapy (namely rate of stimulus detection and shift of the transition zone: Poggel *et al.*, 2008a; Mueller *et al.*, 2007).

On the contrary, the patient's age seems to be correlated with the improvement of stimulus detection and with the shift of the transition zone after VRT (Poggel *et al.*, 2008a, but see Kasten *et al.*, 2006, p. 24 and Mueller *et al.*, 2007, p. 566).

The size of the spared visual field before the training is positively correlated with the shift of the visual field border after the training but not with the improvement of the detection threshold at standard automated perimetry (Tübinger automated perimetry, TAP).

The eccentricity of the transition zone at baseline is positively correlated with the shift of the visual field border after the training.

The number of loci of abolished vision (absolute defect) at baseline is negatively correlated with the enlargement of the visual field after the training, *i.e.* with the shift of the transition zone (the higher the number of loci with absolute defect at baseline, the smaller the shift).

The extent of the transition zone is the most important predictor of recovery after treatment: the larger the transition zone at a given eccentricity on the vertical meridian, the higher the rate of stimulus detection after the training, and the greater the shift of the visual field border at that eccentricity. It should be noted that the effect of the size of the transition zone on the rate of improvement is topographically specific so a larger transition zone in the upper quadrant is not predictive of the outcome after training in the corresponding lower quadrant and *vice versa* (table 8.2).

To be considered, however, that some of the significant findings at HRP did not reach significance at standard automated perimetry (Tübinger Automated Perimeter, TAP-2000). Finally, the co-occurrence of neglect worsens the rehabilitative outcome.

VRT is generally administered over 6 months, according to the procedure devised by Kasten and Sabel. A longer duration of the training (*i.e.* 12 months) does not further increase the effects obtained at the end of the 6th month (Mueller *et al.*, 2008; Gall *et al.*, 2006)[16]. However, the possibility that using different stimuli (*e.g.* moving targets) or more intense luminance levels may lead to further improvement even after this period cannot be ruled out.

[16]Mueller anbd colleagues evaluated the effect of prolonged VRT in a sample of 17 hemianopic patients comparing the outcome of High-Resolution Perimetry (HRP, binocular conditions) and standard automated perimetry (Rodenstock Perimat 206, monocular conditions). VRT was administered at home twice a day for 30 min each, five days a week for 6 months (the current training period) and 12 months (long-term training period). At the end of the current training period, the number of missed stimuli at HRP decreased by 13% and the number of perimetric loci with absolute defect at SAP decreased by 9%. After the additional 6 months of training, no further improvement was observed in the two outcomes.

TAB. 8.2 – Predictors of the outcome of vision restoration therapy.

Independent variable (predictor)	Dependent variable (outcome)
Sex	NO effect on the rate of stimulus detection and shift of the transition zone (Poggel *et al.*, 2008a; Mueller *et al.*, 2007)
Time since lesion	NO effect on the rate of stimulus detection and shift of the transition zone (Poggel *et al.*, 2008a; Mueller *et al.*, 2007; Sabel *et al.*, 2004; Zihl and von Cramon, 1985)
Spontaneous recovery before training	NO effect on recovery (Poggel *et al.*, 2008a)
Age of the patient	Patients aged >65 years showed greater improvement than patients aged <65 years (Poggel *et al.*, 2008a; Mueller *et al.*, 2007; Kasten *et al.*, 2006)
Etiology	NO effect on the rate of stimulus detection and shift of the transition zone (Poggel *et al.*, 2008a; Mueller *et al.*, 2007)
Side of defect	NO effect on the rate of stimulus detection and shift of the transition zone (Poggel *et al.*, 2008a); however, right-sided hemianopia requires more training sessions to achieve the same results as left hemianopes
Extent of the transition zone (gradient)	Positive correlation with the shift of the visual field border after the training
Eccentricity of the transition zone	Positive correlation with the shift of the visual field border after the training
Number of loci of abolished vision (absolute defects)	Negative correlation with the shift of the visual field border after the training, thereby with the enlargement of the visual field after the training

8.2.12 The Discrepancy between Objective vs. Subjective Improvement

Even when the improvement in terms of visual field enlargement is negligible after vision restitution, many patients declare to benefit from the treatment. This discrepancy between the objective modest results after vision restoration training, namely the limited visual field enlargement (if any), and the subjective improvement in daily living activities often reported by patients has been discussed By Poggel and colleagues (2007, 2010). The authors considered that a shift of the visual field border (the transition zone) at the level of the fixation point leads to a greater benefit compared to a more eccentric shift of the same size along the vertical meridian. So, the subjective improvement yielded by vision restoration therapy cannot be inferred from the overall objective (perimetric) results. In their prospective study, Poggel and colleagues investigated the subjective effect of visual restoration therapy and compared subjective *vs.* objective outcomes (detection rate and shift of the transition zone). Visual restitution training was performed by presenting static stimuli at different intensities, slowly increasing over time, in the transition zone of the patient. Training consisted of the detection of the stimuli and lasted about 6 months (two sessions of 30–35 min per day). After each month of training, the transition zone was re-evaluated and presentations were adapted to the performance achieved by the trainee. The subjective outcome after the training was evaluated with a semi-structured questionnaire made of general and more specific open questions about reading, navigation, and orientation, and a rating scale[17].

The average number of detected stimuli in 19 patients with homonymous hemianopia increased by 4% and the transition zone shifted toward the affected hemifield by about 1.4°, with high intersubject variability (that depended on the extent of the transition zone, as already reported). At the end of the rehabilitation period, most of the patients were satisfied with the training and many of them described their scotoma as "less solid", or "more transparent" (58% of cases), with improved navigation (74% of cases), better self-confidence (47%), more efficient visual scanning (21%), more confidence when driving (37%), and easier reading (37%). Still, the increase in the rating score on the ability to cope with daily activities after the training was not significant. Likewise, the correlation between the number of detected stimuli and the subjective sensation that the training was helpful was not significant, as well as the correlation with the rating scale. Yet, it is worth considering that those patients who did not show objective improvement after the training did not report amelioration in daily activities. The authors argued that other factors and not just the improvement of the visual field influence the satisfaction of the patients: for example, reduced reaction times to visual inputs.

The group of Poggel (2008b) observed that the perimetric defect does not necessarily correspond to the way patients are aware of it. In other terms, a discrepancy may exist between the scotoma evaluated at perimetry and its subjective description by the patient. To clarify the way a post-training[18] visual field enlargement affects the patients' awareness of it, nineteen subjects with stable hemianopia were asked to draw on a perimetric map their visual field border (in monocular condition). The correlation between automated perimetry[19] and the visual field drawn by the patients was significant, but the central (normal or scotomatous) regions of the visual field were overrepresented. So, the subjective enlargement of their visual field close to the fixation point was more "sensed" by the patients than the same enlargement at more eccentric regions.

Overall, these results suggest that subjects become more aware of their visual field defects at the end of the training period and that even small improvements in the central visual field may be felt as clinically relevant in daily activities.

[17]See Poggel *et al.* (2010, table 1, p. 178), for content, categories, and responses of the interview.

[18]VRT was carried out with the High-Resolution Perimeter (HRP) (Kasten *et al.*, 1998a, 1998b, 1999). The overall rehabilitation period was administered in two sessions per day and lasted about six months.

[19]Tübinger automated perimetry, performed in monocular conditions.

In sum, the key factor to define the rehabilitation as successful is the patient's awareness of a visual field enlargement rather than the objective reduction of the scotomatous region.

8.3 Vision Restitution in Humans: Training of the Blind Hemifield

The principle underlying the visual training of the transition zone (*i.e.* the *hypothesis of the minimal residual structure* of Sabel) makes a visual restitution program aimed at the inner part of the hemianopic field counter-intuitive. Yet, there is evidence that the affected hemifield, which is traditionally considered lost, *i.e.* blind, in some cases retains a sort of unconscious visual processing. This phenomenon is called *blindsight.*

Studies in animals and humans suggest that blindsight can be trained. This finding, indeed, justifies a rehabilitative approach focused on the blind region (see section 8.1.5).

8.3.1 Blindsight and Its Training-Rationale

Since the fifties, a bulk of research showed that in the presence of striate deafferentiation a coarse and, most of the times, unconscious form of perception may persist in the blind region: this phenomenon is known as *blindsight.* Patients who show blindsight can localize very brief flashes of light in their blind hemifield (*e.g.* Weiskrantz *et al.*, 1974), to discriminate, or even better *to guess* colors and colored stimuli (Boyer *et al.*, 2005; Stoerig and Cowey, 1989, 1992), orientation (Boyer *et al.*, 2005; Weiskrantz, 1986), form (Weiskrantz, 1987; Weiskrantz *et al.*, 1974), and especially motion (*e.g.* Perenin, 1991; Ptito *et al.*, 1991; Barbur *et al.*, 1980). The prevalence of this phenomenon among patients with visual field defects due to occipital lesions is highly variable, ranging from 5% (Marzi *et al.*, 1986) to 64% (Weiskrantz, 1980). The different criteria adopted for the diagnosis may partly account for the variability of this estimate.

Blindsight has been attributed to a mere effect of light scattering (Campion *et al.*, 1983) or spared islands of intact function in area 17 (Wessinger *et al.*, 1997, 1999; Fendrich *et al.*, 1992; Celesia *et al.*, 1991), and yet both hypotheses seem unlikely (Stoerig *et al.*, 1998; Kentridge *et al.*, 1997; Barbur *et al.*, 1993; Lutzemberger *et al.*, 1985). Instead, there is consistent evidence that "blind vision", is mediated by extrastriate circuits, namely a geniculate extrastriate pathway (Schmid *et al.*, 2010; Boyer *et al.*, 2005; Sincich *et al.*, 2004) and/or a retinotectal route that involves the superior colliculus (Boyer *et al.*, 2005; Ro *et al.*, 2004). Indeed, a direct geniculate-extrastriate pathway has been described in the macaque monkey: the pathway starts from all the layers of the LGN and projects to V2, V3, and V4 (Bullier and Kennedy, 1983; Fries, 1981; Yukie and Iwai, 1981), and to the medial temporal region (MT or V5 area: Bridge *et al.*, 2008; Sincich *et al.*, 2004), bypassing V1. Alternatively, blindsight is the result of a retinotectal (extrageniculate) pathway, from the retina to the superior colliculus, and from here to the extrastriate cortex.

Subjects with blindsight may be completely unaware of the stimulus (blindsight type I) or may have a feeling of its presence (blindsight type II: Weiskrantz, 1998).

Whatever the type, the repeated stimulation inside the scotomatous region is reported to improve the unconscious (or, to a certain extent, conscious) perception in the trained region. Upon this basis, a training procedure focused on the scotomatous region may be used as a complementary form of visual restitution. Huxlin *et al.* (2009) provide two mutually non-exclusive explanations for the recovery of visual functions (in their specific study global motion discrimination) in the affected field of hemianopic patients:

1- visual training in the scotoma may increase or reactivate the functional response of intact islands of cortex localized in the damaged region, whose responsiveness is at a subthreshold level. This result would depend on enhanced cortical plasticity. There is some evidence, indeed, that cortical plasticity takes place not only at the border between the seen and not seen region but even deeper in the scotomatous area. Dilks and colleagues reported the case of a subject who suffered from damage to the optic radiation leading to cortical deafferentation with upper quadrantanopia. Of note, the correspondent cortical region was not destroyed but disconnected, thereby silenced (Dilks *et al.*, 2007). Six months after the onset, the patient experienced a distorted perception of space, with stimuli presented in his spared quadrant that appeared stretched into the blind region and grasping deviated toward the same direction. Functional magnetic resonance demonstrated that the deafferentiated region of the cortex had become responsive to adjacent retinotopic locations, revealing plastic changes in the functional cortical cytoarchitecture.

2- according to the reverse–hierarchy model (Ahissar and Hochstein, 1997), perceptual learning takes place from higher-level to lower-level visual areas. Within this framework, higher-level cortical activation induced by training drives perceptual learning of lower-level, intact visual areas, enhancing or taking over their function. In the case of damage to V1, the repetitive stimulation of higher-level visual areas (*e.g.* V2, V3, V4, and V5) that receive direct inputs from the retina *via* extrastriate pathways, could be the target of perceptual learning, in other terms the functional substrate of visual training. Perceptual learning, indeed, would make the extrastriate areas suitable to take over the lost striate cortex.

Whatever the reason, there is evidence that the constant stimulation of the blind region with spots of light of different wavelengths leads to specific neuronal modifications (Potthoff, 1995).

Here are summarized some representative studies on visual restoration training performed in the blind region of hemianopic patients.

8.3.2 The Flickering Rehabilitation Protocol of Hyvärinen, Raninen, and Colleagues (2002, 2007)

The group of Hyvärinen and Raninen (Raninen *et al.*, 2007; Hyvärinen *et al.*, 2002) described a visual rehabilitation program administered to 5 patients with long-standing homonymous hemianopia due to damage to the geniculocalcarine pathway and to the striate and extrastriate cortex. Patients, who had macular sparing of 10–12° and retained motion perception in their blind hemifield[20], underwent a two-step training program that made use of flickering discs and, subsequently, letters.

The first step aimed at rehabilitating detection: 4 deg wide sinusoidally flickering discs were presented on an equiluminant background at a temporal frequency of 1, 2, 5, 10, 15, 20, and 35 Hz, with an exposure duration of 2 s. The stimuli were displayed at 30 degrees of eccentricity from the midline in the blind hemifield along the horizontal meridian. A transformed staircase method (1U4DTR) was coupled with a 2AFC response model to estimate the contrast sensitivity of the discs at each temporal frequency[21]. The subject had to decide which of the two intervals contained the stimulus. The rehabilitation consisted of repeated measures of contrast threshold at each temporal frequency. The training was administered for 12 months.

The second step aimed at rehabilitating discrimination (or identification): sinusoidally flickering letters (T, L, H, and U) were presented on an equiluminant background at a temporal frequency of 0.1 (stationary stimuli), 1, 2, 5, 10, 15, and 20 Hz. For each subject, the size of the letter was at a threshold (2–8 degrees). Exposure time was 2 s (3 s for stationary stimuli). The targets were displayed at 10 and 20 degrees of eccentricity from the midline in the blind hemifield along the horizontal meridian. A transformed staircase method (1U4DTR) was coupled with a 4AFC response model (implicit version: Aleci, 2021) to estimate contrast sensitivity at each temporal frequency. At each trial, the subject had to decide which of the four letters was presented. The rehabilitation consisted of repeated measures of contrast threshold at each temporal frequency.

Hyvärinen and colleagues (2002) described the results obtained from one of their patients (MR) after completion of the first program of rehabilitation. Flicker sensitivity in the affected hemifield, which was up to 17 times lower than in the normal hemifield at the beginning of the rehabilitation, normalized (*i.e.* was equal to

---

[20]Estimated with Goldmann stimuli moving at speed >20°/s.

[21]Contrast of the flickering discs was expressed as root mean square contrast; $C_{RMS} = \sqrt{\int c^2(t)dt/T}$, where:

- c(t) is the contrast waveform: $c(t) = (L(t) - L_0)/L_0$. (L(t) is the temporal luminance waveform, L_0 is the mean luminance);
- T is the duration of the stimulus.

After each miss response, C_{RMS} was increased by 1.26, whereas after 4 consecutive hit responses C_{RMS} was decreased by the same amount. The subject had to choose which one of two temporal intervals contained the signal. The viewing distance was 115 cm.

the normal hemifield) at the end of the treatment. The normalization in the affected hemifield took place at all the temporal frequencies but 35 Hz (figure 8.7). The improvement decreased after 1.5 years but it returned to the post-training value after 4 additional rehabilitative sessions.

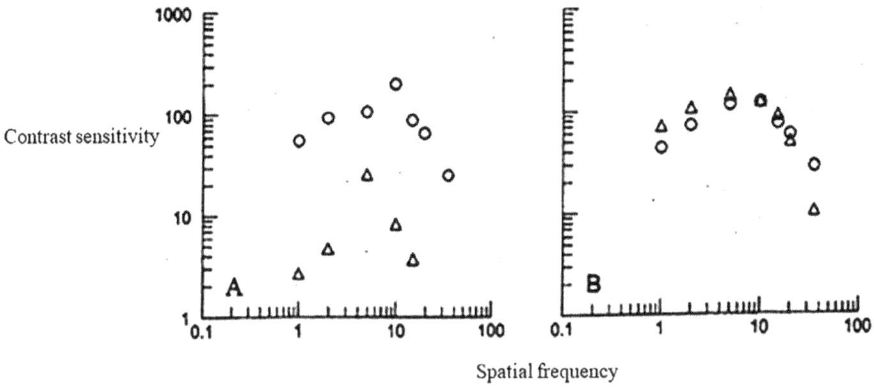

FIG. 8.7 – Contrast sensitivity to the flickering discs before (left panel) and after (right panel) the training in the spared (circles) and blind hemifield (triangles) at 30° of eccentricity as a function of temporal frequency. Patient MR. To be noted that after the training the sensitivity in the blind hemifield was equal to that in the spared hemifield at all the temporal frequencies but the highest (35 Hz). From Hyvärinen *et al.* (2002). With permission of Taylor & Francis publisher.

The second protocol was then administered to MR. In the pre-training phase, the identification of flickering letters in the affected hemifield was limited to those of greater size (8 deg) presented quite close to the border of the scotomatous region (10 degrees of eccentricity). On the contrary, in the normal hemifield letters 2 deg wide were identifiable at all the frequencies not only at 10 degrees but also at 20 degrees of eccentricity.

After five months of training, the patient was able to recognize letters 2 deg wide at 20 deg of eccentricity in the blind hemifield at all the frequencies (1–20 Hz) but not static (non-flickering) letters. After eleven months of training, the patient was able to recognize 2-degrees static letters at 20 degrees of eccentricity provided they were presented for 3 s. After an additional month of training, the presentation time required to identify static letters at the same eccentricity was reduced to 2 s: MR's performance in the affected hemifield, therefore, was normalized (figure 8.8).

At the end of the training, the patient could perceive a V/4 Goldmann stimulus here and there in his blind hemifield.

Interestingly, the rate of improvement was not linear but was slow at the beginning of the training then it increased and persisted even during the intervals between sessions: this trend suggests that once the process of cortical reorganization has been prompted by the treatment, it may proceed even in the absence of additional stimulation.

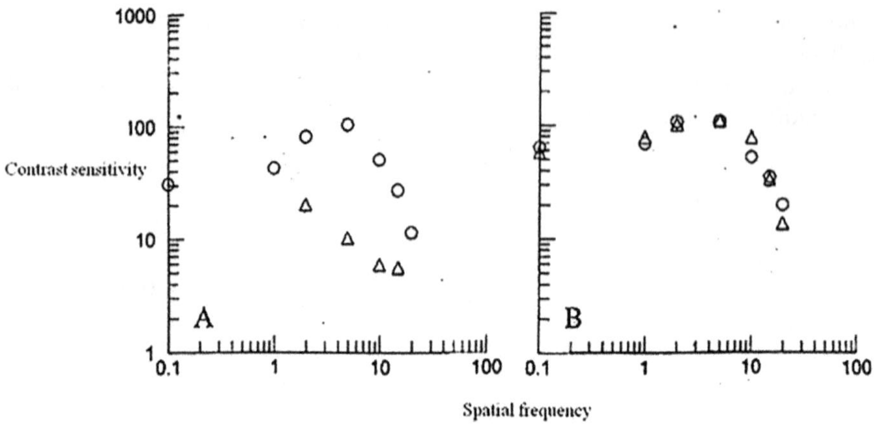

FIG. 8.8 – Contrast sensitivity to the flickering letters after five months (left panel) and after 12 months (right panel) of training in the spared (circles) and blind hemifield (triangles) at 20° of eccentricity as a function of temporal frequency in patient MR. To be noted that after the training the sensitivity in the blind hemifield (triangles) to letters 2° in size was equal to that in the spared hemifield (circles) at all temporal frequencies but the highest (35 Hz). From Hyvärinen *et al.* (2002). With permission of Taylor & Francis publisher.

In a subsequent study, the same group trained with the same procedure two subjects suffering from stable homonymous hemianopia (Raninen *et al.*, 2007). Both patients had macular sparing of about 2–3°.

Before training, the detection threshold of flickering discs at 30 deg of eccentricity in the affected hemifield was higher than in the spared hemifield by 1–1.8 log units at the low (but not at the highest) frequencies. After 5 months of training (*i.e.* 40 training sessions) the detection threshold normalized (*i.e.* it was the same as in the spared hemifield) at all the temporal frequencies at the same eccentricity.

Before training, flickering letters could be recognized only at 5 deg of eccentricity. After 3 months of training (*i.e.* 32 sessions) in one subject and after 7 months of training (*i.e.* 56 sessions) in the other, the identification threshold of letters presented at 10 deg of eccentricity in the affected hemifield was the same as in the spared hemifield at the same eccentricity.

Visual field, measured with kinetic Goldmann perimetry, did not change after the training, but patients reported subjective improvement and felt more confident when navigating in crowded places and crossing the street.

According to the authors, neither light scattering nor eccentric or unstable fixation may have biased the results.

8.3.3 The Effect of the Flickering Stimulation of the Blind Field on the Cortex

Using fMRI, Nelles and colleagues (2002) reported that in normal subjects the stimulation of each hemifield with a black-and-white checkerboard generates a strong pattern of activation of the contralateral V1 extending to V2/V3 associated with a weaker activation of V2/V3 *ipsilateral* to the side of stimulation[22]. This is in line with the finding of Tootell *et al.* (1998) who mapped the ipsilateral cortical representation of the visual hemifield in 12 healthy subjects with functional magnetic resonance. Hemifield stimulation activated an ipsilateral region anterior to the areas with well-defined contralateral retinotopy (*i.e.* V1, V2, V3). The activated region showed two branches that begin at the anterior boundary of V3: a superior branch that extends superiorly and borders the anterior portion of V3, and an inferior branch that extends anteriorly, passing through and beyond MT (figure 8.9).

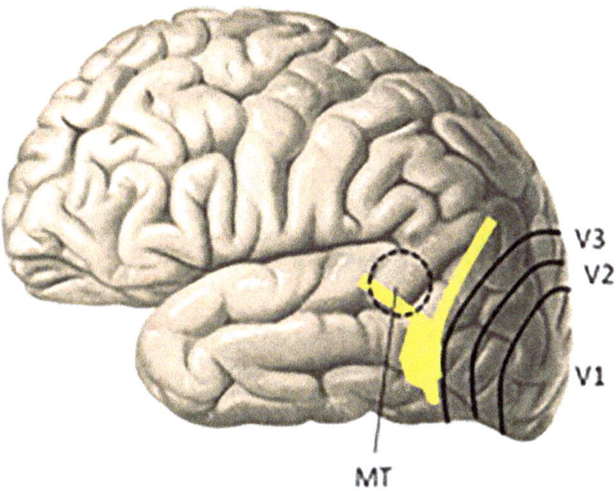

FIG. 8.9 – Ipsilateral activation of the visual areas anterior to V3. Based on the data from Tootell *et al.* (1998).

The authors concluded that visual information is processed first in the contralateral visual area, then it extends into the ipsilateral hemisphere (Tootell *et al.*, 1998).

The activation of V2 and V3 ipsilateral to the stimulated hemifield can be explained as a transcallosal transfer. Such a transfer seems to be enhanced in hemianopic patients: in these cases, in fact, the group of Nelles showed that the stimulation of the spared hemifield led to activation of the contralateral V1 extending to V2/V3 and a weaker ipsilateral activation of V2/V3. Most interestingly, the stimulation of the affected hemifield led to activation of the contralateral V2/V3 (whereas V1 remained silent) and to a stronger ipsilateral activation of V2/V3 (Nelles *et al.*, 2002: figure 8.10).

[22]The study was conducted on 7 normal subjects and 7 hemianopic patients with no neglect (time since lesion: minimum 6 months).

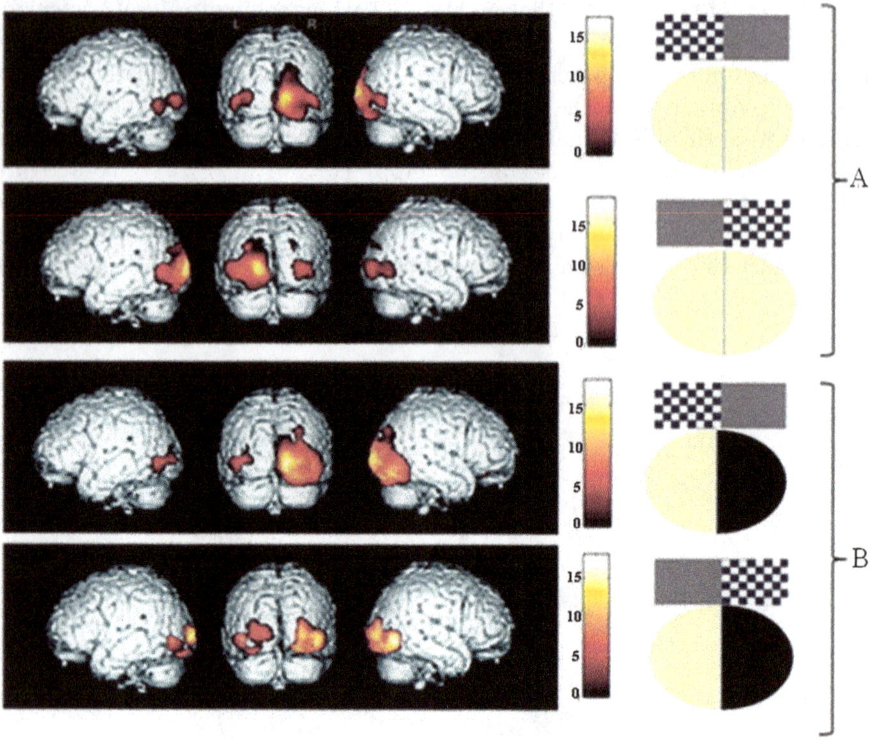

FIG. 8.10 – A: activation during hemifield stimulation in normal subjects. B: activation during hemifield stimulation in patients. Upper panel: stimulation of the unaffected hemifield; lower panel: stimulation of the affected hemifield. From Nelles *et al.* (2002). With permission of Wolters Kluwer Health Publisher.

In a subsequent study on 13 patients, the same authors confirmed their previous findings: the stimulation of the blind hemifield induced activation of the extrastriate cortex in the contralateral and ipsilateral hemifield of hemianopic patients who suffered from a unilateral occipital stroke of the primary visual cortex (Nelles *et al.*, 2007b). The pattern of activation was studied in detail in 13 patients with homonymous hemianopia and no neglect. At fMRI, the stimulation of the normal hemifield[23] led to activation of the contralateral striate and extrastriate cortex, and, even if to a lesser extent, the ipsilateral extrastriate cortex. In turn, the stimulation of the affected hemifield led to activation of the extrastriate cortex bilaterally, stronger in the ipsilateral hemisphere (Nelles *et al.*, 2007b; table 8.3). The ipsilateral activation in patients was stronger than the ipsilateral activation in normal subjects.

[23]With a black-and-white checkerboard pattern reversal.

TAB. 8.3 – The effect of stimulation of the blind field on the occipital cortex (data from Nelles *et al.*, 2007b).

Stimulation ↓	Striate cortex (a.17) CONTRALATERAL	Extrastriate cortex (a.18/19) CONTRALATERAL	Striate cortex (a.17) IPSILATERAL	Extrastriate cortex (a.18/19) IPSILATERAL
Spared hemifield	XX	XX	NO	(x)
Affected hemifield	NO	X	NO	XX

Magnetoencephalographic recordings performed in one of the two patients studied by the group of Henriksson demonstrated that before the training no response could be recorded when the affected (right) hemifield was stimulated with a checkerboard pattern, but after two years of rehabilitation a sudden response was found in the ipsilesional (right) posterior hemisphere (Henriksson *et al.*, 2007).

Functional magnetic resonance showed that the activation was mainly located in the ipsilesional V3a, V3, V5/MT, and, V1. So, at the end of the training visual information from both hemifields was processed in the intact hemisphere.

To confirm the ipsilateral activation, spontaneous cortical oscillations, which generally attenuate after stimulation (Hari and Salmenlin, 1997), were examined before and after the training (flickering stimulation). As expected, before the practice spontaneous oscillation was observed in both hemispheres when stimulating the blind hemifield, confirming that no cerebral activation was evoked in the subject. After the rehabilitation, the spontaneous oscillation was reduced in the right (ipsilateral) hemisphere (Henriksson *et al.*, 2007). At the same time, the patient had become aware of most of the stimuli projected in his blind hemifield.

In sum, the stimulation of the blind hemifield in hemianopic patients activates the ipsilateral and, to a lesser extent, the contralateral peri/parastriate cortex.

The ipsilateral extrastriate activation can be explained by:

i- Pre-existing transcallosal pathways that transfer visual information from the contralateral (stimulated) hemisphere to the ipsilateral (non-stimulated) hemisphere. The transcallosal pathway can be enhanced *via* axonal sprouting in response to striate cortical damage, accounting for the stronger ipsilateral activation of V2 and V3 when the blind hemifield of the hemianopic patients was stimulated.

ii- Multitasking ability of the visual areas, so that a cross-modal reorganization in the extrastriate cortex would take place after striate injury.

According to Henriksson and co-workers (2007), the ipsilateral activation in the hemianopic subject is unlikely to depend on callosal connections from the affected hemisphere as the recording of spontaneous oscillations demonstrated functional disconnection of the contralateral occipital region. Instead, the ipsilateral activation would depend on the activation of a subcortical pathway involving the superior colliculus. This subcortical route would transfer the left (contralateral) cerebral activation to the right (ipsilateral) extrastriate visual areas. Indeed, there is evidence that the visual information crosses at the cullicular level to the opposite hemisphere (Tardif and Clarke, 2002).

As an alternative to the collicular pathway, a direct extrastriate geniculo-cortical pathway connecting the lateral geniculate nucleus to V5 (MT), bypassing V1, has been demonstrated in animals and is likely to be present in humans as well (Schoenfeld *et al.*, 2002a, 2002b; Barbur *et al.*, 1993).

In both cases, the unexpected ipsilateral representation of both hemifields would depend on the disconnection of the lesioned visual cortex and subsequent plastic changes that enhance the transmission along these subcortical routes (Raninen *et al.*, 2007). Overall, this finding suggests that visual areas in the intact hemifield may contribute to post-training recovery.

8.3.4 Flickering Rehabilitation of the Blind Field: The Study of Roth and Colleagues (2009)

In a subsequent study (Roth *et al.*, 2009), a training procedure derived from that adopted by the group of Hyvärinen and Raninen (Hyvärinen *et al.*, 2002) was administered to a group of 15 patients with homonymous hemianopia. Sinusoidally flickering letters (A, H, K, or T) were presented individually at 21.8 degrees of eccentricity from the midline in the blind hemifield along the horizontal meridian at a temporal frequency of 10 Hz. The size of the letter was at the threshold for each subject (2–8 degrees). Exposure time was 2 s (3 s for stationary stimuli). In the intact region of the visual field, the four letters were presented vertically arranged. The testee had to choose which one corresponded to the letter just presented in the blind hemifield according to a 4AFC response model (Roth *et al.*, 2009).

The training was performed at home for 60 min per day, 5 days a week for 6 weeks.

The outcome of interest was visual search time, estimated with the same paradigm used during the training before, immediately after, and after 6 weeks from the end of the rehabilitation.

In addition, natural search time was evaluated by asking the subject to find on a table 20 distinct objects presented in succession in each hemifield. Finally, fixation stability, reading speed, and static automated perimetry (measured with a Tübinger perimeter, 30°, and SLO) were considered.

After the training, visual search time decreased in both hemifields and the improvement persisted during the third month of follow-up. It should be noted that the improvement was weaker compared to the visual search training performed in the same study on a parallel group (see section 9.5). Fixations during the exploration of natural scenes remained unchanged, the training did not yield any improvement in reading speed, and, finally, no perimetric differences were found, in line with the previous investigation by the group of Hyvärinen (2002).

8.3.5 *The Selective Stimulation Training of Sahraie et al. (2006)*

The training protocol devised by the group of Sahraie aims at the spatial channels that remain functional in blindsight.

According to the studies of Saharaie and colleagues and Barbur and associates, blindsight is mediated by a channel modulated within the range 0.5–3.5 c/deg (maximal response at 1 c/deg) and a peak of activation at a temporal frequency of 10 Hz (Sahraie *et al.*, 2003, 2006; Barbur *et al.*, 1994). At spatial frequency 1 c/deg, the proportion of correct detection was above chance with stimuli with contrast ≥25% (from 25% to 98%), showing a monotonic rise with the increase of contrast.

Upon this basis, Saharaie and associates devised a specific training aimed at this channel, stimulating the blind hemifield with black circular patches 6° wide made of a vertical sinusoidal grating flickering at a temporal frequency of 10 Hz and spatial frequency of 1 c/deg (Sahraie *et al.*, 2003).

A temporal 2-AFC paradigm was used so that an interval containing the signal and another with a "null" stimulus were presented in randomized order, Null stimuli were uniform patches with the same luminance as the background.

The observer had to indicate at each trial:

i- which of the two intervals contained the signal (interval 1/interval 2: each interval was signaled by an audible beep);
ii- whether he/she had any awareness of the stimulus (yes/no).

Two field locations in the blind hemifield were repeatedly stimulated. In addition, the targets were displayed at a position straddling the transition zone. The stimulation at the transition zone served to keep the patient alerted during the repetitive presentation in the affected region.

During the training, the stimuli were initially presented at Michelson contrast 90% on a uniform gray background. According to a 1-up, 3-down staircase procedure (1U3DTR), if the proportion of detected stimuli was >84% in three consecutive sessions, the contrast was decreased by 10% at the next session. If the proportion of detected stimuli was <66% in a session, the contrast was increased by 10% in the next session. Each interval was signaled by a beep and no feedback was given to the patient.

Each session was made up of 50 trials at each visual field location ($3 \times 50 =$ total: 150 trials). The whole training lasted 3 three months and was self-administered by patients at home.

During the first sessions (30–40 in the two cases reported as examples by the authors) of the rehabilitation period, grating detection in the blind region remained at the chance level, then the performance rose above the chance level in the two stimulated regions. When the detection rate reached 84% (this occurred after about 60–80 sessions in the two recruited patients), the contrast of the gratings was reduced, as planned, as long as the detection rate remained unchanged. Contrary to the increase in detection rate, the awareness remained low, confirming that patients had type 1 blindsight (figure 8.11).

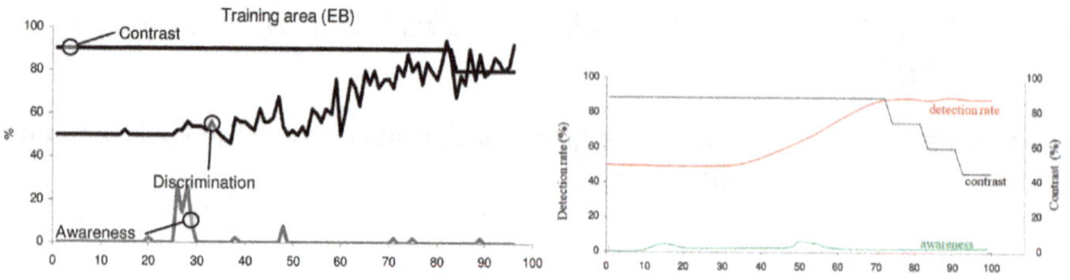

FIG. 8.11 – Change in detection rate at baseline for 1 c/deg gratings as a function of the number of trials. See text for explanation. Panel to the left: from Sahraie *et al.* (2006). Copyright (2006) National Academy of Sciences, U.S.A.

At the end of the training, detection rate was re-evaluated with the same procedure used at the baseline. A higher detection rate was observed for high-contrast (50%) gratings with spatial frequency from 0.5 to 3.5 c/deg. The improvement was accompanied by increased awareness of gratings with a spatial frequency of 0.5 and 1 c/deg (figure 8.12).

After the training, differential light sensitivity was higher in both the 30° and 10° wide tested region of the visual field, and patients reported a subjective binocular reduction of their blind region.

In some of the non-trained regions, an improvement was observed for stimuli with medium contrast (50%) and spatial frequency from 0.5 to 2 c/deg, but the awareness remained absent.

Even if the increase in sensitivity was overall restricted to the trained locations, it led to improved navigation skills.

As considered by the authors, the improvement in visual attention directed toward the blind field (in everyday life the affected region is typically ignored) may have a role in increasing the sensitivity in the blind region, both in the stimulated and unstimulated areas.

8.3.6 *The Saccadic Stimulation of the Blind Hemifield of Zihl and von Cramon (1980, 1981, 1985)*

Fourteen hemianopic patients with damage to the geniculo-striate visual pathways were trained by stimulating their saccadic movements toward targets presented in their blind hemifield (Zihl, 1980). The recruited patients showed clear difficulty in avoiding obstacles, orientation, and reading. Training sessions (each lasting 45 min) were performed three times daily or at least once a week.

Monocular and binocular kinetic perimetry and binocular static perimetry were carried out before and after the treatment using a modified Tübinger perimeter.

During the practice session, carried out with the same perimeter, targets were displayed for 100 ms at different random positions along a particular meridian in the blind hemifield. The patients, who were informed along which meridian the targets would be displayed, had to look at the fixation point, and, whenever they heard a click signal, had to shift their gaze toward the region of the blind hemifield where the

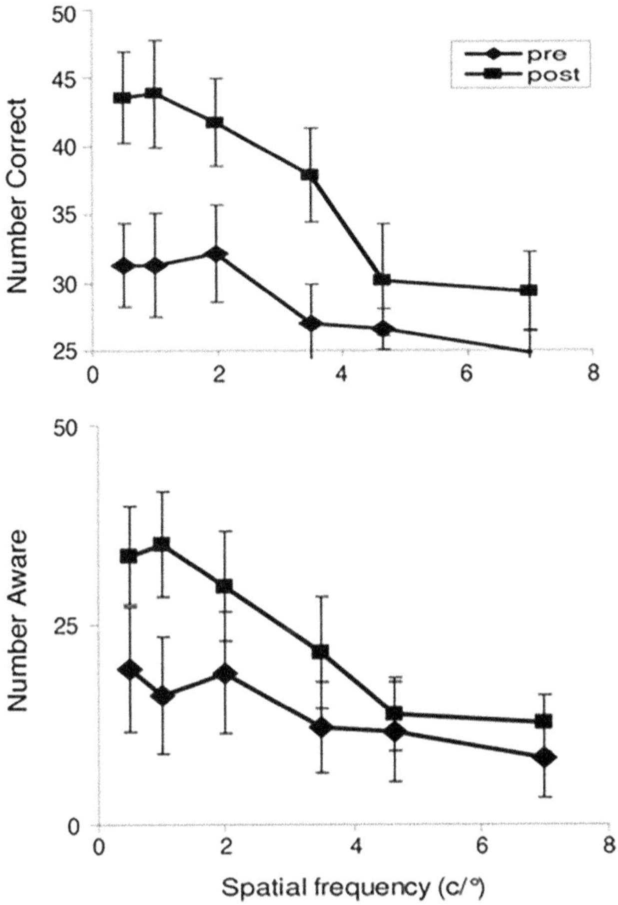

FIG. 8.12 – Change in detection rate and related awareness before and after the training for high-contrast (50%) gratings as a function of spatial frequency Temporal modulation: 10 Hz. From Sahraie *et al.* (2006). Copyright (2006) National Academy of Sciences, U.S.A.

target was supposed to be. The author pinpointed that they were instructed to "localize" the target with a single saccadic sweep and not with several searching eye movements. During the training eye movements were recorded.

At the end of the rehabilitation period (5, 7, 9, 11, and 12 sessions), increased visual field size in the trained region was observed in most of the patients. The extent of the enlargement was variable (from 5° up to 27°), and was related to the width of the transition zone since steep gradients led to poorer improvement. Interocular transfer was reported. The same correlation applied to the number of trials required to achieve 1° of visual field enlargement. Interestingly, the transition zone was always narrower after the training. The position of the stimuli inside the scotomatous region was not crucial as well as age and time since onset: all the variables were not correlated with the number of trials required to obtain a visual field enlargement and with the amount of the latter. The results were stable after 6 months.

Visual acuity[24] and color perception[25] improved in the trained regions as well. Reading was subjectively better, and vision within the restored part of the visual field did not differ qualitatively from vision in the intact region.

The authors concluded that even in the absence of the striate cortex the detection and localization of stimuli was possible, being probably mediated by the retino-tectal-extrastriate pathway.

Indeed, according to Mohler and Wurtz (1977), the superior colliculus and its projection onto the extrastriate cortex play an important role in the recovery of visual function following saccadic training like this in patients with damage to the striate cortex. Visual restitution, in fact, is related to an increase in the ipsilesional neuronal collicular population corresponding to the blind region. So, damage to the superior colliculus prevents rehabilitating the visual function of subjects with occipital lesions *via* saccadic training (Mohler and Wurtz, 1977). The suprasylvian gyrus needs to be preserved as well (Baumann and Spear, 1977; Fischman and Meikle, 1965).

In two subsequent studies, Zihl administered his saccadic localization training to a sample of hemianopic patients. In the first investigation 14 patients with stable homonymous hemianopic defects (differing in extent) after damage to the geniculostriate pathway were recruited. In their visual field, the border of the scotoma was close to the fixation point (Zihl, 1981).

In the second investigation Zihl and von Cramon trained with the same procedure 55 patients with stable homonymous hemianopia (44, *i.e.* 80%) or quadrantanopia (11, *i.e.* 20%). Patients suffered from infarction of the territory of the posterior cerebral artery or closed head trauma (Zihl and von Cramon, 1985). All the rehabilitated patients in these studies complained of bumping into obstacles and reading difficulty (Zihl and von Cramon, 1985; Zihl, 1981).

The visual functions tested before and after the training were:

- Static and dynamic binocular conventional perimetry (Zihl and von Cramon, 1985; Zihl, 1981).
- Color recognition, measured with binocular perimetry performed with red, green, and blue stimuli (320 cd m^{-2}). Patients were asked to press a key as soon as they could recognize the color of the perimetric target (Zihl and von Cramon, 1985; Zihl, 1981).
- Visual acuity at different eccentricities. Circles and diamonds of different sizes were used as targets and displayed for 1 s at different eccentricities along the meridian selected for the training. The subject had to report

[24]Binocular visual acuity was tested by presenting in randomized order a circle or a diamond-shaped target of seven different sizes, ranging from 7 min arc (equivalent to 1.00 decimal acuity, or 20/20 Snellen acuity) to 116 min arc (0.06 decimal acuity, or 20/333 Snellen acuity). The patient had to report which target (circle or diamond) was displayed.

[25]Color perception was assessed by presenting colored targets (blue, green, and red) and asking the subject to identify the hue of the stimulus.

which of the two targets was presented (Zihl and von Cramon, 1985; Zihl, 1981).
- Form recognition, measured with binocular kinetic perimetry performed with a diamond-shaped target of different sizes. Patients were asked to press a key as soon as they could identify the stimulus (Zihl and von Cramon, 1985).
- Light detection: pairs of spots of light were presented symmetrically to three patients, one in the spared hemifield, the other in the blind hemifield along the horizontal axis or 10° above or below (presentation time: 10 ms, luminance 1.3 cd m^{-2}). Patients had to fixate on a central red spot and report if they saw one or two stimuli after each presentation (Zihl and von Cramon, 1985).
- Recognition task: a series of black numerals randomly arranged was presented to the left or to the right of the fixation point, along the horizontal axis, or 10° above or below (presentation time: 80 ms). The series began at the vertical meridian. Patients had to report the numerals (Zihl and von Cramon, 1985).

The training consisted of the presentation of light targets in the blind hemifield accompanied by a sound. Using a Tübinger perimeter, light targets were displayed at a given eccentricity (at least 3° away from the border of the scotoma) along one meridian (known by the subject) in the blind field for 100 ms (Zihl, 1981) or 1000 ms (Zihl and von Cramon, 1985). At the onset of an acoustic signal, the subject had to move his gaze toward the target. The training was administered three times daily or at least once a week in the first study (Zihl, 1981), and daily or at least three times a week in the second experiment (Zihl and von Cramon, 1985).

After the training:

- A visual field enlargement ranging from 2° to 24° was observed (Zihl, 1981). In the subsequent study, a widening >1.5° was found in 80% of the patients: of these, 32% showed an enlargement >10°[26] (Zihl and von Cramon, 1985).
- The perimetric improvement was limited to the region corresponding to the trained meridian and did not involve the whole field border (*e.g.* only the superior or the inferior quadrant: Zihl and von Cramon, 1985; Zihl, 1981). The improvement was not correlated with age, time since onset, duration of each stimulation, laterality, or type of cerebral damage (Zihl and von Cramon, 1985; Zihl, 1981). The improvement was observed during the training periods and it was negligible (no more than 2°:

[26]This enlargement of the visual field after saccadic localization training has not been confirmed (Pambakian *et al.*, 2004; Nelles *et al.*, 2001; Balliet *et al.*, 1985): Balliet and colleagues administered a saccadic training similar to that used by Zihl (1981) and Zihl and von Cramon (1985), consisting in a repeated saccadic localization task presented in the affected hemifield of three hemianopic patients who had previously demonstrated to be nonresponsive to a visual restoration training. Patients had to look centrally at a fixation spot, then move their eye toward a stimulus presented monocularly on a Goldmann perimeter at different locations (3–50° from the visual field border) on preselected meridians in the hemianopic field (presentation time: 1 s). The rehabilitation period was 1 month. Visual field enlargement was less than 1° toward the affected hemifield (Balliet *et al.*, 1985).

Zihl, 1981) or absent (Zihl and von Cramon, 1985) during the intervals (1–6 weeks) between subsequent rehabilitation sessions. Finally, the gain remained stable for at least four (Zihl and von Cramon, 1985) or six months (Zihl, 1981) after the end of the training. Additional rehabilitation after the end of the treatment did not produce further enlargement of the visual field.
- The visual field enlargement was positively correlated with the extent of the transition zone (the wider the transition zone, the greater the enlargement and the smaller the number of trials needed for its achievement): it is indicative, indeed, that the width of the transition zone was reduced after the training. In addition, a transition zone close to the fovea seems related to a poorer recovery compared to a transition zone ≥10° away from the fixation point.
- The number of trials required to achieve 1° of visual field enlargement was highly variable (from 25 up to 400) and was not correlated with the age of the patient:
- color perception and eccentric visual acuity improved in the recovered regions (Zihl, 1981). The same was observed for shape recognition (Zihl and von Cramon, 1985) in 94% of the patients who showed perimetric enlargement. The subjects who improved were those with posterior cerebral artery infarction and not those with closed head trauma.

According to subjective reports, the daily activities of patients (orientation, navigation, and reading) improved after the training:

- 96% of the patients who complained of severe to moderate problems in avoiding obstacles dropped to 49% after the rehabilitation (Zihl and von Cramon, 1985).
- The patients with reading difficulties (*i.e.* those with a macular sparing ≤3°) decreased from 58% to 22%. Those who improved showed faster reading rates and reduced number of errors (even if both variables remained below normal). Reading improvement in terms of reading rate and accuracy took place irrespective of whether training had determined or not a visual field enlargement even if, in the second case, worse results were observed. The authors suggested that the relative independence of reading performance from visual field enlargement depended on enhanced searching strategies when scanning the text (Zihl and von Cramon, 1985).
- The recognition rate of numerals in tachistoscopic conditions in the blind hemifield increased in two of the patients who showed post-training visual field enlargement[27]. In a third patient, who did not benefit from a perimetric enlargement after rehabilitation, numerals' recognition remained unchanged (Zihl and von Cramon, 1985).
- Finally, when a single eye was treated, interocular transfer could be demonstrated in the fellow (occluded, *i.e.* not treated) eye.

The authors posited that the effect of the training takes place in the regions of the striate area with reversible damage (functionally depressed but not abolished regions.

[27]Since patients reported to have perceived the numerals, the recovery applies to conscious vision and not to blindsight.

8.3.7 Visual Restitution Associated with Pharmacotherapy (Widdig et al., 2003)

The group of Widdig investigated the effect of visual restitution training associated with the administration of amphetamine (Widdig *et al.*, 2003). A 58-year-old man with complete cortical blindness due to bilateral occipital infarction that occurred 12 weeks earlier was stimulated with white light flashes projected alternatively onto his left/right hemifield at 45 deg of eccentricity. After two weeks, the detection task with white flashes was replaced with an identification task of simple shapes (circles, squares, and triangles), colors (red, blue, yellow, green, and white), and finally colored shapes.

This first phase of training lasted 139 days. In the end, amphetamine[28] was administered in association with the training for an additional period of 85 days. At the baseline VEP amplitude was deeply depressed and shape and color perception was virtually null.

After the first period of training, an improvement in shape perception[29] was observed when the presentation time was 5 s, even if the proportion of correct discrimination remained very low. At the end of the second period (with amphetamine), the proportion of correct discrimination was about 70% for colors and almost 100% for shapes. Increased vision ability was specific for the trained function, even if a visual field enlargement was observed in the inferior regions. The experimental gain of visual function was paralleled by improvement of vision in daily life after the 90th day of treatment, with recognition of faces, persons, and simple objects; in addition, the patient was able to read words and sentences after 170 days of treatment (Widdig *et al.*, 2003). The authors supposed that the training associated with amphetamine induces specific synaptic plastic changes in the cortical regions with decreased or dysfunctional neuronal activity. Their hypothesis is supported by an fMRI study that showed increased striate cortical activation parallel to the functional improvement in the trained subject (Pleger *et al.*, 2003).

8.3.8 Visual Restitution via Training of Motion Perception (Huxlin et al., 2009)

The group of Huxlin trained motion perception in the blind hemifield of seven subjects with post-stroke damage to the striate cortex occurred 8–40 months before their recruitment (Huxlin *et al.*, 2009). All patients suffered from homonymous quadrantanopia or hemianopia but the ipsilesional MT+ area was intact.

Before the training, the visual field was tested with static perimetry and motion perception was measured with a procedure devised on purpose.

[28]Initial dosage: 10 mg, then gradually increased to 20 mg administered three hours before each treatment. Since the sixties, the effect of low-dosage amphetamine in facilitating the restablishemnt of visual discrimination was reported in animal studies (Braun *et al.*, 1966).

[29]Exposure time of 5 and 10 s.

The discrimination of motion direction along the horizontal axis was studied by asking patients to report the left *vs.* right displacement of random dot stimuli or sine-wave gratings. The threshold was estimated with a transformed up-down staircase procedure at different visual field locations. A forced-choice 2-AFC (left/right) response design was adopted.

Global motion discrimination was examined by presenting an array of random dots, with the range of displacement of the array around the right or leftward vector as the independent variable. Stimulus duration was 500 ms (see Huxlin *et al.*, 2009 for more details). The range of motion direction was varied according to the response of the observer by a transformed 1-up, 3-down staircase procedure.

Local motion discrimination was estimated with sinewave gratings drifting either to the left or to the right, with contrast as the independent variable.

The discrimination of motion direction was severely impaired in the blind hemifield: the threshold was 9° around the horizontal vector *vs.* 309° in the intact hemifield[30]. In addition, the signal coherence required for ≥75% correct responses was significantly higher (coherent signal: 70% *vs.* 12% in the intact hemifield). Likewise, the amount of contrast required to discriminate the direction of the gratings was significantly higher in the affected hemifield (contrast sensitivity: 15 *vs.* 121 in the intact hemifield).

The training was carried out daily (one session made up of 300 trials a day, lasting about 30 min, training period: 9–18 months) with the initial stimulus setting based on the optimal performance obtained during the testing phase. The type of stimulation was the same as in the pre-training testing, with an array of random dots moving left- or rightwards; the range of direction was varied based on the response of the observer according to a staircase procedure. The stimulation started at the transition zone and moved toward the blind region as the threshold improved. The authors paid particular attention to the control of fixation by using an integrated pupillometer.

Training gradually widened the motion discrimination range in the affected hemifield from 9° (pre-training) up to 293 ± 12°, which is comparable to the discrimination range threshold estimated in the contralateral (intact) hemifield. The number of sessions required to reach this level of performance varied greatly from patient to patient, ranging between 20 and 100.

No transfer was observed across different regions of the affected hemifield: in fact, loci only 2° away from a trained location did not show any threshold improvement[31]. In turn, in the trained locations of the affected hemifield the recovery of motion discrimination transferred to other visual tasks, namely contrast sensitivity and light detection.

[30]This means that in the normal hemifield the array of dots moving to the upper or lower left within a range of orientations of 309° was correctly identified as moving leftward (the same applies to rightward displacements), whereas in the affected hemifield the tolerance to deviation from the horizontal meridian was restricted to 9°.

[31]On the contrary, in the intact hemifield the results of global motion discrimination training in a location transferred to the neighbournig regions.

Contrast sensitivity improved at the spatial frequency of 0.5–1 c/deg and temporal frequency of 10 Hz, corresponding to the spatiotemporal channels that mediate blindsight (Sahraie *et al.*, 2003; Barbur *et al.*, 1994): so, these channels may be involved in training-induced plasticity of motion perception after damage to the striate cortex. Upon these bases, the authors argued that the target of the rehabilitation was the extrastriate pathway (from the dorsal lateral geniculate nucleus and the superior colliculus to the extrastriate areas) and not V1. Light detection threshold decreased as well so that regions with less than 5 dB of sensitivity in the affected hemifield (as measured at automated perimetry) decreased in size, and light sensitivity in each eye on average increased by 13 dB around the trained regions.

The correlation between these experimental findings and the subjective improvement of vision supports the potential usefulness of this rehabilitative approach within the clinical setting.

8.3.9 Vision Restitution via Extrastriate Stimulation (Jobke et al., 2009)

The effect of stimulating the extrastriate pathway related to the blind hemifield was evaluated by Jobke, Kasten, and Sabel, and the outcome was compared to the "conventional" VRT aimed at the transition zone (Jobke *et al.*, 2009). The rationale of this approach relies on the enhancement of the direct (magnocellular) extrastriate geniculo-cortical pathway that connects the lateral geniculate nucleus directly to V5 (MT), bypassing V1 (Sincich *et al.*, 2004; Fries, 1981; Yukie and Iwai, 1981). The main function of MT is detecting the presence and direction of visual motion (Zeki, 2015). This route, demonstrated in animals, is likely to be present in humans as well (Schoenfeld *et al.*, 2002a, 2002b; Barbur *et al.*, 1993), and would explain the so-called Riddoch phenomenon and blindsight in general. The authors stimulated the extrastriate cortex in the blind hemifield of 18 patients with stable hemianopia or quadrantanopia with a massive moving spiral made of concentric moving rings. The results after extrastriate stimulation of the blind hemifield and after conventional VRT (directed toward the transition zone) were analyzed in terms of detection at high-resolution perimetry (HRP)[32]. A small but significant increase in detection rate was found after both extrastriate training (4.2% on average) and conventional VRT (2.4% on average, $p = .036$). Contrary to VRT, the improvement in detection rate after the extrastriate stimulation was observed not only in the transition zone but also in the blind region.

Even if standard perimetry did not confirm the slight gain in sensitivity found at HRP, the authors concluded that extrastriate stimulation may add benefits if associated with "conventional" vision restoration therapy.

[32]See section 8.2.7.

Target of the training	Study	Sample	Stimuli	Modality	Training duration	Results	Follow-up
Transition zone	*Zihl and von Cramon, 1979, 1982*	12 patients with post-stroke, homonymous hemianopia, quadrantanopia, or central scotoma of cortical origin.	- Static perimetry, white stimuli presented with the method of limits; - Background 3.2 cd m^{-2}.	- Monocular repetitive assessment of contrast threshold at the transition zone at constant eccentricities along the horizontal meridian; - no control group.	- 15–20 threshold estimates per session; - frequency of sessions: daily; - duration of each session: one hour.	- Increase in sensitivity after 3–5 sessions, greater for the peripheral loci (up to 0.5 log units) than for the central loci (0.2 log units); - enlargement of the visual field ranging from 1 to 8–15 degrees (it depended on the gradient of the transition zone) after 9–37 sessions; - intraocular transfer when the training was peripheral, (improvement not restricted to the trained region but extended over an area of 8–10 deg); - no interocular transfer when the stimulated loci were more central; - almost total interocular transfer (the improvement was observed also in the non-treated eye).	- The improvement persisted at least 6 months after the end of the training.
Transition zone	*Van der Wildt and Bergsma, 1998*	2 patients: a male (58 years old) with left-side hemianopia and a female (58 years old) with upper right quadrantanopia.	Phase 1: binocular automated perimetry, procedure similar to that adopted by Zihl and von Cramon (1979); - targets: circular stimuli with four contrast levels.	Phase 1: binocular repetitive assessment of threshold in 68 different points from the transition zone to the more peripheral regions of the blind hemifield.	Phase 1: 28 training sessions (each session lasting one hour). Phase 2: 33 training sessions (each session lasting one hour).	Phase 1: - proportion of detections increased from 61% to 90%; - proportion of detections of the lowest contrast stimuli increased from 0% to 66%;	- The improvement persisted after two months.

(continued).

Target of the training	Study	Sample	Stimuli	Modality	Training duration	Results	Follow-up
			Phase 2: - targets: circular stimuli with contrast 100%.	Phase 2: binocular repetitive induction of saccadic movements with stimuli presented at the transition zone and in the blind hemifield: - the subject looks centrally at a fixation point and makes a saccade toward the stimulus reporting its detection and the corresponding meridian; - no control group.		- enlargement of the binocular visual field by 5–12° (*i.e.* the transition zone shifted by 5–12° toward the blind region). Phase 2: - proportion of localized stimuli increased from 60 to 95%; - no additional visual field enlargement.	
Transition zone	*Bergsma and van der Wildt, 2010*	11 subjects with hemianopia or quadrantanopia and no neglect.	Static Goldmann perimetry, background 10 cd m^{-2}; - stimulus: Goldmann V; - luminance from 4 cd m^{-2} to 318 cd m^{-2}.	Monocular repetitive static threshold estimation along the transition zone at different eccentricities from the central vertical axis.	40 days, one hour per day.	- Enlargement of the visual field (4–13°) due to a gradual shift of the transition zone; - increased reading rate in the patients who showed visual field enlargement after the training (mean improvement: 33 words/min with fewer regressions).	
Transition zone	*Poggel et al. 2004, 2008a*	19 patients with postgeniculate lesions and no neglect or other neuro-ophthalmological disorders.	Stimuli with increasing luminance from 30 to 96 cd m^{-2} over 2000 ms.	Repetitive stimulation of the transition zone; - task: to report detection by pressing a key.	Two sessions of about 30–35 min per day; - overall duration: about six months; - training done at home.	- Decrease of the absolute defect within the 30 central degrees of the visual field; - shift of the transition zone toward the blind field by 1.31 deg on average; - increased size of the transition zone;	

(continued).

Target of the training	Study	Sample	Stimuli	Modality	Training duration	Results	Follow-up
						- decreased reaction time to stimuli presented across the visual field → faster visual search; - training judged helpful by 58% of the patients, with more confidence in traffic situations, easier reading, and improved visually-guided navigation.	
Transition zone	*Julkunen et al., 2003*	5 patients with chronic stroke and homonymous quadrantanopia without neglect.	White blinking dots (luminance: 110 cd m^{-2}, duration 490 ms) randomly presented 2°, 1°, or 0.5° wide; - background: 0.13 cd m^{-2}.	Training program Silmäpeli (University of Turku), carried out on a 17″ PC screen; - stimulation with white blinking dots randomly presented at the transition zone; - at each locus, presentation iterated 3–5 times, the size of the stimuli decreased after each correct detection; - no control group.	33–47 h (3 sessions a week, each session lasting 1 h; - overall duration of the training: three months on average.	- Reduction of the loci with absolute defect at static perimetry in 3 patients (no improvement in the remaining 2 subjects); - reduction of the scotoma by 8 up to 15 degrees along the transition zone at kinetic perimetry in 3 patients (no improvement in the remaining 2 subjects); - VEP improvement in terms of P100 amplitude and/or latency in 3 patients.	3 months after the end of the training: Reduction of the loci with absolute defect at static perimetry in 3 patients.
Transition zone	*Schmielau and Wong, 2007*	20 hemianopic patients with no neglect.	Small green LEDs with luminance varying in steps of 0.2 log units (maximum luminance: 3200 cd m^{-2}) projected onto a bowl (background: 0.014 cd m^{-2}).	Binocular (13 patients) or monocular (7 patients) repetitive stimulations of the transition zone starting in the intact field and moving to the defective region performed with	2 sessions per week (from 34 to 169 sessions in total), each session lasting on average 45 min (about 500 stimulations per session);	- Visual field increased by 11.3 ± 8.1°; - improvement of detection rate: 18.6 ± 13.5% (restricted to the stimulated region);	Improvement still observable after 6 months in 86% of the patients.

(continued).

Target of the training	Study	Sample	Stimuli	Modality	Training duration	Results	Follow-up
				the Lubeck Reaction Perimeter (LRP); - after two miss responses: next stimulus presented 12 deg toward the intact region; - repetition of the procedure at each eccentricity across the vertical meridian in correspondence to the transition zone; - indicator of performance level: reaction time; - no control group.	- total training period: from 2 to 27 months.	- binocular training three to four times more effective than monocular training; - monocular stimulation: interocular transfer in 70% of the sample; - subjective improvement of daily activity in 70% of the sample.	
Transition zone	*Kasten et al., 1998a*	19 patients with post-chiasmatic injury.	White suprathreshold stimuli, luminance: 95 cd m^{-2}, background <1 cd m^{-2}.	VRT: binocular repetitive stimulation of the transition zone with squares of different sizes presented at different locations at the transition zone (500 stimuli in each session); - the difficulty of the training parameters adjusted and customized once or twice a month based on the improvement of the patient; - home training; - controlled with a placebo group.	One hour per day divided into two 30-min sessions, 6 days a week for 6 months.	After 50–100 h of practice: higher frequency of perceived stimuli and enlargement of the spared visual field (shift of the visual field border): 4.9 ± 1.7) deg as measured by the perimeter developed by the authors (HRP), but only by 0.43 ± 0.3 deg at standard automated perimetry; - subjective improvement of daily activity in 72% of the sample.	Improvement persisted at least 6 months after the end of the training.

(continued).

Target of the training	Study	Sample	Stimuli	Modality	Training duration	Results	Follow-up
Transition zone	*Sabel et al., 2004*	16 patients with homonymous hemianopia.	VRT: see Kasten *et al.*, 1998a.	VRT: see Kasten *et al.*, 1998a.	One hour per day divided into two 30-min sessions, 6 days a week for 6 months.	- Proportion of stimuli detected at high-resolution perimetry increased by 6.59% of the total visual field; - disappearance of absolute defects at conventional perimetry on average in 8 tested loci; - peripheral shift of the border of the absolute scotoma at conventional perimetry by 0.98–1.94°. Changes more evident in the peripheral regions of the transition zone than centrally; - improvement of visual confidence and mobility in 75.4% of cases; - improvement of reading in 43.5% of cases, bumping into objects less frequently in 31.9% of cases.	Improvement persisted at least 6 months after the end of the training.
Transition zone	*Schreiber et al., 2006*	16 patients with stable complete or incomplete homonymous hemianopia.	VRT: see Kasten *et al.*, 1998a; No control group.	VRT: see Kasten *et al.*, 1998a.	One hour per day, 6 days a week for 6 months.	- On average, improvement of eight loci with absolute defect at monocular perimetry (TAP); - mean training effect (difference in the proportion of absolute loci before and after the	

(continued).

Target of the training	Study	Sample	Stimuli	Modality	Training duration	Results	Follow-up
						training) relevant in only 2 patients; - average shift of the border of the scotoma by 1.62° with only two patients with a shift of more than 2 degrees in the central region; No control group.	
Inside the scotoma. Flicker rehabilitation	*Hyvärinen et al., 2002*	5 patients (age: 38–78 y) who had previously shown unexpected improvement of performance at visual field follow-up and retained motion perception in their blind hemifield; - onset: 6–16 years before the treatment; - in all the subjects: macular sparing (10–12°).	First protocol (detection task): 4 deg wide flickering discs presented on an equiluminant background (50 cd m^{-2}) at a temporal frequency of 1, 2, 5, 10, 15, 20, and 35 Hz (sinusoidal temporal modulation); - exposure time 2 s at 30 degrees of eccentricity along the horizontal meridian in the blind hemifield. Second protocol (recognition task): flickering letters (T, L, H, and U) presented on an equiluminant background (luminance: 50 cd m^{-2}) at a temporal frequency of 0.1 (stationary stimuli) 1, 2, 5, 10, 15, and 20 Hz (sinusoidal temporal modulation);	First protocol: repeated measures of contrast sensitivity of the discs at each temporal frequency; - psychophysical procedure: transformed staircase method (1U4DTR) coupled with a 2AFC response model; - the subject had to decide which of the two intervals contained the stimulus. Second protocol: repeated letter identification at each temporal frequency as a function of letter contrast; - psychophysical procedure: transformed staircase method (1U4DTR) coupled with a 4AFC response model; - the subject had to decide which of the	First and second protocol: twice a week for a year, each session lasted 1–2 h.	Results from a patient (MR). First protocol: flicker sensitivity in the affected hemifield normalized (*i.e.* equal to the spared hemifield) at all the temporal frequencies but 35 Hz. Second protocol: letter identification in the affected hemifield normalized at all the temporal frequencies so that the patient was able to recognize 2-degree letters at 20 degrees of eccentricity at all the temporal frequencies (1–20 Hz) but not static (non-flickering) letters; - after eleven months of training: patient able to recognize 2-degrees static letters at 20 degrees	First protocol: The improvement decreased 1.5 years after the end of the training, but it returned to the post-training value after 4 additional rehabilitative sessions; - it seems that once the process of cortical reorganization has been prompted by the training, it may somehow proceed even in the absence of additional stimulation.

(continued).

Target of the training	Study	Sample	Stimuli	Modality	Training duration	Results	Follow-up
			- size of the letter: at threshold for each subject (2–8 degrees): - exposure time: 2 s (3 s for stationary stimuli) at 10 and 20 degrees of eccentricity from the midline in the blind hemifield along the horizontal meridian.	four letters was presented.		of eccentricity when presented for 3 s; - after an additional month of training: the required presentation time for static letter identification at the same eccentricity reduced to 2 s: performance in the affected hemifield, therefore, normalized; - at the end of the training: the patient could perceive a V/4 Goldmann stimulus here and there in his blind hemifield.	
Inside the scotoma. Flicker rehabilitation	*Raninen et al., 2007*	Two subjects (61 and 64 years old) with homonymous hemianopia and macular sparing of about 2–3°; - time since onset: 22 and 11 months.	The same stimuli adopted by Hyvärinen *et al.*, 2002.	The same procedure of Hyvärinen *et al.*, 2002.	First protocol: 5 months of training (*i.e.* 40 training sessions). Second protocol: 3 months (*i.e.* 32 sessions) and 7 months (*i.e.* 56 sessions) of training.	First protocol: after the training, the detection threshold of flickering discs at 30 deg of eccentricity in the affected hemifield was the same as in the spared hemifield at the same eccentricity at all the temporal frequencies. Second protocol: after the training, the identification threshold of letters presented at 10 deg of eccentricity in the affected hemifield was the same as in	

(continued).

Target of the training	Study	Sample	Stimuli	Modality	Training duration	Results	Follow-up
						the spared hemifield at the same eccentricity; - no change in the visual field at kinetic Goldmann perimetry after the training; - subjective improvement and more confidence when navigating in crowded places and crossing the street.	
Inside the scotoma. Flicker rehabilitation	*Roth et al., 2009*	15 patients with homonymous hemianopia (age 31–71, time since onset 6 months–19 years).	Stimuli similar to those adopted by Hyvärinen *et al.*, 2002, and by Raninen *et al.*, 2007: sinusoidally flickering letters (10 Hz) (A, H, K, or T) presented individually at 21.8 degrees of eccentricity from the midline in the blind hemifield along the horizontal meridian; - size of the letters at threshold for each subject (2–8 degrees); - exposure time: 2 s (3 s for stationary stimuli).	Flicker training procedure derived from that used by the group of Hyvärinen and Raninen (Hyvärinen *et al.*, 2002): A 4AFC response model used by presenting on the intact region of the visual field the four letters arranged vertically. The testee had to choose which letter corresponded to that just presented in the blind hemifield; - training performed at home.	60 min per day, 5 days a week for 6 weeks; - training performed at home.	- Visual search time: decreased in both hemifields; - visual search time and fixation during exploration of natural scenes: unchanged; - reading speed: unchanged; - static automated perimetry: unchanged.	- Visual search time improvement persisted after 6 weeks from the end of the treatment.
Inside the scotoma. Channel stimulation	*Sahraie et al., 2006*	Twelve cortically blind subjects (age: 40–83 years, time since onset: 4–47 months).	Black circular patches 6° wide made of a vertical sinusoidal grating with spatial frequency: 1 c/deg, temporal modulation: 10 Hz, duration 2 s;	Training carried out at home. Two field locations stimulated, deep in the blind hemifield. Subjects had to report the interval that contained the stimulus according to a temporal	Training daily for 3 months: - each session made up of 50 trials at each visual field location (3×50 = total: 150 trials).	- Increased detection rate of high-contrast (50%) gratings with spatial frequency from 0.5 to 3.5 c/deg. Improvement accompanied by increased awareness	

(continued).

Target of the training	Study	Sample	Stimuli	Modality	Training duration	Results	Follow-up
			- contrast progressively reduced starting from 90%; - space-average luminance of the stimuli: the same as the background ($37\ cd\ m^{-2}$); - null stimuli: uniform patches with the same luminance as the background; - each presentation preceded by an acoustic signal; - no feedback provided to the patient.	2-AFC detection task and whether they had any awareness of the stimulus (yes/no); - stimuli initially presented at Michelson contrast 90% according to a 1-up, 3-down staircase procedure: - i proportion of detected stimuli w > 84% in three consecutive sessions → contrast decreased by 10% at the next session. - ii proportion of detected stimuli < 66% iIn a session → contrast increased by 10% at the next session; - additional presentations at the transition zone to keep the patient alerted during the repetitive stimulation of the blind field; - training carried out at home by the patient.		of gratings with spatial frequency of 0.5 and 1 c/deg; - increased detection rate of low-spatial frequency gratings (1 c/deg) with contrast >5%. improvement accompanied by increased awareness of gratings with contrast >5%; - in some of the non-trained regions: improvement for stimuli with medium contrast (50%) and spatial frequency from 0.5 to 2 c/deg, but the awareness of the stimulation remained absent; - improved visual field sensitivity with subjective binocular reduction of the blind region; - even if the increase in sensitivity was restricted to the trained locations: improved navigation skills.	
Inside the scotoma. Saccadic stimulation	*Zihl, 1980, 1981; Zihl and von Cramon, 1985*	(Zihl, 1980): 14 hemianopic patients with damage to the geniculo-striate visual pathways and a clear difficulty in avoiding obstacles,	(Zihl, 1980): Targets 116 min arc in size; - luminance: $32\ cd/m^{-2}$ displayed for 100 ms at different random positions along a	(Zihl and von Cramon, 1985; Zihl, 1980, 1981): stimulation of the saccadic movements toward targets presented in the blind hemifield. Patients,	(Zihl, 1980): training sessions of 45 min; - 3 sessions per day or at least one training session a week.	(Zihl, 1980): - Increased visual field size in the trained region in most of the patients. Extent of the enlargement variable	(Zihl, 1980): Improvement of the visual field stable after 6 months of follow-up.

(continued).

Target of the training	Study	Sample	Stimuli	Modality	Training duration	Results	Follow-up
		orientation, and reading; - interval between training and onset: from 1 to 21 months. (Zihl, 1981): 14 patients with stable homonymous hemianopic defects (differing in extent) after damage to the geniculostriate pathway with the border of the scotoma was close to the fixation point; - evident difficulty in avoiding obstacles and reading; - time interval after onset: from 1 to 21 months. (Zihl and von Cramon, 1985): 55 patients with stable homonymous hemianopia (44, *i.e.* 80%) or quadrantanopia (11, *i.e.* 20%) following infarction of the territory of the posterior cerebral artery or closed head trauma. - evident difficulty in avoiding obstacles and reading;	particular meridian in the blind hemifield. (Zihl, 1981) Light targets presented with a Tübinger perimeter at a given eccentricity (at least 3° away from the border of the scotoma) along one meridian (known by the subject) in the blind field for 100 ms. (Zihl and von Cramon, 1985): light targets presented with a Tübinger perimeter at a given eccentricity (at least 3° away from the border of the scotoma) along one meridian (known by the subject) in the blind field for 1000 ms.	who were informed along which meridian the targets would be displayed, had to look at the fixation point, and, whenever a click signal was heard, they were required to shift their gaze toward the region of the blind hemifield where the target was supposed to be; - localization of the target to be done with a single saccadic sweep and not with several searching eye movements.	(Zihl, 1981): 3 sessions per day or at least once a week in the first study; - session duration: about 45 min. (Zihl and von Cramon, 1985): 3 sessions per day or at least three times a week: - session duration: about 45 min.	(from 5° up to 27°), and related to the width of the transition zone (steep gradients ⇒ poorer improvement); -interocular transfer reported; - age and time since onset not correlated with the visual field enlargement and with the number of trials required to achieve it; - improved visual acuity and color perception in the trained regions; - subjective reading improvement. (Zihl, 1981): - visual field enlargement ranging from 2° to 24°. Perimetric improvement limited to the region corresponding to the trained meridian and not involving the whole field border; - improvement of color and eccentric visual acuity in the recovered regions.	(Zihl, 1981): Gain stable for at least six months after the end of the training; - additional rehabilitation after the end of the treatment did not produce further enlargement of the visual field. (Zihl and von Cramon, 1985): Gain stable for at least four months]; - additional rehabilitation after the end of the treatment did not produce further enlargement of the visual field.

(continued).

Target of the training	Study	Sample	Stimuli	Modality	Training duration	Results	Follow-up
		- time interval after onset: from 4 weeks to 26 months.				(Zihl and von Cramon, 1985): - visual field enlargement >1.5° in 80% of the patients; visual field enlargement >10° in 32% of the cases. Perimetric improvement limited to the region corresponding to the trained meridian and not involving the whole field border; - improvement of color and shape recognition in 94% of the patients who showed perimetric enlargement; - increased recognition rate of numerals in tachistoscopic conditions in the blind hemifield of the patients who showed post-training visual field enlargement; - patients who complained of severe to moderate problems in avoiding obstacles dropped from 96% to 49%; - patients with reading difficulties (*i.e.* those with a macular sparing ≤3°) decreased from 58% to 22% with faster reading rate and	

(continued).

Target of the training	Study	Sample	Stimuli	Modality	Training duration	Results	Follow-up
						reduced number of errors (even if both variables remained below normal); - presence of interocular transfer.	
Inside the scotoma. Visual restitution + pharmacological treatment	*Widdig et al., 2003*	A 58-year-old man with complete cortical blindness due to bilateral occipital infarction occurred 12 weeks earlier.	- First period: white flashes (100–150 ms) with luminance: 910 cd m^{-2} projected alternatively to the left/right hemifield at 45 deg of eccentricity. - Second and third period: shapes (circles, squares and triangles; luminance: 900 cd m^{-2}), colors (red, blue, yellow, green, and white; luminance: 350 cd m^{-2}), and, finally, colored shapes.	1st–2nd week: detection of light flashes; - Day 14th until day 139: identification of shapes and colors added; - subsequent 85 days: amphetamine administered in addition to the training (initial dosage: 10 mg, then gradually increased to 20 mg administered three hours before each treatment).	No amphetamine-period of training: 139 days; - amphetamine-period of training: 85 days; - frequency: 5 days a week, 2 h a day.	- At the end of the no-amphetamine period: mild improvement of color, and especially of shape perception (presentation duration: 5 s); - after the amphetamine period: further improvement of color and shape perception (proportion of correct discriminations about 70% for colors and almost 100% for shapes); - improvement specific for the trained function, even if the visual field was enlarged in the inferior regions; - experimental amelioration paralleled by improvement in face and object recognition (after 90 days of training) and reading (after 170 days of treatment).	

(continued).

Target of the training	Study	Sample	Stimuli	Modality	Training duration	Results	Follow-up
Inside the scotoma. Training motion	*Huxlin et al., 2009*	Seven subjects with post-stroke damage to the striate cortex occurred 8–40 months before the recruitment. In all patients: homonymous quadrantanopia or hemianopia but intact ipsilesional MT+ area.	*1) Global discrimination of motion:* array of random dots; - independent variable: range of displacement around the right or leftward vector; - stimulus duration: 500 ms. *2) Local discrimination of motion:* sinewave gratings drifting either to the left or to the right, with contrast as the independent variable.	*1) Global discrimination of motion:* task: discrimination of the left or right direction of motion of an array of random dots; - range of displacement around the right or leftward vector varied based on the response of the observer by a staircase procedure. *2) Local discrimination of motion:* task: discrimination of the direction of sine-wave gratings drifting either to the left or to the right. Contrast varied based on the response of the observer. In both experimental conditions: - response model: 2-AFC (left/right direction); - psychophysical procedure: transformed 1-up, 3-down staircase; - training started at the transition zone and moved into the blind region as the threshold improved; - initial stimulus setting based on the optimal	Training carried out daily (one 300-trail session a day, lasting about 30 min; - training period: 9–18 months; - number of sessions required to reach the maximum level of performance: greatly variable, ranging between 20 and 100, according to the patient.	1) *Global Discrimination of motion:* after a variable number of sessions (between 20 and 100): range in the affected hemifield widened from 9° (pre-training) up to 293 ± 12°, which is comparable to the discrimination range threshold estimated in the contralateral (intact) hemifield (300°). *2) Local discrimination of motion:* increased contrast sensitivity of the moving gratings at the spatial frequency of 0.5–1 c/deg and temporal frequency of 10 Hz; - increased light sensitivity by 13 dB around the trained regions after the treatment. - regions with less than 5 dB of sensitivity decreased in size; - no transfer of the training across different regions of the affected hemifield;	

(continued).

Target of the training	Study	Sample	Stimuli	Modality	Training duration	Results	Follow-up
				performance obtained during the testing phase.		- transfer of motion training to contrast sensitivity and light detection in the trained locations of the affected hemifield; - correlation between the experimental findings and subjective improvement of vision.	
Inside the scotoma. Extrastriate stimulation	*Jobke et al., 2009*	18 patients with stable hemianopia or quadrantanopia.	Massive moving spiral made of concentric moving rings.	Massive moving spiral made of concentric moving rings.	Duration: 30 min a day for three months.	- Small but significant increase in detection rate (4.2% on average); - improvement observed not only in the transition zone but also in the blind region.	

8.4 Training Blindsight with Audiovisual Stimulation

A strand of research investigates the effect of auditory stimulation to make visual rehabilitation more effective. The rationale of audiovisual training relies on the existence of an integrated audiovisual system that, when activated, may enhance visual performance in normal subjects as well as in patients with visual field defects (Bolognini *et al.*, 2005a, 2005b; Frassinetti *et al.*, 2002b, 2005). It seems that this audiovisual integration takes place in the superior colliculus (Leo *et al.*, 2008; Stein, 1998), an anatomical structure involved in spatial orientation and attention, that contains "multisensory" or "multimodal" neurons organized to form multiple unimodal receptive fields, spatially overlapped. In addition, specific multisensory cortical regions like the ectosylvian sulcal cortex in the cat (Wallace *et al.*, 1992) or the frontotemporal areas in humans (Giard and Peronnet, 1999) seem involved in this function.

In audiovisual interaction, auditive and visual inputs combine so that auditory stimuli administered in close temporal and spatial proximity to visual stimuli enhance the neural response to the latter; on the contrary, temporally and/or spatially disparate bimodal stimulations do not provide an additive effect compared to unimodal stimulation.

According to the *spatial rule* of multisensory integration (Stein *et al.*, 1996; Stein and Meredith, 1993; Meredith and Stein, 1986), the enhancement takes place when the visual and acoustical input stimulate the same multisensory receptive field. If the visual and auditory inputs stimulate different receptive fields, the enhancement does not take place. Finally, if the visual input stimulates the center and the auditory input stimulates the peripheral, inhibitory region of the multisensory receptive field, the visual response is depressed[33].

According to the *temporal rule* of multisensory integration (Stein and Meredith, 1993), the enhancement occurs when the visual and acoustical stimulation take place simultaneously. Finally, the weaker the visual stimulation, the greater the response in bimodal conditions (*inverse effectiveness rule*: Stein *et al.*, 1996; Stein and Meredith, 1993; Meredith and Stein, 1986).

Cross-modal visuo-auditory interaction has been studied in humans (Bolognini *et al.*, 2005b; Frassinetti *et al.*, 2002b). The group of Frassinetti and Bolognini used a semicircular structure made of green LEDs and loudspeakers positioned in front of the subject at eight eccentricities along the azimuth (four to the left and four to the right of a central fixation point). At each location, the target (the green LEDs, 90 cd m^{-2}) was surrounded by four red LEDs (80 cd m^{-2}). Flashing red LEDs during the presentation of the target acted as a mask, reducing the visibility of the green LED (thereby making it optimal for cross-modal enhancement according to the *inverse effectiveness rule*). The subject was instructed to keep the gaze fixed on a

[33]Cross-modal interaction is spatially asymmetric: the stimulation of the temporal hemifield is more effective than the stimulation of the nasal hemifield in virtue of a more direct connection of the nasal hemiretina to the superior culliculus compared to the temporal retina (Passamonti *et al.*, 2009; Bertini *et al.*, 2008).

central point and to detect the target presented in unimodal condition (no audio-visual stimulation) and bimodal condition (with a sound emitted simultaneously with the visual stimulus, for the same duration, and at the same spatial location). Visual sensitivity was higher in the bimodal condition compared to the unimodal visual condition at all the eccentricities. When the auditory and visual stimuli were presented at spatially disparate loci or not simultaneously, the improvement was not observed, following the *spatial* and *temporal rule* of crossmodal integration.

Frassinetti and colleagues (2005) examined 7 patients with hemianopia and no neglect (mean age: 46 years), 7 patients with hemianopia and neglect (mean age: 67 years), and 7 neglect patients with lesions restricted to the fronto-temporo-parietal areas and spared visual areas (thereby no hemianopia: mean age: 70 years).

In a semicircular structure, a loudspeaker coupled with a LED (luminance: 80 cd m^{-2}) was positioned at eight horizontal locations (8°, 24°, 40°, and 56° to the left and right side of a central fixation point) in front of the trainee. Visual stimuli were presented in association with a synchronous white noise burst of the same duration (100 ms). When audiovisual stimuli were presented, the spatial localization of the auditory stimulus could be the same or different from the spatial localization of the visual stimulus. The subject was asked to look at the fixation point and to report the detection of the visual stimuli. In addition to the audiovisual stimuli (cross-modal condition), visual and auditory stimuli were presented in isolation in a given proportion of cases (unimodal condition). Tests with more than 10% of false positive trials (more than 10% of responses to auditory stimuli in the absence of the visual presentation) were discarded.

In the cross-modal condition, the accuracy of patients with hemianopia but without neglect improved compared to the unimodal visual condition when the auditory and visual stimuli were spatially coincident and, in the temporal hemifield, also in the case of spatial disparity of 16° (as expected by the cross-modal asymmetry. See previous footnote). A negative correlation between the percentage of correct responses in unimodal visual conditions and the magnitude of the sensory enhancement confirmed that multisensory enhancement is inversely related to the visibility of the visual stimulus, as expected by the inverse effectiveness rule. The magnitude of the cross-modal enhancement was negatively correlated with the size of the cerebral lesion: the smaller the lesion, the greater the enhancement.

On the contrary, the accuracy of patients with hemianopia *with* neglect was not affected by cross-modal stimulation.

According to these results, audiovisual stimulation has therefore been considered for rehabilitation purposes.

The group of Bolognini (Bolognini *et al.*, 2005a) trained visual search of seven hemianopic patients and one quadrantanopic subject (time since onset: 4–24 months) with an audiovisual procedure similar to that used by Frassinetti and colleagues (2005).

In a semicircular structure, a loudspeaker coupled with a red LED (luminance: 90 cd m^{-2}) was positioned at six horizontal locations in front of the trainee at 24°, 40°, and 56° to the left and right side of a central fixation point. The subject was asked to look at the fixation point and, at the onset of the stimulus, to search for the target that appeared more often in his/her blind hemifield (stimulus duration:

100 ms). In the unimodal condition, only the visual target was presented. In the cross-modal condition, the visual target was accompanied by a noise burst at the same or at a different spatial position.

The training was administered 4 h daily for 2 weeks and the effect of the treatment was assessed considering the following parameters:

- perimetric visual detection, measured as the proportion of detected visual stimuli along the horizontal meridian in unimodal conditions, at 8°, 24°, 40°, and 56°. In addition, the proportion of visual stimuli detected in the four meridians was measured. As it occurs in perimetric examinations, the subject had to look straight ahead at a fixation point, and eye movements were not allowed;
- visual search (*i.e.* visual detection with eye movements allowed), evaluated as before but allowing eye movements (the same as during the training phase);
- visual scanning, measured with the E–F test, the Triangles test, and the Number test (Zihl, 2000). In the E–F test a green "F" (the target) is embedded in an array of "Es" distractors, projected on a black background. The patient is asked to search for the target, and the proportion of correct responses as well as reaction time was recorded. In the Triangles test the subject is required to find yellow triangles embedded in an array of yellow squares. In the Number test, arrays of 15 numbers are randomly presented on a black background. The task is pointing to numbers in ascending order. Time required by the patient to complete the task without errors is recorded;
- reading, evaluated presenting words and non-words;
- daily activities, assessed with an ADL questionnaire (Kerkhoff *et al.*, 1994).

After the audiovisual rehabilitation, the mean percentage of visual detections in the unimodal condition was greater compared to the baseline. The improvement of visual search in the blind hemifield was significant and persisted one month after the end of the treatment, whereas no significant change was found in perimetric visual detection. Following the enlargement of the search field, visual scanning was more efficient, as shown by the higher accuracy and lower time required to perform the E–F, the Triangles test, and the Number test compared to the pre-training baseline. The effect persisted for 1 month after the end of the treatment.

At the reading test, an increased percentage of words and non-words correctly read was observed, and the improvement was still present 1 month after the end of the treatment.

Finally, according to the results from the ADL questionnaire, these experimental results transfer to daily living activities.

Based upon the discrepancy between improved visual search field and unchanged visual field, the authors concluded that the improvement of visual perception obtained after treatment did not depend on an enlargement of the latter. This is in accordance with what was previously found by Nelles *et al.* (2001).

Passamonti and colleagues (2009) trained twelve hemianopic patients (age: 22–65 years) with stable field defects (time since onset 5 months–30 years) with a procedure similar to that used by Frasinetti and Bolognini. In a semicircular structure, a loudspeaker coupled with a LED (luminance: 80 cd m^{-2}) was positioned at eight horizontal locations in front of the trainee at 8°, 24°, 40°, and 56° to the left and right sides of a central fixation point. The subject was asked to look at the fixation point and to move his/her eyes toward the visual target (stimulus duration: 100 ms), which appeared more often in the blind hemifield. In some cases, the visual target was accompanied by a noise burst at the same or at a different spatial position. The temporal interval between visual and auditory stimuli was progressively decreased from 300 to 0 ms. The training was administered 4 h daily for 2 weeks.

To compare the effect of the audiovisual stimulation with that of standard visual training, patients underwent an additional visual stimulation with the same procedure and for the same time, but in the absence of the auditory stimuli.

A series of oculomotor parameters related to visual exploration[34] and reading were evaluated before the audiovisual training, immediately after the audiovisual training, three months and 1 year later, and after unimodal (conventional) visual training.

After the unimodal visual training, no changes in fixations/refixations number and saccadic amplitude were observed during visual search. On the contrary, at the end of the audiovisual training, patients showed fewer fixations and refixations, and increased saccadic amplitude. The improvement in the number of refixations and saccadic amplitude made them comparable to normal subjects. As a consequence, search time was reduced. The ameliorative effect persisted for up to 1 year. Accuracy in visual exploration improved after the audiovisual training but not after the unimodal visual training.

Likewise, after the unimodal visual training no changes were observed in the number of forward and backward saccades, duration of fixations, and saccadic amplitude at the reading task[35]. On the contrary, at the end of the bimodal training right-sided hemianopes showed fewer forward and backward saccades, shorter fixation duration, and increased saccadic amplitude and velocity. In turn, left-sided hemianopes showed a normalized (less fragmented) return sweep. Following the oculomotor improvement, reading time decreased and accuracy increased after the audiovisual rehabilitation. The ameliorative effect persisted for up to 1 year.

The affected visual hemifield did not show enlargement after the audiovisual procedure whereas the field of view (or search field) improved and the ameliorative effect persisted up to 1 year after the audiovisual training (whereas it was unchanged after the unimodal visual rehabilitation). This suggests that the subjective improvement reported in the ADL[36] (persistent up to 1 year after the audiovisual training) depended on the acquisition of a more efficient oculomotor compensatory behavior.

---

[34]The visual search task consisted of arrays of 15 numbers randomly presented over a black background. The observer had to count the number in ascending order.

[35]The reading task consisted of a brief passage of 330 syllables to be read aloud.

[36]ADL is the questionnaire that evaluates efficiency in daily life activities.

The author concluded that the audiovisual stimulation allows for optimally combining the properties of visually elicited saccades (responsible for saccadic accuracy) and auditory-elicited saccades (responsible for saccadic latency). This combination improves the saccadic spatial and temporal aspects, explaining the post-training increase in saccadic amplitude and velocity. The authors considered testing a *trimodal* training that, in addition to visual and auditory inputs, makes use of tactile stimulation.

Audiovisual rehabilitation

- **Bolognini *et al.*, 2005a**

SAMPLE:
7 hemianopic patients and 1 quadrantanopic patient (age 40–77, time since onset: 4–24 months).

AIM:
to improve visual search and reading.

PROCEDURE:
in a semicircular structure a loudspeaker coupled with a red LED (luminance: 90 cd m^{-2}) was positioned at six horizontal locations in front of the trainee at 24°, 40°, and 56° to the left and right side of a central fixation point. The subject was asked to look at the fixation point and, at the onset of the stimulus, to search for the target that appeared more often in his/her blind hemifield (stimulus duration: 100 ms). The visual target was accompanied by a noise burst at the same spatial position.

FREQUENCY OF ADMINISTRATION:
4 h daily for 2 weeks.

EXPECTED OUTCOME:
- improvement of visual scanning in the blind hemifield (higher accuracy and lower time required to perform the E–F, the Triangles test, and the Number test compared to pre-training);
- improvement of reading (increased percentage of words and non-words correctly read);
- improvement of the daily living activities measurable with the ADL questionnaire.

FOLLOW-UP (Y/N):
1 month, the improvement persisted.

- **Passamonti *et al.*, 2009**

SAMPLE:
12 hemianopic patients (age: 22–65 years) with stable visual field defects (time since onset 5 months–30 years).

AIM:
to improve visual exploration and reading.

PROCEDURE:
in a semicircular structure a loudspeaker coupled with a LED (luminance: 80 cd m^{-2}) was positioned at eight horizontal locations in front of the trainee at 8°, 24°, 40°, and 56° to the left and right side of a central fixation point. The subject was asked to look at the fixation point and to move his/her eyes toward the visual target, (stimulus duration: 100 ms), which appeared more often in the blind hemifield. In some cases, the visual target was accompanied by a noise burst at the same or at a different spatial position. The temporal interval between visual and auditory stimuli was progressively decreased from 300 to 0 ms.

FREQUENCY OF ADMINISTRATION:
4 h daily for 2 weeks

EXPECTED OUTCOME:
- reduced search time;
- higher accuracy in visual exploration with enlargement of the field of view;
- decreased reading time and increased accuracy;
- improvement of the daily living activities measurable with the ADL questionnaire.

FOLLOW-UP (Y/N):
three months later and one year. The improvement persisted.

Chapter 9

Rehabilitation of Hemianopia: Visual Compensation

Visual compensation is an alternative (or complementary) rehabilitative approach to visual restoration. Saccadic training strengthens the ability of patients to compensate for their visual field loss using eye movements.

9.1 The Visual Search Training of Kerkhoff and Colleagues (Kerkhoff *et al.*, 1994, 1992b)

Kerkhoff and colleagues (1992b) examined the effect of a systematic procedure in 122 hemianopic subjects, of whom 30 had additional left-sided visual neglect. The rehabilitation consisted of large saccadic movements directed to targets of variable duration presented in the affected hemifield. Unlike the training of Zihl and Zihl and von Cramon,[1] patients were instructed to perform horizontal and vertical scanning to localize the target. After six weeks, the mean visual search field in the scotomatous region widened by 20 deg (from 15 to 35°) and the improvement remained stable at follow-up (22 months). However, in some cases the effect of training, albeit significant, was marginal. Patients with additional neglect needed some 25% more rehabilitation sessions (2–3 additional months) to achieve the same enlargement of the visual search field. The effect of the treatment was independent of aetiology, time since lesion, age, and amount of field sparing. Unwanted head movements had a deleterious effect on training progress.

Two years later, the same authors reported the results of a three-step visual search training (Kerkhoff *et al.*, 1994). First, patients were trained to perform large saccades in the blind field. For this purpose, stimuli with different durations were presented on a large screen at various eccentricities in the affected hemifield, and the subject had to direct his/her gaze toward the target without moving the head.

In a second step, the same patients were taught a systematic visual search strategy (horizontal and vertical scanning) to inspect two hundred slides containing

[1]See section 8.3.6.

DOI: 10.1051/978-2-7598-3493-8.c009

an array of stimuli. The slides differed in number, size, and similarity of the stimuli as well as their spatial arrangement (ordered in rows and columns or mixed). Patients were recommended to start searching in the peripheral parts of their blind hemifield.

The training was administered at least 30 min per day 5 days a week for 4–12 weeks (the termination criterion depended on the improvement obtained in each subject).

In the third step, patients were prompted to apply the trained search strategies to situations of everyday life.

Twenty-two left/right hemianopes (mean age 46) underwent the treatment (Kerkhoff *et al.*, 1994). The time since the onset of stroke was 1–37 months.

The binocular search field was estimated with the Tübinger perimeter (kinetic perimetry). Subjects were asked to fixate a small central red spot while the operator moved a target from the periphery toward the center of the visual field at a velocity of about 2°/s. The trainee had to search for the target by moving the eye but not the head.

In addition;

- the accuracy of the visual search was tested with three slides containing symbols (circles in the first, triangles in the second, and squares in the third) among distractors (the remaining two types of symbols), projected at a distance of 86 cm. The subject had to indicate with a pointer when the symbol of a specific class was presented (targets/distractors ratio: 0.5);
- search time was measured by presenting an object and asking the subject to find the same object on a table representing 40 objects as quickly as possible ("table test");
- the subjective visual impairment was rated with a questionnaire based on 11 items.

After the training:

- on average, the visual field increased by 6.6° (range 2–24°) in 54% of the patients;
- visual search field improved from 10–20°[2] before treatment to about 35° at the end of the training in all the patients. The improvement persisted three weeks after the end of the rehabilitation. To be noted that visual search improvement was not correlated with visual field enlargement;
- visual search accuracy improved after the training with fewer errors (average number of errors in the blind hemifield: 4.6 before, 0.7 after the treatment, stable at follow-up), and decreased average search time (from 96.2 s to 75.8 s, stable at follow up). In addition, search time was reduced by about 50% in all the patients at the *table test.*

The questionnaire revealed consistent improvement in daily activities, with significant transfer effect of the training.

The improvement was not correlated with the side of the defect, age, time after onset, site of cerebral lesion, and sex.

Despite a control group was not included, the authors ruled out a placebo effect since the ameliorative effect was specific (visual search improved whereas the untrained visual functions remained unchanged).

[2]For comparison, the size of a normal visual search field is about 46°.

9.2 The Saccadic Search Training of Zihl (Zihl, 1995b)

Zihl devised a two-step procedure to improve visual search and visual scanning of hemianopic patients who complain of orientation difficulty. Fourteen patients with left- and right-sided homonymous hemianopia with orienting and navigating problems were trained.

In the first phase, a spot of light was presented for 1000 (subsequently 500) ms at different positions in the blind hemifield along the horizontal axis. Patients had to shift their eyes toward the affected region while keeping the head still and press a key as soon as the target was perceived.

In the second phase, slides with 5–30 different letters or shapes of equal size randomly distributed were displayed. The observer was informed on which type of item to search for. He/she must keep her head still and find the targets. In each session, the targets to be identified were 3–5, then, as the training progressed, they increased up to 12–15, embedded in an array of 10–20 non-targets. The treatment ended when the patient's performance matched that of the hemianopic patients who did not show orienting or navigating problems (*i.e.* those whose performance in everyday life was similar to that of normal subjects).

After the training, the author reported shorter search time (within the normal range in 78.5% of the cases) due to optimization and reduced repetitions of the scanpath in both hemifields and to fewer fixations in the affected hemifield, and wider saccadic amplitude.

Quality of life was subjectively better in 78.5% of cases (figure 9.1).

It should be considered that the prognosis after the treatment was poorer in patients with involvement of the parietal cortex and the posterior thalamus.

9.3 The Saccadic Search Training of Nelles and Colleagues (Nelles *et al.*, 2001)

The group of Nelles administered a saccadic training to twenty-one patients with homonymous hemianopia (Nelles *et al.*, 2001). Forty red lights distributed across a board in four horizontal lines were placed 1.5 mt in front of the patient. The patients had to systematically scan horizontally the board and report, in the presence of multiple stimuli, a target (a horizontal line of three lights) presented for 3 s. The visual field was assessed before, after the training, and after 8 months from the end of the rehabilitation. In addition, before and after the rehabilitation detection rate and reaction time were measured. The training was administered in two daily sessions, each session lasting about 30 min for 4 weeks. Head movement was not allowed.

An increased number of detected stimuli and reduced reaction time were found after the treatment and persisted at the follow-up. On the contrary, the visual field size remained unchanged. The activity of daily living scored with a questionnaire, improved after the rehabilitation.

The authors concluded that saccadic training improves the visual function of hemianopes *via* increased saccadic efficiency without changing the visual field.

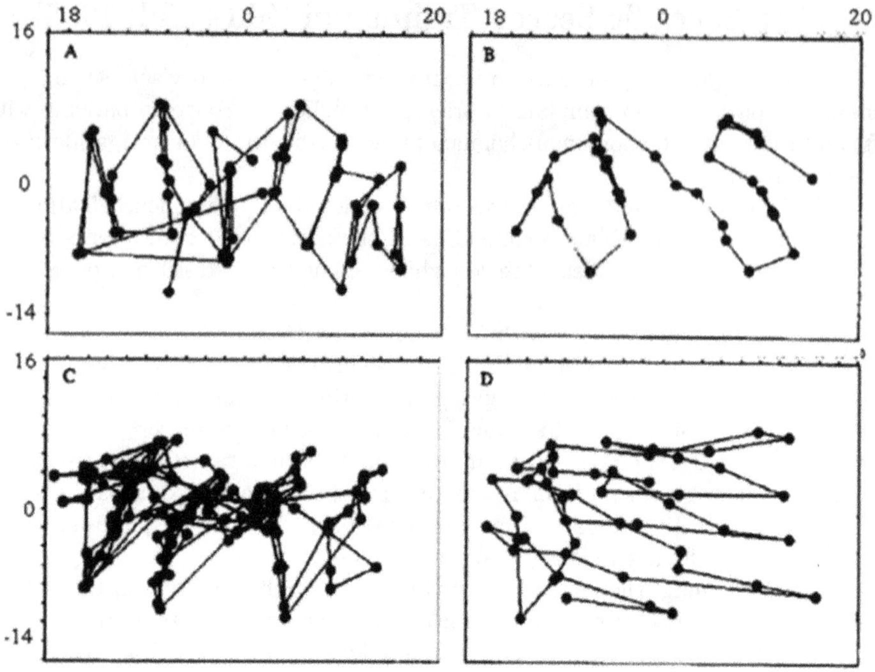

FIG. 9.1 – The scanpath of two hemianopic patients who complained of orienting and navigating problems before (left) and after the training. From Zihl (1995b), with permission of Elsevier.

9.4 The Portable Search Training System of Pambakian *et al.* (2004)

The group of Pambakian devised a portable system to allow home visual search rehabilitation (Pambakian *et al.*, 2004). Visual search was trained by presenting on a $25° \times 20°$ screen a target (line, square, or triangle) intermingled amid an array of distractors that differed from the target by orientation or size. Search time was limited to 3 s after the disappearance of a central fixation cross. The duration of the training was 1 month, with 20 sessions in total, each lasting 40 min.

At the end of the training, the visual search time of 29 patients with stable homonymous hemianopia or quadrantanopia (and no neglect) decreased by 46% in 76% of the cases and a small enlargement (4°) of the search field was recorded. On the contrary, the extent of the visual field remained unchanged. The faster search time was accompanied by improvement in completion time for tasks related to the activity of daily life like collecting coins, posting shapes in posting boxes, bead threading, ordering elements in a row, and sorting plumber's nuts by size. This means that the post-training reduction in visual search time observed in experimental conditions transferred to daily activities.

In the remaining 24% of the patients, visual search time remained unchanged; of these, 14% were faster in detecting targets that fell initially in the blind hemifield but slower in the seeing hemifield. This difference in the response to treatment suggests that the effect of the training depends on the patients: a generalized improvement of attention across the whole visual field (76% of the cases) or a selective improvement of attention in the blind hemifield, with reduced visual search time limited to the affected region.

The magnitude of improvement after the visual search training increased with age. Results were stable over 1 month.

9.5 The Digits Search Training of Roth *et al.* (2009)

An explorative saccadic rehabilitation was devised by the group of Roth and tested in a sample of 15 subjects with homonymous hemianopia (age 34–76, time since onset >6 months) and no neglect (Roth *et al.*, 2009). Patients were presented with a random array of digits (0–9) distributed with the same probability on the blind and spared sides. They were required to move the cursor over a predefined digit. In case of a correct response the digit turned into a "$" accompanied by a "beep". The procedure was repeated for all the digits, then the screen cleared and a new trial began.

The training was performed at home twice for 30 min per day, 5 days a week for 6 weeks. A follow-up (6 weeks) was considered.

The outcome variables were:

- search time, estimated with the same paradigm used during the training;
- natural search time, evaluated by asking the subject to find on a table 20 distinct objects presented in succession in each hemifield;
- number of fixations and fixation stability during exploration of natural scenes (landscapes, street scenes);
- static automated perimetry (Tübinger perimeter, 30°);
- reading speed;
- quality of life, assessed with a questionnaire.

After the training:

- visual search time decreased by 47% in both hemifields but was more evident in the blind hemifield. The improvement persisted at the follow-up;
- natural search time decreased in the blind hemifield by 23% and the improvement persisted at the follow-up;
- fixations during free exploration of natural scenes increased in the blind hemifield and decreased in the normal hemifield, even more after 6 weeks of follow-up. Fixation stability was reduced by 43% in the blind hemifield. Overall, these findings indicate an enhanced "readiness" to perform eye movements toward the affected side;
- no perimetric differences were found;
- no differences in reading speed were found;
- the quality of life was improved according to the questionnaire.

As a control group, 13 patients with homonymous hemianopia were recruited. A flicker stimulation training (vision restitution), which is unlikely to affect visual search, was administered to these subjects. Flickering letters were presented on the normal and blind hemifield and patients had to identify them. In the control group, the flickering stimulation led to a weaker reduction in visual search time compared to the previous sample, no decrease in natural search time, and no differences in the number and stability of fixations. The improvement in quality of life was less evident compared to the group treated with the digit search paradigm.

Visual compensation

- Kerkhoff *et al.*, 1994, 1992b

SAMPLE:
122 hemianopic patients, of whom 30 had additional left-sided visual neglect (Kerkhoff *et al.*, 1992b);
22 hemianopic patients (mean age 46) with left- or right-sided hemianopia and no neglect;
time after onset: 1–37 months (Kerkhoff *et al.*, 1994).

PROCEDURE:
(Kerkhoff *et al.*, 1992b) Large saccadic movements directed to targets of variable duration presented in the affected hemifield. Patients were instructed to perform horizontal and vertical scanning to localize the target

(Kerkhoff *et al.*, 1994) *First step*: patients are trained to perform large saccades in the blind field. Targets are presented on a large screen. The trainee has to direct his/her gaze toward the target presented with different durations and at various eccentricities in the affected hemifield without moving the head.
Second step: stimuli presented in two hundred slides. The slides differed in number, size, and similarity of the stimuli as well as their spatial arrangement (ordered in rows and columns or mixed). Subjects are taught a systematic visual search strategy (horizontal and vertical scanning) to scan each slide, starting searching from the peripheral parts of the blind hemifield.
Third step: patients are prompted to apply the trained search strategies to situations of everyday life.

TERMINATION RULE:
variable, depending on the improvement obtained in each subject (Kerkhoff *et al.*, 1994).

FREQUENCY OF ADMINISTRATION:
at least 30 min per day 5 days a week for 4–12 weeks (Kerkhoff *et al.*, 1994).

EXPECTED DURATION OF THE TRAINING:
6 weeks (15–25 training sessions) (Kerkhoff *et al.*, 1992b).

EXPECTED OUTCOME:
(Kerkhoff *et al.*, 1992b): - Average widening of the visual search field in the scotomatous region by 20 deg (from 15 to 35°). Effect of training, albeit significant, marginal in some patients;
- some 25% more rehabilitation sessions (2–3 additional months) are required in patients with additional neglect to achieve the same improvement in the visual search field;
- effect of training independent of aetiology, time since lesion, age, and amount of field sparing;
- head movements: deleterious effect;

(Kerkhoff *et al.*, 1994):- average visual field enlargement by 6.6° (range 2–24°) in 54% of the patients;
- visual search field enlargement (from 10 to 20° before treatment to about 35° at the end of the training) in all the patients. Improvement stable after three weeks from the end of the rehabilitation;
- increase in visual search accuracy with fewer errors (average number of errors in the blind hemifield: from 4.6 before the treatment to 0.7 after the treatment, stable at follow- up), and decreased average search time (from 96.2 s to 75.8 s, stable at follow-up). Search time was reduced by about 50% in all the patients at the *table test*;
- consistent improvement in daily activities as revealed with a questionnaire;
- improvement not correlated with the side of the defect, age, time after onset, site of cerebral lesion, and sex.

FOLLOW-UP (Y/N):
improvement stable at 22 months (Kerkhoff *et al.*, 1992b).

- Zihl, 1995b

SAMPLE:
14 patients with homonymous hemianopia (LH: 6, RH:8, no neglect; range: 23–73 years) with orienting and navigating difficulties (problems in avoiding obstacles and other problems related to visual perception in everyday life);
- macular sparing ranging from 1 to 5 deg;
- time since lesion: 6–18 weeks.

PROCEDURE: Treatment subdivided into two phases:

Phase 1: Spot of light (luminance of the target and of the background not provided, size of the stimuli not provided) presented for 1 s (subsequently 500 ms) at different positions in the affected hemifield at 10, 20, 30, and 40 degrees along the horizontal axis, in random order. Task: pressing a button when, after shifting the eyes toward the affected region, the target is detected. Click associated with the stimulation. Presentation time is halved (500 ms) when the patient can see all the stimuli. Generally, the patient can detect all the 500 ms targets after 5–6 sessions, each made of 60–90 presentations. The observer must keep the head still.

Phase 2: Presentation of slides (52′ × 45″) with 5–30 different letters or shapes (stars, triangles, circles, squares) of equal size randomly distributed. The patient is informed on which type of item to search for. Task: finding the target while keeping the head still. In each session, which lasted 30 min, 20–30 slides are presented. In the first sessions, the targets to identify are 3–5, then, as the training progresses, the targets increase to 12–15 embedded in an array of 10–20 non-targets.

TERMINATION RULE:
phase 1: detection of all the targets at a presentation time of 500 ms; phase 2: performance equal to that of hemianopic subjects with no navigation and orientation problems.

FREQUENCY OF ADMINISTRATION:
phase 1: 5–6 sessions each made up of 90–120 presentations; phase 2: 8–23 sessions, each lasting 30 min.

EXPECTED DURATION OF THE TRAINING:
left-sided hemianopic patients require on average fewer sessions than the right hemianopes.

EXPECTED OUTCOME:
shorter search time (within the normal range in 78.5% of the cases) due to fewer repetitions of the scanpath (from 17% of repetitions to 8% of repetitions) in both hemifields, to fewer fixations (from 44% to 22%) in the affected hemifield and to increased saccadic amplitude;
- improvement of quality of life in 78.5% of the patients;
- prognosis after the treatment poorer in patients with involvement of the parietal cortex and the posterior thalamus.

FOLLOW-UP (Y/N): NO

- Nelles *et al.*, 2001

SAMPLE:
21 patients with homonymous hemianopia.

PROCEDURE:
board with 40 red lights distributed in four horizontal lines that could be turned on independently placed 1.5 mt in front of the patient. Task: systematically scanning horizontally the board and reporting, in the presence of multiple stimuli, a target (a horizontal line of three lights) presented for 3 s.

TERMINATION RULE:
fixed, after 4 weeks.

FREQUENCY OF ADMINISTRATION:
two daily sessions, each session lasting about 30 min.

EXPECTED DURATION OF THE TRAINING:
4 weeks.

EXPECTED OUTCOME:
- increased number of detected stimuli and reduced reaction time;
- visual field size unchanged;
- the activity of daily living, scored with a questionnaire, improved.

FOLLOW-UP (Y/N):
results stable after 8 months.

Pambakian *et al.*, 2004

SAMPLE:
29 patients with stable homonymous hemianopia or quadrantanopia (and no neglect).

PROCEDURE:
Portable system to allow home visual search training. A target (line, square, or triangle) intermingled amid an array of distractors differing from the target by orientation or size presented on a $25° \times 20°$ screen;
search time limited to 3 s after the disappearance of a central fixation cross.

TERMINATION RULE:
fixed, 1 month,

FREQUENCY OF ADMINISTRATION:
20 sessions in total, each lasting 40 min.

EXPECTED DURATION OF THE TRAINING:
1 month.

EXPECTED OUTCOME:
- in 76% of the cases decrease of visual search time by 46% with a small enlargement (4°) of the visual search field;
- post-training decrease of visual search time estimated in experimental conditions transferred to daily activities as suggested by the reduced completion time for tasks related to the activity of daily life, like collecting coins, posting shapes in posting boxes, bead threading, ordering elements in a row, and sorting plumber's nuts by size;
- in 24% of the cases visual search time is unchanged, but in most of these cases visual search is faster for targets that fell initially in the blind hemifield, albeit it remains slower than in the seeing hemifield.
- extent of the visual field unchanged;

FOLLOW-UP (Y/N):
Results stable over 1 month after the end of the training.

Roth *et al.*, 2009

SAMPLE:
15 patients with homonymous hemianopia (age 34–76, time since onset >6 months) and no neglect.

PROCEDURE:
random array of digits (0–9) distributed with the same probability on the blind and spared sides. Task: moving the cursor over a predefined digit. In case of correct response, the digit turned into a "$" accompanied by a "beep". Procedure repeated for all the digits then the screen cleared and a new trial was started. Training performed at home.

TERMINATION RULE:
fixed, 6 weeks.

FREQUENCY OF ADMINISTRATION:
twice for 30 min per day, 5 days a week for 6 weeks.

EXPECTED DURATION OF THE TRAINING:
6 weeks.

EXPECTED OUTCOME:
- visual search time decreased by 47% in both hemifields, more evident in the blind hemifield;
- natural search time decreased in the blind hemifield by 23%;
- fixations during free exploration of natural scenes increased in the blind hemifield and decreased in the normal hemifield, even more after 6 weeks of follow-up. Fixation stability reduced by 43% in the blind hemifield. Overall, these findings

indicate an enhanced "readiness" to perform eye movements toward the affected side;
- no perimetric differences;
- no differences in reading speed;
- quality of life improved according to the questionnaire.

FOLLOW-UP (Y/N):
6 weeks. Decreased search time persisting at the follow-up. Decreased natural search time in the blind hemifield persisting at the follow-up.

9.6 The Effect of Visual Search Training on Saccade and Fixations

The effect of visual search training on the eye movements of hemianopic subjects has been investigated by the group of Mannan and Pambakian (Mannan *et al.*, 2010), who administered a visual search rehabilitation paradigm devised some years before (Pambakian *et al.*, 2004) to 29 hemianopic patients with no neglect. After the training, the saccadic/fixation pattern changed in the sample as follows:

a) fixations:
- overall fewer fixations;
- fewer initial fixations in the hemifield not containing the target and more fixations in the hemifield (hemianopic or spared) containing the target. In other terms patients made fewer "wrong fixations" after the training;
- faster switch of "wrong fixations": when an initial fixation occurred in the hemifield not containing the target ("wrong fixation"), the latency of the next fixation into the hemifield containing the target was shorter;
- shorter duration of "right" fixations (*i.e.* fixation occurring in the spared hemifield when the target is in that hemifield);

b) saccades:
- overall fewer saccades;
- higher proportion of saccades in the direction of the target, be it in the affected or spared hemifield;
- lower latency of the first saccade;
- more initial saccades directed toward the hemifield (hemianopic or spared) containing the target. This means that the training facilitates saccadic orientation toward the hemifield containing the target, be it the spared or the affected one;
- wider initial saccade, especially when the target is in the intact hemifield;

In sum, after the training patients required fewer saccades to locate the target, made more "useful" fixations into the hemispace containing the target, and were faster to switch the next fixation into the hemifield containing the target. These changes were long-lasting.

9.7 The Effect of Visual Rehabilitation (Saccadic Training) on the Cortex

In an fMRI study, the group of Nelles recruited eight stroke patients with hemianopia and no neglect[3] and evaluated the difference in brain activation during visually-guided saccadic movements before and after the saccadic training described in section 9.3 (Nelles *et al.*, 2001).

In a control sample, bilateral activation induced by saccadic movements was recorded in the:

- FEF and SEF (Brodmann area 6);
- PEF (Brodmann area 7);
- striate/parastriate (area 17/18) and peristriate (area 19) cortex.

The same areas (except for the striate/parastriate cortex) were bilaterally activated in the hemianopic sample during saccadic movements before, immediately after, and 4 weeks after the saccadic training. However:

i- Immediately after the training, the ipsilesional peristriate cortex (area 19) showed increased activation compared to the baseline.
ii- Four weeks after the training an additional area, *i.e.* the contralesional striate/parastriate cortex (area 17/18), and SEF showed increased activation compared to the baseline.

[3]Time from onset was 8 weeks. Neglect was evaluated at the line bisection task and cancellation task.

Chapter 10

Rehabilitation of Hemianopic Alexia

Research is dealing with the problem of how to improve the reading function of hemianopic alexics. Visual restoration, aimed at reducing the hemianopic scotoma, would be the most straightforward solution, but, as seen, visual restoration is time-consuming and the gain in terms of paracentral visual field enlargement is very limited.

So, since the past decades, studies have been focusing on oculomotor compensation aimed at optimally adapting the saccadic pattern to the hemianopic reading condition.

The saccadic pattern of hemianopic dyslexics can be optimized by adopting two different rehabilitation strategies, depending on the way the ocular movements are trained: directly or *via* the optokinetic reflex.

10.1 Optokinetic Reading Training (ORT)

As explained by Spitzyna and colleagues, <<patients with HA [Author's note: hemianopic alexia] make smaller amplitude rightward reading saccades compared to normal subjects but have a similar mean amplitude for the saccadic component of their induced OKN [Author's note: optokinetic nystagmus] [...]>> (Spitzyna *et al.*, 2007, p. 1929). Repeatedly inducing OKN in hemianopic alexics, therefore, would increase the size of rightward saccades so to make them as wide as the saccadic component of the OKN. In turn, wider rightward saccades means a faster reading rate and better accuracy. The induced optokinetic response, called *small-field optokinetic nystagmus*, can be triggered with right-left scrolling text (Ong *et al.*, 2012): the induction of small-field optokinetic nystagmus has therefore been used to train the saccadic pattern during reading in hemianopic patients.

In substance, words, then sentences, and finally short passages shifting horizontally in the opposite direction of reading are presented to induce small-field optokinetic nystagmus. Speed, print size, and interletter spacing are generally customized for each patient, who is required to read without moving the head while keeping the fixation at the center of the screen. As the training goes on, the reading samples are made longer (from simple words to complex words, to sentences up to

DOI: 10.1051/978-2-7598-3493-8.c010

brief stories), the speed of the shift is increased, and the interletter spacing is reduced.

The results achieved with this visual compensation strategy have been described in a series of studies (Ong *et al.*, 2012; Spitzyna *et al.*, 2007; Zihl, 1995a, 2000; Kerkhoff *et al.*, 1992a).

Kerhkoff *et al.* (1992a) obtained overall stable results in terms of reading rate in a sample of 56 patients with hemianopic alexia and no hemineglect. Training consisted of the presentation of lines of single words and short sentences moving from right to left on a screen. As the reading rate of the trainee got faster, line speed and word difficulty were increased, and interletter distance was reduced. Improvement after the training was attributed by the authors to fixation optimization (reduced duration and number of fixations), and not to the slight enlargement of the central visual field found in 34% of the patients.

Zihl (1995a) used a paradigm similar to that described by Kerkhoff. Left-sided hemianopes (LH) were forced to shift their fixation to the beginning of the word in each line of text, which moved slowly from right to left. In turn, right-sided hemianopes (RH) were forced to shift their fixation to the end of the word. In substance, both groups were forced to perceive the whole word before reading it.

The method was tested in a sample of 20 patients (mean age: 39 years). The author reported that after 8–16 (LH) or 9–29 (RH) sessions, the reading rate improved by 32% in LH and by 45% in RH, with a complete absence of errors in both classes. The oculomotor pattern became more regular and systematic, with fewer fixations (thereby reduced number of forward saccades) in LH and RH, and reduced duration of fixations in RH. The number of backward saccades decreased in both classes of patients (LH: from 42% to 32%; RH: from 49% to 35%). Zihl pinpointed that the amelioration was not due to the enlargement of the paracentral visual field (table 10.1).

TAB. 10.1 – Data from Zihl (1995a).

Class	Reading rate	Errors	Fixation nb	Fixation duration	Backward sacc (nb)	Forward sacc (nb)	Forward sacc (ampl)
LH	↑ from 76 wpm (±25) to 113 wpm (±29)	↓ from 0–6 to 0	↓	ns (from 319 ms to 294 ms)	↓ from 42% to 32%	↓	ns
RH	↑ from 53 wpm (±31) to 96 wpm (±46)	↓ from 4–16 to 0	↓	↓ from 526 ms to 372 ms	↓ from 49% to 35%	↓	↑

Spitzyna *et al.* (2007) trained a sample of right-sided hemianopic subjects using sentences moving from right to left on a screen to induce a small-field optokinetic response directed toward the blind field. After the training (performed at home by the patients[1]: 400 min over 4 weeks), reading speed improved by 18%–23%. After 6–8 weeks of follow-up, a mild decrease in reading speed was observed compared to a placebo group. The gain in reading rate was lower compared to that obtained by Kerkhoff *et al.* (1992a) (54%) and by Zihl (1995a) (45%); according to the authors, the difference depends on the shorter time from the onset in the study of Kerkhoff and in the study of Zihl (on average 40 and 6 weeks, respectively, *vs.* 96 weeks in the study of Spitzyna *et al.*). The oculomotor pattern improved, with longer forward saccades (*i.e.* directed toward the blind hemifield), thereby fewer fixations, and fewer refixations. Longer forward saccades and fewer refixations, indeed, were considered by the authors the main factors responsible for reading improvement. Contrary to the finding of Zihl (1995a), in the study of Spitzyna fixation duration remained stable after the training, with no reduction in the number of backward saccades (contrary to Kerkhoff *et al.* (1992a)). In addition, no enlargement of the central visual field at static and kinetic perimetry was observed.

Finally, the group Ong trained 33 right-sided hemianopic patients (mean age: 62 years, median time since stroke: 15.7 months). The rehabilitation software consisted of laterally scrolling text (from right to left) and was freely available to patients so that they could treat themselves at home.[2] Patients underwent domiciliary rehabilitation for at least 20 min a day (more than 5 h of therapy: Ong *et al.*, 2012). The reading rate improved after 5, 10, 15, and 20 h of therapy by 10.4%, 19.6%, 39.3%, and 45.9%, respectively. The effect after 5 and 10 h of training did not correlate with the extent of the visual field and with patients' age.

To be noted that:

i- a significant variability of the effect of the training among individuals was observed, with 27% of patients who remained unresponsive after 5 h of treatment and 18% who did not show improvement after 10 h of training;
ii- no enlargement of the visual field was found.

Overall, the gain obtained after ORT was stable over time (Spitzyna *et al.*, 2007; Kerkoff *et al.*, 1992a) and was task-specific (the training improved reading but was not effective on visual exploration and *vice versa*: Schuett *et al.*, 2008b; Spitzyna *et al.*, 2007).

10.2 Saccadic Reading Training (SRT)

Single words of different lengths and sentences are presented tachistoscopically at the center of the screen and the patient is required (without moving the head) to

[1] http://www.ucl.ac.uk/mediares/mm/mm-projects/neurology/read_right/.

[2] http://www.readright.ucl.ac.uk.

read each of them after accomplishing a saccadic scanning. Word length and presentation time are customized for each subject. As the training goes on, reading samples are made longer (short words, then long words, and finally, sentences), and presentation time is reduced (Schuett *et al.*, 2008a).

In their study, Schuett and associates displayed tachistoscopically single short words at the center of a screen, and the patient was asked to shift the gaze as quickly as possible from the center of the screen to the beginning (in the case of LH) or to the end (in case of RH) of the word. This way, the patient learns to project the word located in the blind hemifield onto the spared hemifield. As the training progressed and the saccadic movements of the patient improved, the length of the words was increased and presentation time was reduced. In a sample made up of 20 LH and RH subjects, reading rate increased from 140 to 166 words per minute, and errors were no longer present (Schuett *et al.*, 2008b). The gain in reading rate was associated with improved oculomotor pattern, as examined in a subgroup of 7 patients, with reduced fixations and fixation duration, fewer re-fixations (backward saccades), and fewer forward saccades with increased amplitude. A slight improvement in reading performance continued and the oculomotor amelioration persisted at the follow-up.

To ascertain that the results did not depend on the recruitment of higher-order linguistic processes, the authors administered the same rehabilitation protocol replacing letters with digits, and found overlapping results. Despite the similar outcome, the authors advised using digits instead of lexical material, as this avoids the cognitive load associated with word processing.

Finally, the improvement was specific to reading so no transfer effect to visual search and visual orientation/navigation was observed.

A summary of the most representative studies is reported below.

Optokinetic Reading Training (ORT)

- Kerkhoff *et al.*, 1992a

SAMPLE:

56 patients with hemianopic alexia (LH: 60.7%, RH: 16%, diffuse defect: 23.2%, range: 13–74 years) and no neglect. Macular sparing ranging from 0.25 to 4.1 deg, time since onset: 3–220 weeks (average: 40 weeks).

PROCEDURE:

32 reading samples, from simple words to short texts, each made up of 1024 characters (yellow words on a black background). Each sample is displayed as a string smoothly scrolling from the right to the left side on a window 10 cm wide at the center of the screen. The subject is asked to read aloud. Whenever the patient reads the sample without errors, speed is increased, the interletter distance is reduced, and the text is made more complex (from short single words to simple three-word sentences whose length word was progressively increased). Errors, whenever occur, are corrected by the operator.

TERMINATION RULE:
- when a plateau in performance is reached and lasts for at least five sessions;
- alternatively, when reading is normalized.

FREQUENCY OF ADMINISTRATION:
once for 40 min a day, 5 days per week.

EXPECTED DURATION OF THE TRAINING:
14 sessions (4–6 weeks) on average.

EXPECTED OUTCOME:
- reduced reading time by 52% due to lower fixations and fixation durations, and fewer reading errors. The highest improvement takes place in those patients who show more severe reading difficulty;
- visual field recovery of 1.6° (on average) as a consequence of the drifting words that stimulate the transition zone of the visual field.

FOLLOW-UP (Y/N):
follow up reported for 46% of the treated patients (mean interval: 22 months, range: 6 months–5 years). In the follow-up, reading time tends to increase but remains lower compared to the pre-training level. Regression occurs in those patients who did not practice daily reading after the end of the treatment. In turn, reading errors remain stable.

- Zihl, 1995a

SAMPLE:
20 patients (mean age: 37 years in RH and 39 years in the LH group). Macular sparing ≤3°.

PROCEDURE:
paradigm similar to that described by Kerkhoff *et al.* (1992a). Left-sided hemianopes (LH) were forced to shift their fixation to the beginning of the word in each line of text while it moved slowly from right to left. In turn, right-sided hemianopes (RH) were forced to shift their fixation to the end of the word. In substance, both groups were forced to perceive the whole word before reading it.

TERMINATION RULE:
reading performance reaches the range of age-matched normal subjects.

FREQUENCY OF ADMINISTRATION:
two sessions per day (total duration: 1–2 weeks in LH, 2–3 weeks in RH).

EXPECTED DURATION OF THE TRAINING:
8–16 (LH) or 9–29 (RH) sessions.

EXPECTED OUTCOME:
- reading rate improvement by 32% in LH and by 45% in RH, with a complete absence of errors in both classes;
- fewer fixations (reduced number of forward saccades) in LH and RH, and shorter fixations in RH;
- fewer backward saccades in both classes of patients (reduction by 24% in LH and 28% in RH).

FOLLOW-UP (Y/N): not assessed.

- Spitzyna *et al.*, 2007

SAMPLE:
19 patients with right-sided hemianopic alexia (range: 20–78 years) mainly due to stroke in the posterior cerebral artery territory. Macular splitting or macular sparing of 2° (range: 0.25–4.1 deg). Time since onset at least 4 months. No information on hemineglect was provided.

PROCEDURE:
sentences moving across the middle of the screen from right to left (*i.e.* from the blind side to the spared hemifield) at 7 different speeds (85, 105, 143, 173, 205, 240, 275 words per minute in Times New Roman, 24 points). Black characters are presented on a white background. Patients self-train at home, and whenever they feel confident enough to read the actual block of sentence, they require a faster block to the operator.

TERMINATION RULE:
fixed (*i.e.* irrespective of the obtained results), after 4 weeks of training.

FREQUENCY OF ADMINISTRATION:
one session of 20 min per day, 5 days a week.

EXPECTED DURATION OF THE TRAINING:
total rehabilitation program: on average four weeks (400 min of training).

EXPECTED OUTCOME:
reduced reading time by 18%–23% due to longer forward saccades (thereby fewer fixations), and fewer refixations. Reading errors are not considered.

FOLLOW-UP (Y/N):
at a follow-up of 6–8 weeks reading time tends to increase slightly but it remains lower compared to the pre-training level.

- Ong *et al.*, 2012

SAMPLE:
33 right-sided hemianopic patients (mean age: 62 years, median time since stroke: 15.7 months). No information on hemineglect was provided.

PROCEDURE:
laterally scrolling text (from right to left) is freely available to patients so that they can treat themselves at home.

TERMINATION RULE:
- after at least 5 h of therapy. Maximum: 20 h of therapy.

FREQUENCY OF ADMINISTRATION:
at least 20 min a day.

EXPECTED DURATION OF THE TRAINING:
at least 5 h of therapy.

EXPECTED OUTCOME:
- reading rate improvement after 5, 10, 15, and 20 h of therapy by 10.4%, 19.6%, 39.3%, and 45.9%, respectively, irrespective of the extent of the visual field or patient's age. Reading errors are not considered;
- no improvement of the visual field after treatment;
- significant variability of the effect of the training among individuals was observed.

FOLLOW-UP (Y/N):
not assessed.

Saccadic Reading Training (SRT)

- Schuett *et al.*, 2008b

SAMPLE:
20 patients with left- or right-sided hemianopic alexia (range: 28–80 years) due to stroke of the posterior cerebral artery. Macular sparing ranging from 1 to 4 deg. Average time between the occurrence of brain damage and the beginning of the treatment: 29 weeks (range: 5–97). None of the patients had hemineglect.

AIM:
to improve reading rate and visual orientation and navigation.

PROCEDURE:
single words, 3–13 letters long, yellow in color, presented for 1 s at the center of the screen on a blue background. Letter size: 2 deg, interletter spacing: 0.4 deg. The patient is asked to shift the gaze as quickly as possible from the center of the screen to the beginning (in case of LH) or the end (in case of RH) of the word. As the training progresses and the saccadic movements of the patient improve, the length of the words is increased from 3 to 13 letters. When the correct identification of a word with a given length is 90%, presentation time is reduced from 1 s up to 300–400 ms. In a subsequent phase, the length of the word is increased and the procedure is repeated. In the final phase, words of different lengths are randomly presented. Reading errors are immediately corrected by the operator.

TERMINATION RULE:
90% of correct responses for any level of difficulty (presentation time × word length).

FREQUENCY OF ADMINISTRATION:
on average, 11 sessions are to be completed within 2 weeks. Each session (made up of 300 presentations) lasts about 45 min.

EXPECTED DURATION OF THE TRAINING:
two weeks.

EXPECTED OUTCOME:
reduced reading time by 18.5% due to longer forward saccades, reduced fixations, fixation duration, backward saccades, and forward saccades.

FOLLOW-UP (Y/N):
6–15 weeks. The reading rate tends to increase further but to a small extent. Overall, the improvement is stable for at least 12 weeks.

Even if the ORT and SRT are equally effective in increasing the reading performance of hemianopic patients, the latter requires less time commitment (7–9 h: Schuett *et al.*, 2008a *vs.* 10–20 h: Spitzyna *et al.*, 2007). In both cases, sessions of 30–45 min should be carried out daily or every other day over 2–3 weeks (Schuett *et al.*, 2008b; Spitzyna *et al.*, 2007; Zihl, 1995a; Kerkhoff *et al.*, 1992a), in the presence of a supervisor that provides verbal feedback and prevents the subject from making head movements, as recommended by Schuett (2009). Non-text material like couples of digits can effectively substitute words, making the sessions less distressing (Schuett *et al.*, 2008b).

The mechanism underlying the rehabilitation outcome is unclear. It has been advanced that saccadic training induces activation of the frontoparietal network (Nelles *et al.*, 2007), in line with the poor outcome in patients with associated lesions of the parietal region (Zihl, 1995a).

10.3 Factors Influencing the Outcome

The duration of the compensatory therapy and the level of improvement (found to a certain extent in almost all the patients) depend (Schuett, 2009):

- on the location and extent of brain injury. The rehabilitation duration is longer and the outcome is poorer in patients with additional white matter damage in the occipital or occipitoparietal region (Zihl, 1995a). On the contrary, in the presence of *isolated* lesions of the occipital cortex the top-down attentional control is preserved so that in these cases the training is expected to be more effective;
- on the type of visual field defect: hemianopic patients require more training sessions compared to quadrantanopic patients, and right hemianopia, often associated with contralesional neglect, requires twice as much training than left hemianopia, with a poorer outcome (Zihl, 1995a). Moreover, absolute defects are more difficult to rehabilitate compared to relative defects;
- on the awareness of the visual deficit. Hemianopic patients with anosognosia[3] (Vallar and Ronchi, 2006; Celesia *et al.*, 1997; Bisiach *et al.*, 1986; Koehler *et al.*, 1986) have worse rehabilitative results (Ownsworth and Clare, 2006). Likewise, Halligan and colleagues (1991) pinpointed the relationship between neglect and lack of rehabilitation success;
- on the presence of secondary oculomotor disorders. Secondary oculomotor disorders reduce the successful outcome of the rehabilitation (Anderson, 2003);
- on the presence of a depressive state. Depression after brain injury decreases the benefits of the treatment (Hadidi *et al.*, 2009);
- on the association of cognitive disorders. Cognitive disorders are a negative prognostic factor for rehabilitation (Anderson, 2003).

Instead, time onset and age seem not relevant (Zihl, 1995a; Kerkhoff *et al.*, 1992b).

[3]Hemianopic anosognosia (HAN) is the unawareness of visual loss in the homonymous hemifield (or hemiquadrant). In their prospectic study of 32 patients, Celesia and colleagues (1997) reported a HAN prevalence of 62%. In almost two-thirds of the cases, anosognosia occurs in right-sided hemianopes. The authors suggested that hemianopic anosoagnosia may be related to severe visual hemineglect, sometimes to generalized cognitive impairment, or to a combination of both. Anatomically, anosoagnosia is related to larger and more anterior lesions, involving the parietal cortex (Koehler *et al.*, 1986). To be noted that, when present, visual hallucinations, phosphenes, and photopsias are generally experienced by patients without hemianopic anosoagnosia (Celesia *et al.*, 1997). Bisiach and colleagues (1986) graded anosognosia as: grade 0 (the disorder is spontaneously reported by patients when questioned about their problems), grade 1 (the disorder is reported only after a specific question), grade 2 (the disorder is acknowledged only after demonstration), and grade 3 (the disorder is not acknowledged).

Finally, a small ameliorative effect on reading has been observed by Reinhard *et al.* (2005) after vision restitution therapy (VRT) with an improvement of reading rate by about 3%–10%. Likewise, in a sample of 11 hemianopes, (all but three with left hemianopia), Gall and Sabel reported a reading rate improvement of about 12% after VRT[4] (Gall and Sabel, 2012). The lexical gain was correlated with the shift of the seen/not seen zone toward the blind side (enlargement of the paracentral visual field: Gall and Sabel, 2012). However, compensatory therapy focused on the ocular movements should be preferred to restorative training as it is less costly, less time-consuming (7–20 h), and more effective in ameliorating both reading and visual exploration (Schuett, 2009). Vision restoration therapy, indeed, is not so effective in treating hemianopic alexics as it does not train the oculomotor function which is, indeed, the main factor responsible for their reading disability (Schuett, 2009).

In conclusion, two points should be kept in mind when rehabilitating hemianopic patients with the training of visual compensation:

a- training for visual exploration and reading is task-specific: reading improvement after rehabilitation does not transfer to visual exploration and *vice versa.* As a matter of fact, rehabilitation of reading requires practicing the use of small and precise horizontal saccades, whereas rehabilitation of visual exploration requires practicing organized scanpath and large saccadic movements (Schuett *et al.*, 2009a). This lack of carry-over effect requires specific protocols aimed at the lexical function and at improving visual exploration, whereas the sequence of these interventions is not decisive for the outcome (Schuett *et al.*, 2009b);

b- attention is a main requirement for responsiveness to treatment. Patients with low or misdirected attention will obtain poor or no results (Zangemeister and Utz, 2002).

[4]No neglect. Two sessions (30 + 30 min) a day, 6 days a week for 6 months.

Chapter 11

Rehabilitation of Hemianopia: Visual Substitution

Visual substitution procedures have been developed to supply the loss of function in the hemianopic region with the spared visual hemifield. Visual substitution makes use of optic devices (essentially prismatic lenses or, less commonly, small mirrors to be mounted over the spectacle frames) that determine *relocation*, *i.e.* a shift of the spared hemifield toward the blind side, or *expansion* (*i.e.* enlargement) of the field of view. Expansion is, evidently, more desirable and can be intermittent, occurring only when the gaze intercepts the system and interacts with it, or constant, occurring in any direction of gaze.

According to Lawton Smith and colleagues, the best candidates for visual substitution (in their specific case pursued with monocular Fresnel prismatic sectors) are hemianopic patients whose visual field defect is their main complaint (Lawton Smith *et al.*, 1982). It should be considered that the co-occurrence of neglect is a detrimental factor for the rehabilitation of hemianopia with visual substitution as neglect patients, being unaware of the perimetric loss, do not feel the need to compensate, that is to exploit the prism. It remains that binocular sector prisms may improve their inattention (Rossi *et al.*, 1990).

11.1 Mirrors

Bailey (1978) explained that the classic mirror system is a planar reflector mounted on the frame of the glass on the same side of the field loss at the nasal eye wire. To this purpose, small adjustable mirrors mounted on a clip have been devised (Mintz, 1979). In the case of right hemianopia, for example, the mirror is mounted on the nasal eyewire of the right eye. In primary position, a small reduction of the spared hemifield as the result of the masking effect of the mirror on the left side takes place, but part of the right visual field, blind, becomes visible as it is reflected by the mirror onto the nasal side of the fixation point. Adaptation to the mirror is the key to success, as seeing a region on the right side projected, thereby superimposed,

DOI: 10.1051/978-2-7598-3493-8.c011

to the left side of the fixation point generates confusion, even more so considering that the reflected image is reversed.

The two variables of the system are the width of the mirror and its inclination toward the side of the loss. Increasing the inclination of the mirror makes peripheral parts of the blind hemifield more perceivable, but at the same time it reduces the extent of the spared hemifield to the nasal side (that is the area seen by direct view) when the gaze is in primary position. The adduction of the eye with the mirror causes a reduction of the area seen by direct view. Bailey (1978) explained that a mirror not inclined toward the eye (*i.e.* parallel to the medial plane) reflects up to 50° of the hemianopic field, and up to 90° for an inclination of 20°. This system intends to increase the awareness of objects and obstacles in the blind hemifield. Head rotation is expected when an object of interest is spotted *via* the mirror reflection so to see it by direct view.

Nooney described the use of a mirror mounted on the inner edge of the frame, on the eye with the temporal homonymous defect, facing the scotomatous side (Nooney, 1986). The orientation of the mirror varied from 35 to 40° to the horizontal axis. The orientation within this range was trimmed based on individual characteristics: the mirror was judged well fitted if the examiner, standing to the side of the patient, saw his/her iris into the mirror and the pupil centered vertically when the patient looked straight ahead (figure 11.1). The author reported that adaptation was fast in a cohort of 69 patients.

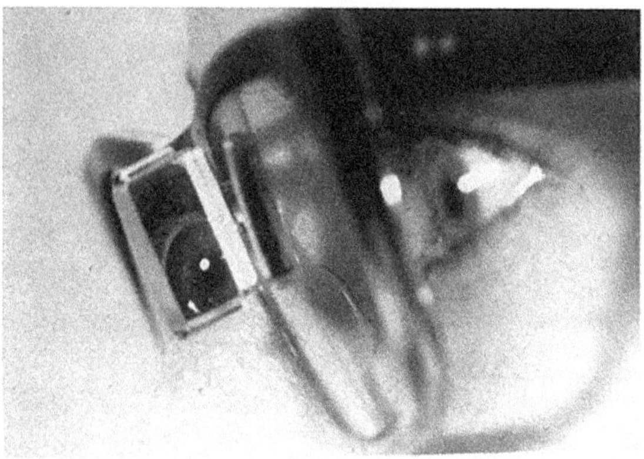

FIG. 11.1 – The appearance of the mirror according to the method of Nooney in a patient with left homonymous hemianopia. From Nooney (1986). With permission of Wolters Kluwer Health publisher.

A similar procedure had been previously described by Nerenberg. In his case, the mirror was removable (Nerenberg, 1980). Variations to the original method are the use of dichroic mirrors that, making the patient more aware of the reflected image, should reduce confusion (Duszynski, 1955), and the positioning of the mirror within the hemianopic hemifield, namely temporal to the pupil of the eye to the side of the loss. This way, in the primary position the mirror has no effect, whereas it comes into action when the subject decides to examine the hemianopic side, rotating the eyes toward the blind hemifield (Weiss, 1969).

Despite the efforts made to make mirrors a suitable solution, they are rarely used in clinical practice for the disorienting effect experienced by patients due to the reversal of images and the fact they are cosmetically unacceptable.

11.2 Prisms. Premise: The Apical Scotoma

Prisms are wedge-shaped lenses that deviate the light beam toward the base by an angle proportional to the angle of the apex. When using a prismatic correction, an undesirable effect takes place: the so-called *apical scotoma*. The apical scotoma is the gap between the last deviated and the first non-deviated light ray at the apex of the prism. The spatial extent of the visual field corresponding to the gap is abolished. When a prism is placed in the peripheral portion of the visual field (base out), the peripheral visual field is shifted centrally and the spatial gap induced by the apical scotoma takes place medially to the apex of the prism (figure 11.2).

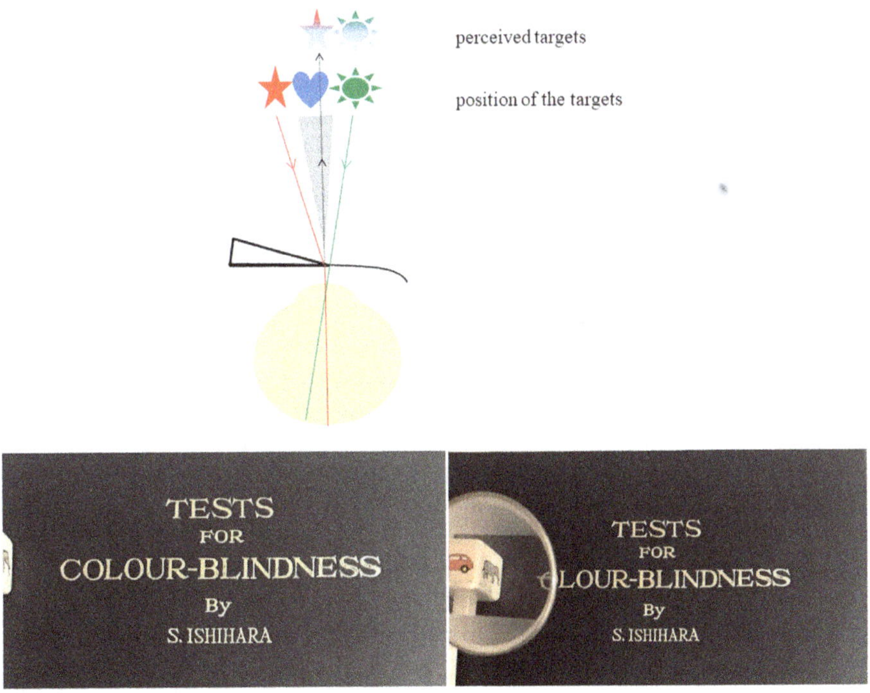

FIG. 11.2 – Upper panel: the apical scotoma (gray) is the gap in the visual world between the last deviated (red) and the first non-deviated (green) light ray at the apex of the prism. Due to the apical scotoma, the blue heart is no more visible; lower panel: a prism (base out) placed to the left of the visual field determines a shift of the visual field toward the left, and an apical scotoma that "cuts" a vertical portion of the visual field at the apex.

The extent of the apical scotoma corresponds to the prism power in degrees[1] (Jung and Peli, 2018).

11.3 Binocular Full-Field Prisms

Relocation of the whole field of view from the non-seeing toward the seeing field by about 10° is obtained with 20Δ full-diameter binocular prismatic lenses mounted with the base toward the side of the field loss (Cohen and Wass, 1996).[2] However, the power of full-field binocular prisms is generally limited to less than 15Δ as higher powers are associated with spatial distortion, light scattering, and chromatic dispersion. Binocular full-field prisms relocate the field of view but do not produce visual field expansion. True expansion, indeed, is prevented by:

i- the apical scotoma, which reduces the visual field. It is worth considering that the apical scotoma is located at 45–60°: this is, indeed, a critical position as a lack of perception in this region of the visual field increases the risk of collisions (Jung and Peli, 2018).
ii- the eye and head rotation toward the seeing side for refixation of the target: eye and head rotation reduces or even neutralizes the shift of the field of view when its cumulative angular extent is grossly the same as the power of the prism.

For these reasons, Jung and Peli do not recommend the use of binocular full-field prisms for rehabilitating hemianopic patients (Jung and Peli, 2018). However, as reported in section 5.5, this solution can be useful in the presence of hemineglect.

11.4 Binocular Sector Prisms

Binocular sector prisms (generally 20 diopters) fitted to cover the full height of the lens and with the base in the direction of the field loss, determine field relocation of about 11° (Apfelbaum *et al.*, 2013), with no expansion.

When the patient looks straight ahead, the prism does not affect the visual field as the sector is placed completely in the blind hemifield. When the patient moves the gaze toward the hemianopic field, *i.e.* looks through the prism, the binocular visual field is shifted toward the blind hemifield by an extent in degrees that can be computed as about half the prism power in diopters; in addition, a gap close to the fixation point, the *apical scotoma,* takes place (Apfelbaum *et al.*, 2013).

When, for example, a patient with left homonymous hemianopia gazes to the left, *i.e.* through the prism, the visual field is shifted toward the left and, correspondingly, the visual field to the right is lost. In addition, an apical scotoma appears in the paracentral region to the left of the apex of the prism. Since the apical scotoma involves both eyes, it will persist in binocular vision. The apical scotoma

---

[1] $P^{\circ} = \tan^{-1}\left(\frac{P^{\Delta}}{100}\right)$ (Apfelbaum *et al.*, 2013).

[2] According to Jung and Peli the field shift in degrees is roughly equal the power of the prism (Jung and Peli, 2018).

precludes true expansion of the visual field since the part of the visual field gained by the shift is neutralized by the loss due to the bilateral apical scotoma (figure 11.3). In substance, bilateral sectors help "grab" portions of the world in the blind hemifield with a smaller ocular versional movement compared to the no-prism condition but do not provide expansion of the binocular visual field.

A major limitation of the procedure is that significant displacements can be obtained only at the cost of high diopter values, but high diopter values determine visual distortion and chromatic aberrations (Morgan, 1963).

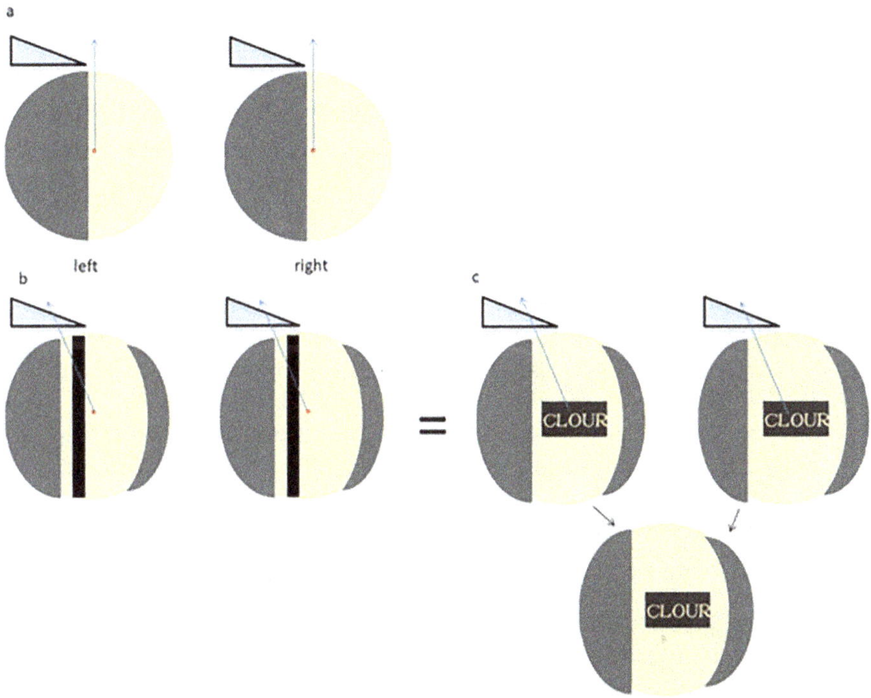

FIG. 11.3 – Binocular sector prisms left homonymous hemianopia. Panel a primary position: the prisms have no effect on the visual field as the sectors cover only the blind hemifield. Panel b: gaze turned 20° leftward through the prisms: the visual field is shifted toward the left and, correspondingly, the most eccentric visual field to the right is lost. In addition, an apical scotoma appears as a vertical gap in the paracentral region to the left of the apex of the prism. Panel c: the effect of the apical scotoma.

Lee and Perez applied binocular sector prisms in nine hemianopic patients. Of these, seven reported subjective improvement in activities of daily living, as evaluated with a questionnaire, so the authors concluded that the use of binocular prisms may enhance peripheral awareness in hemianopic patients through more efficient visual scanning (Lee and Perez, 1999).

Likewise, Rossi and colleagues evaluated the effect of binocular sector prisms on visual perception of patients with post-stroke hemianopia or visual hemineglect.

Binocular half-circle sector Fresnel prisms, 15Δ, were fitted to the part of the lenses corresponding to the blind hemifield and the base oriented to the side of the field loss, with the straight margin placed approximately 2 mm from the pupil to avoid diplopia in primary position.[3] Prisms were worn all day and were well tolerated by most of the patients after a day or two. Relocation of the field of view takes place when the patient moves the gaze and looks through the prism, whereas it is absent when the subject looks through the other parts of the spectacles (Rossi *et al.*, 1990). The shift of the field of view with prisms of 12, 18, or 20Δ is, however, limited to 6°, 9°, or 11°. In addition, as expected, binocular prismatic sectors induce an apical scotoma at the center of the spectacle lens so that the overall field of view is not larger, but even reduced compared to the no-sectors conditions (Cohen and Wass, 1996). In other terms, binocular sector prisms do not expand the visual field in hemianopic patients (Jung and Peli, 2018). Contrary to what was reported by Lee and colleagues, Rossi concluded that binocular prismatic sectors do not provide any improvement in activities of daily living. However, the visuospatial tests focused on spatial neglect improved when wearing the sectors in the recruited sample, suggesting an ameliorative effect on visual heminattention.

The group of Palomar-Mascaró suggested a variant: they positioned bilateral prismatic sectors to the part of the lenses corresponding to the blind hemifield and the base oriented to the side of the field loss in the form of vertical stripes that, contrary to the previous solutions, did not cover the full half-width of the lens to the side of the loss but were attached next to its center (Palomar-Mascaró *et al.*, 2018). The sectors were trimmed between 1.0 and 5.5 mm from the center to the hemianopic side "depending on the homogeneity of the central loss", as reported by the authors (figure 11.4). The prismatic power was 20–25 diopters for far distances and 15–20 diopters for near distances. Even though it is not explicitly described, sectors should determine bilateral relocation of the proximal part of the visual field while moving the gaze toward the blind field should allow direct viewing of the (non-displaced) peripheral region. The effect of the apical scotoma is not discussed in the paper; likewise, the putative advantage (if any) of this procedure over the binocular half-circle sectors is not clarified.

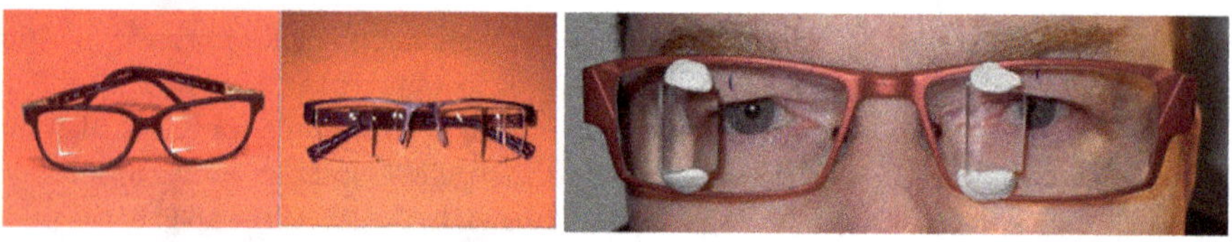

FIG. 11.4 – The Palomar sectors. See text for explanation. From Palomar-Mascaró FJ, Palomar-Mascaró MV, De Miguel Simó Pv. (2018). Rehabilitation of hemianopic patients with Palomar Prisms. Ophthalmology Clinics and Research, **1**(2): 28–34. Distributed under the terms of the Creative Commons Attribution License.

[3]The recommended offset of the prism apex from the pupil varies from 1.5 to 6 mm (Bailey, 2007) but generally the offset is such that a lateral version of 5 degrees into the affected hemifield is required to reach the prism (about 2.3 mm: Apfelbaum *et al.*, 2013).

11.5 Monocular Sector Prisms

Contrary to the binocular sector prisms, monocular sector prisms fitted to the side of the field loss with the base toward the blind hemifield provide true field expansion. In left hemianopia, for example, a sector prism, base out (*i.e.* left), is placed on the temporal half of the left glass. In this condition, the region of no-perception corresponding to the apical scotoma in the eye below the prism is neutralized as it is viewed by the other eye. In the region of expansion, however, visual confusion takes place (figure 11.5).

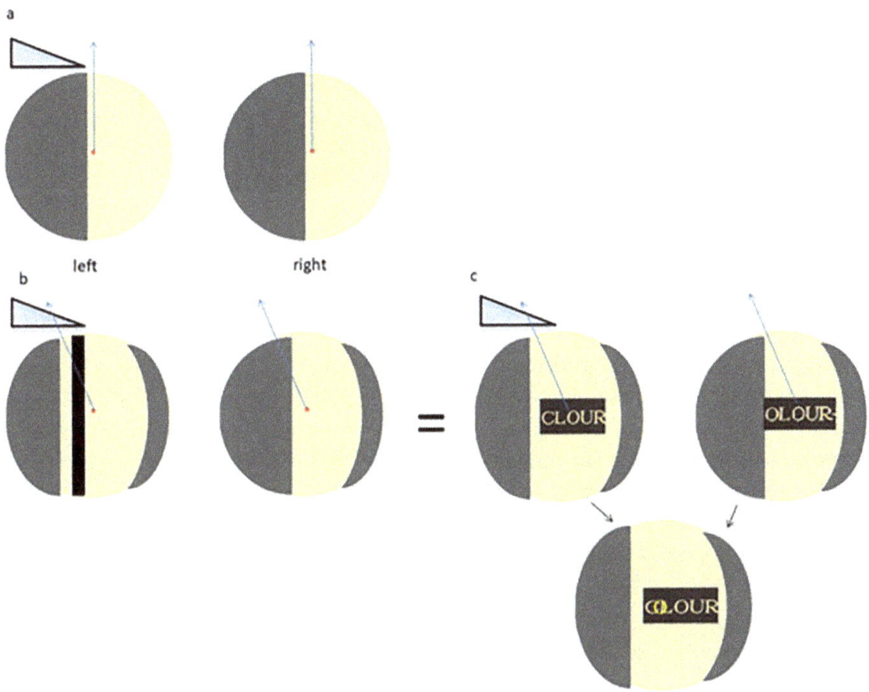

FIG. 11.5 – Monocular sector prisms, left homonymous hemianopia. Panel a, primary position: the prism does not affect the visual field as the sector is placed completely in the blind hemifield. Panel b: gaze turned 20° leftward through the prism: the visual field of the left eye is shifted toward the left and, correspondingly, the most eccentric visual field to the right is lost. In addition, an apical scotoma appears as a vertical gap in the paracentral region to the left of the apex of the prism. In the right eye, the field is not shifted, and the apical scotoma is absent. The region of the apical scotoma in the left eye is seen by the right eye, providing true binocular field expansion, even if a paracentral area of visual confusion inevitably takes place (panel c).

11.5.1 The Trimmed Prismatic Sector of Lawton Smith (Lawton Smith et al., 1982)

Lawton Smith described the case of a young woman with left homonymous hemianopia fitted with a 30 diopters Fresnel prism on the temporal half of her left glass. The sector had a small central area of 1–1.5 mm uncovered by the prims in the optical region corresponding to the pupil, to avoid central diplopia (Lawton Smith *et al.*, 1982: figure 11.6).

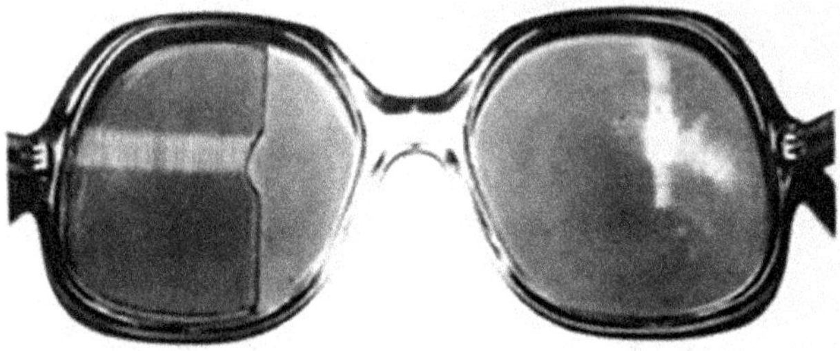

FIG. 11.6 – The trimmed prismatic sector of Lawton Smith. From Lawton Smith *et al.* (1982). With permission of Wolters Kluwer Health publisher.

The authors reckoned empirically a gain of about 15 degrees of useful vision to the left, with satisfaction reported by the patient who did not dismiss wearing the prism after one year from its fitting. The improvement depends on the fact that the prismatic sector deviates the image toward its base, thereby it displaces objects toward its apex: so, a prism base left displaces the objects falling onto the hemianopic (temporal) field (therefore that cannot be seen by the patient) toward the nasal (spared) hemifield, making them visible. This is what happened in the left eye, *i.e.* in the eye wearing the prism in the case described. The authors recommended careful fitting and centering of the prism, with particular attention to the size and position of the central semicircular area, to avoid diplopia and confusion. Moreover, they considered that the use of higher dioptric powers (50, 100, or even 150 diopters) could further enlarge vision in the blind hemifield, but a trade-off must be set between field enlargement and reduction in visual acuity due to the high prismatic power. The prismatic displacement generates confusion in the eye under the prism, but the apical scotoma is neutralized by the contralateral eye.

11.5.2 The Visual Field Awareness System (VFAS: Gottlieb, 1988)

In the Visual Field Awareness System (VFAS) a circular prism (5–35Δ, optimum: 18.5Δ) is mounted on the lens temporally to the pupil or at the temporal limbus (offset: about 6 mm), in correspondence to the affected side, base-out (Gottlieb *et al.*, 1992, 1998; Gottlieb, 1988: figure 11.7). The effect takes place when the

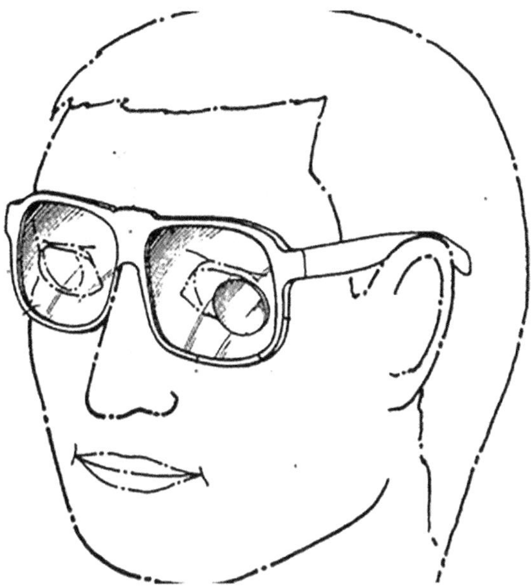

FIG. 11.7 – The Visual Field Awareness System (VFAS). From figure 1, Gottlieb DD. (1988). Method of using a prism in lens for the treatment of visual field loss. U.S. Patent 4 779 972.

patient moves his or her gaze so that the visual axis of the eye behind the prism crosses the sector (Gottlieb, 1988). In this visual condition, the expansion of the field of view takes place in the form of confusion: the patient sees two objects at the same field location: one that falls outside the scotomatous region and is seen by the eye with no prism, and a second that, being located within the blind region, would be invisible in normal (no-prism) conditions. This would make the system uncomfortable, but at a glance through the prism, as soon as an object is spotted in the blind hemifield, the subject should immediately turn his head to view the object of interest through the central (non-prismatic) part of the lens carrier. In other terms, the patient uses the prism-like a driver that glances at the side mirror. The advantage over Fresnel prisms is that the optical quality is not reduced, the prism does not deteriorate, and the cosmetic appearance is acceptable since the sector is mounted on the inner surface of the carrier lens, making it less visible.

Gottlieb reported that 70% of patients benefitted from the Visual Field Awareness System (Gottlieb *et al.*, 1992).

After a training period, Szlyk *et al.* (2005) reported improvement in recognition, mobility, peripheral detection, scanning, and during simulated driving in 10 hemianopic patients: 68% of the sample declared to be "satisfied" with the prism system, 16% were "very satisfied" and 16% were "extremely satisfied". After two years, 57% of the patients continued to use the VFAS frequently and only in one case the use was discontinued.

11.5.3 The Procedure of Peli (EP Prisms: Peli, 2000)

To overcome the problems of central diplopia and confusion related to monocular vertical sector prisms and of the pericentral apical scotoma, Peli proposed a new solution: a monocular horizontal sector prism, base out, placed in the superior and/or inferior part of the lens, ipsilateral to the side of the field loss. This way, the enlargement of the field of view is obtained in all the lateral positions of gaze *via* peripheral confusion. Since in this case, diplopia is not central but peripheral in the upper or/and lower part of the visual field, it is less disturbing. In fact, physiological peripheral diplopia is present in normal vision for objects outside the Panum's area.

On the other hand, confusion (two objects perceived in the same direction), too, is not central but peripheral and is compensated after a period of adaptation by a mechanism similar to anomalous retinal correspondence. It is worth pinpointing that the region of visual confusion is responsible for the visual field expansion.

The prismatic sectors (40Δ) are placed base out at the upper or lower (or both) part of the spectacles, with the border about the limbus, on the side of the hemianopic loss (on the left eye in case of left hemianopia, on the right eye in case of right hemianopia) and encompassing the whole width of the carrier lens. The patient is instructed not to foveate through the sectors, otherwise uncomfortable central diplopia is experienced. This way, when the patient is looking through the carrier lens, a peripheral object projected at the edge of the scotomatous region of the eye without the prism (thereby invisible to that eye) will be seen through the prism in the fellow eye. As a result, a visual field expansion of about 15–20 deg is expected at any position of gaze (and not only when the patient looks through the prism as it occurs with the monolateral prismatic sectors previously described): when viewing both in the direction of the scotoma and to the opposite side. The visual field corresponding to the apical scotoma in the eye with the prism(s) is seen by the fellow eye, but this generates confusion. In this case, however, confusion is less disturbing compared to the "conventional" monocular sector prisms as it is located in more eccentric (upper/upper + lower) positions (figure 11.8).

This solution associates a central image processed by the intact hemifields with a peripheral image diverted by the prism(s) from the blind hemifield to the spared hemifield about 15–20 degrees above and below (in case two sectors were used) the fixation point. In addition, the gain in visual field expansion further increases when the patient scans into the blind side (Peli *et al.*, 2016).

Patients first are fitted with a superior sector that, interacting with the superior visual field, is generally less disturbing in mobility and environmental navigation. After 2–3 weeks of adaptation, the binocular visual field with the prism is examined and if the experience is judged as positive by the patient, another sector is placed in the inferior part of the same carrier lens. Bowers and colleagues (2008) and Giorgi and co-workers (2009) used sectors that cover the full vertical extent of the lens. In this case, if the patient uses progressive lenses, a small semicircular aperture is cut in the bottom part of the lower prism to allow reading for brief periods (figure 11.9).

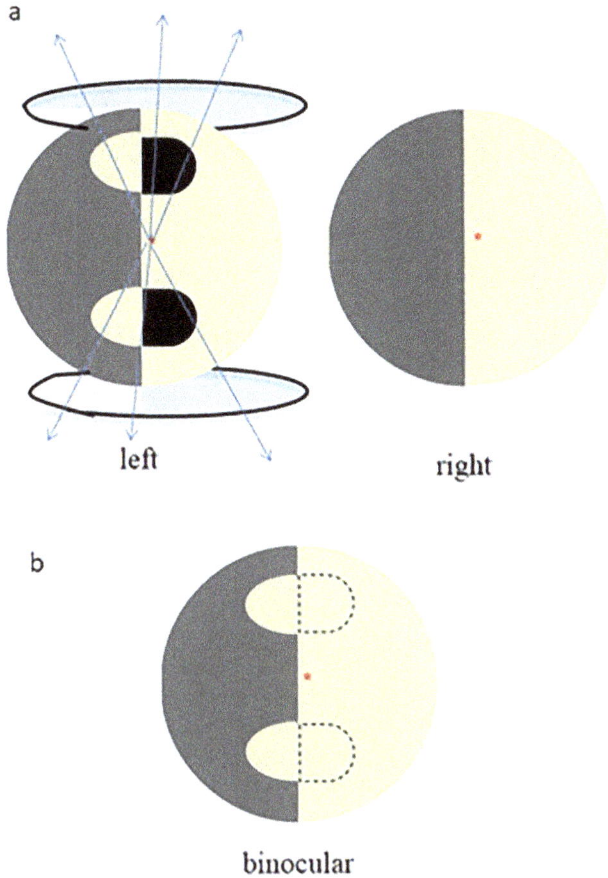

FIG. 11.8 – EP prisms left homonymous hemianopia; a: irrespective of gaze direction, the superior and inferior part of the visual field of the left eye is shifted toward the blind region, but a superior and inferior apical scotoma appears above and below the fixation point in the same eye; b: the two apical scotomata in the left eye are "filled" by the right eye, providing true field expansion. Based on Peli (2000).

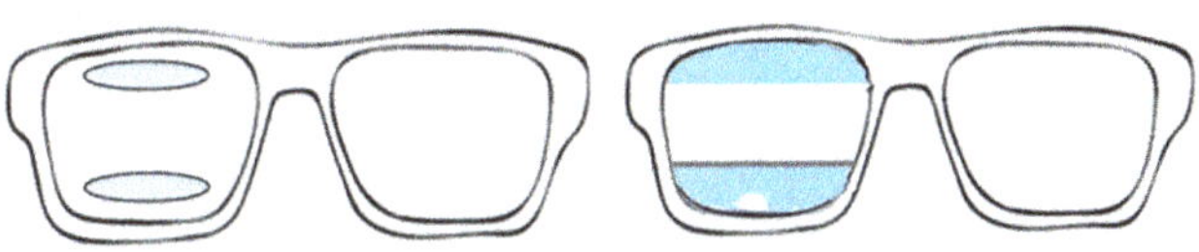

FIG. 11.9 – Left: the EP sectors devised by Peli. Right: the EP sectors used by Bowers *et al.* (2008) and Giorgi *et al.* (2009). Unlike the original design of Peli, Bowers used sectors extending across the whole inferior region of the lens. Contrary to the original EP sectors, this type of fitting may generate diplopia when descending stairs or in the presence of curbs, and in general when looking toward the floor if the subject foveates through the prism. In case patients wear progressive lenses, a small semicircular aperture is cut in the bottom part of the lower prism to allow reading for brief periods.

The optimal inter-sector separation was established in a multicenter evaluation of patients with complete homonymous hemianopia and no physical and cognitive impairment by Bowers and associates (2008). The authors used 40Δ press-on Fresnel prism segments. The optimal interprism distance on average was 11 mm (IQR: 8–11 mm). To avoid time-consuming individual determinations, an interprism separation of 12 mm (the 90th percentile computed on the participants who found useful the use of the prisms after 6 weeks), *i.e.* 6 mm above and below the center of the pupil, can be taken as a standard value (Bowers *et al.*, 2008; Giorgi *et al.*, 2009).

FITTING THE EP SECTORS STEP-BY-STEP

-1: position the superior prism with the lower edge 6 mm above the center of the pupil (Bowers *et al.*, 2008);

-2: assess tolerance:

i- by asking the patient if he/she experiences central diplopia or other problems;

ii- by observing head posture (head elevation means that the prism is placed too low: Bowers *et al.*, 2008);

-3: based on these parameters, displace the upper prism in 2–1 mm steps until reaching the lowest tolerated position (*i.e.* the minimum distance from the pupillary center where no central diplopia or other problems are reported and head posture is not elevated (Bowers *et al.*, 2008);

-4: ask the patient to look at the nose of the operator while the hand is moved on the hemianopic side. The patient has to detect the hand of the operator through the prism, and he is instructed to reach for it (Giorgi *et al.*, 2009);

-5: the patient is explained how to use the prismatic system: when he or she perceives an object through the prism, the eye and head must be moved vertically to foveate it through the carrier lens (and not through the prism) and to avoid diplopia;

-6: ask the patient to walk, paying attention to obstacles, and go up and down stairs (Giorgi *et al.*, 2009; Bowers *et al.*, 2008; Peli, 2000);

-7: the patient is dismissed with reaching-and-touching training to be done at home (Giorgi *et al.*, 2009);

-8: two to three weeks of adaptation (one or two weeks for Giorgi *et al.*, 2009);

-9: perform a binocular visual field with the monocular prism and ask the patient if the experience was judged as positive (Peli, 2000);

-10: position the inferior prism:

i- <<cut the lower prism to fit the lower edge of the lens. The upper edge of the prism must be positioned to intersect the line of gaze from the standing position to a distance of about 4 m on the ground in front of the patient. This is done with the patient standing up, holding the head straight, and looking straight ahead at a target at eye level. An object (a pen or pencil) is placed at the 4 m distance on the floor (on the seeing side of the field). The patient is asked to continue to look at the eye level target. This fixation helps to

maintain the head posture. The patient is asked to note the object on the floor with his peripheral vision…>> (Peli, 2000, p. 458);

ii- <<a piece of paper is brought from below and slowly raised in front of the lens until it obscures the inferior peripheral view of the object on the floor. The paper's edge position on the lens is marked and the mark is used for the upper position of the prism>> (Peli, 2000, p. 458). To avoid time-consuming individual determinations, an interprism separation of 12 mm, *i.e.* 6 mm above and below the center of the pupil, can be taken as a standard value: Bowers *et al.*, 2008; Giorgi *et al.*, 2009);

-11: assess tolerance (see point 2):

i- by asking the patient if he/she experiences central diplopia or other problems;

ii- by observing head posture (head lowering means that the prism is placed too high: Bowers *et al.*, 2008);

-12: based on these parameters, displace the lower prism in 2–1 mm steps until reaching the highest tolerated position (*i.e.* the minimum distance from the pupillary center where no central diplopia or other problems are reported and head posture is not lowered (Bowers *et al.*, 2008);

-13: repeat point 4, 6, and 7.

Using a lower and upper 40Δ prismatic segment, Peli reported a binocular visual field expansion of about 22° across the midline in all but one patient of his sample (9 subjects with homonymous hemianopia and 3 subjects with homonymous quadrantanopia, all with no signs of neglect: figure 11.10). In addition, complete neutralization of the defect in a subject with inferior quadrantanopia was observed (in this case, a single lower segment was fitted). The field expansion was effective in the primary position and at all the other positions of gaze (Peli, 2000).

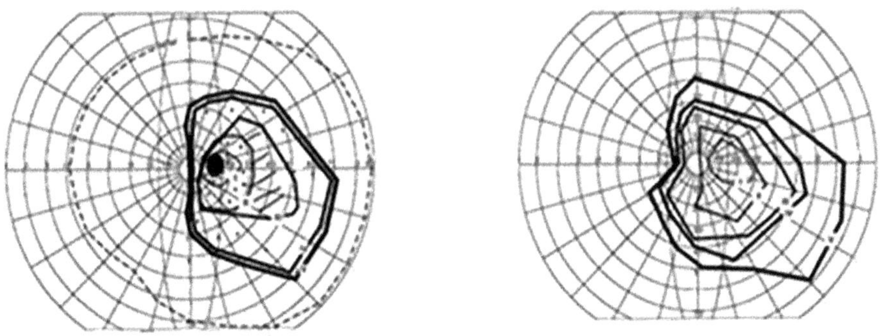

FIG. 11.10 – Left: the Goldmann monocular visual field (right eye) in a patient with left hemianopia; right: the Goldmann visual field measured binocularly with the two EP sectors (40 D) in the left eye. Note the additional field extending about 20° to the left of the midline. The dashed line in the left panel shows the normal visual field. From Peli (2000). With permission of Wolters Kluwer Health publisher.

In a subsequent study by Jamara and colleagues, Fresnel prisms were applied to the patient's spectacle lens of the eye corresponding to the side of the loss, according to the procedure of Peli (upper and lower 40Δ prism segments: Peli, 2000). Four subjects with homonymous hemianopia were treated. The prismatic correction yielded about 20 deg field expansion in three of the patients (Jamara *et al.*, 2003).

Of the 43 patients recruited in the multicenter investigation of Bowers *et al.* (2008), 74% decided to continue wearing the prisms after 2–18 months and 47% were still using the sectors after one year. The main reason for dismissing the prisms was visual confusion, the sudden appearance of images through the prism that caused anxiety in some patients, and no subjective improvement. The EP prisms were found particularly useful in the presence of obstacles, especially in malls or in crowded or unfamiliar areas. On the contrary, as expected, they were not worn when reading or using the computer.

In the study of Giorgi and colleagues, 23 patients with hemianopia and no neglect were fitted with the EP prisms (40Δ), and the benefits were evaluated considering:

i- visual field expansion;
ii- clinical success (*effectiveness*, revealed by the fact that the patient chooses to continue using the prisms);
iii- perceived quality of life, evaluated with two questionnaires (Giorgi *et al.*, 2009).

Prisms provided a visual field horizontal expansion by 22–23°. Two-thirds of the subjects chose not to interrupt wearing the prism (clinical success: 67%, in line with 74% found by Peli (2000)).

The main benefits were reported in walking and in "crowd" situations, like supermarkets, with reduced difficulty in noticing objects off to the side when walking, increased awareness of other persons, and fewer bumps into objects. On the contrary, patients complained about steps and stairs. In this respect, it should be considered that the fitting chosen for the study was the type with sectors extending across the whole inferior region of the lens (see figure 11.9, right panel). This may generate diplopia when descending stairs or in the presence of curbs, and in general when looking toward the floor if the subject foveates through the prism (Giorgi *et al.*, 2009).

11.5.4 The Oblique EP Prismatic Sectors

Using the horizontal EP prisms, the visual field expansion in the blind region takes place above and below the fixation point, with a vertical gap of about 30–40° (Peli *et al.*, 2016). This is undesirable when driving, as the expansion falls well outside the field of view seen through the windshield. Tilting the axis of the prism by rotating the prism bases about 30° toward the horizontal midline[4] enlarges the visual field more centrally than in the horizontal position. The group of Peli reckoned that a 57Δ sector tilted by 30° enlarges horizontally the visual field by 26° and shifts vertically the visual field by 15°, making this solution especially suitable for driving (Peli, 2020; Apfelbaum *et al.*, 2013: figure 11.11; Bowers *et al.*, 2012).

[4]Upper prism: base out and down, lower prism: base out and up.

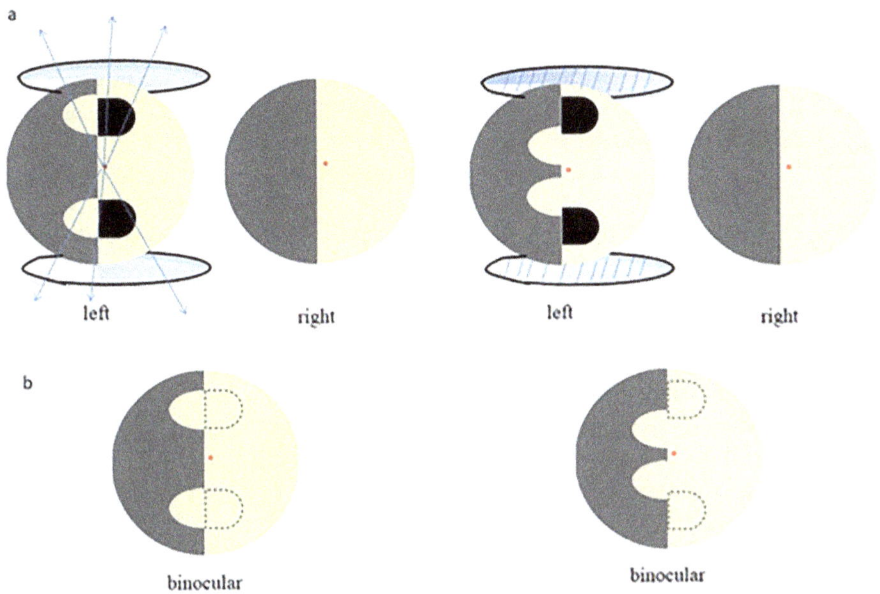

FIG. 11.11 – The EP sector prisms, horizontal and oblique design. Left homonymous hemianopia. Left: horizontal sectors. Right: oblique sectors. As for the horizontal sectors, the superior and inferior part of the visual field of the left eye is shifted toward the blind region, and a superior and inferior apical scotoma appears in peripheral positions. The apical scotoma generated by the prisms in the left eye is "filled" by the right eye. To be noted that the paracentral gap is reduced with the oblique design compared to the horizontal design. Based on Peli *et al.* (2016).

It should be considered that despite the minimization of the vertical gap in the blind region, with the oblique sectors, the extent of the lateral field expansion in the blind hemifield is reduced compared to the horizontal design.

The group of Bowers considered the effect of two 40Δ oblique EP prismatic sectors on the detection of hazardous events (like pedestrians or obstacles) in the blind side when driving in 12 hemianopic subjects with no neglect. The use of oblique EP prisms was found to be beneficial in the detection of hazards in the blind hemifield, without affecting the spared side, so 75% of the patients judged the oblique EP prisms useful when driving: indeed, at the end of the study 10 out of 12 participants decided to continue using the prisms (Bowers *et al.*, 2012).

As a confirmation, Moss and colleagues described the case of two young patients (a 24 and a 31-year-old male) with complete left hemianopia (and no neglect) whose visual field improved consistently when wearing the EP sectors. Two 40-Δ segments were fitted according to the procedure of Peli, oriented obliquely at 45° from the horizontal axis. With the prisms, the visual field enlarged horizontally by 20 and 30° (from 95° to 115° in case 1 and from 82° to 112° in case 2). Patients, who reported significant improvement in their quality of life, re-obtained the driving license (Moss *et al.*, 2014).

Yet, despite the minimization of the vertical gap in the blind region, the extent of the lateral field expansion is reduced with the oblique sectors compared to the horizontal design[5]: a problem that could be prevented by using higher-power prisms. Likewise, to further reduce the vertical gap in the blind region without sacrificing the peripheral field, prisms with higher power can be used. Using 57Δ prisms with a tilt angle of 34° and standard interprism separation of 12 mm, the vertical gap is completely closed with consistent lateral expansion (Peli *et al.*, 2016).

According to a multicenter randomized cross-over trial, the majority of patients with homonymous hemianopia[6] (64%) demonstrate a preference for real EP prism glasses (57Δ, interprism distance: 12 mm) over sham EP prism glasses, judging the former helpful for obstacle avoidance (Bowers *et al.*, 2014). The continuation rate at 6 months was 41%. No preference was expressed between the horizontal *vs.* oblique design, even if the oblique design is more suitable for driving. The side of the loss and duration of hemianopia were not predictive. The authors pinpointed the importance of the training.

O'Neill and co-workers evaluated the improvement of vision-related quality of life (QOL) in a sample of 10 hemianopic patients[7] who were rehabilitated with EP prisms (O'Neill *et al.*, 2011). Patients did not show neglect, had visual acuity equal to or better than 20/50 with or without macular sparing, and were devoid of severe physical disability. By administering the NEI-VFQ-25 questionnaire[8] before and one year after wearing the prisms, the author reported significant improvement in vision-related quality of life, with particular reference to general vision, peripheral vision, and distance vision. As expected, prisms did not affect near vision and color vision. The advantages that emerged from the vision-related items of the questionnaire are reduced dependency, increased social functioning, and improved general health. It remains that the scores of all the subscales of the questionnaire remained lower than normal.

Overall, 83% of the patients were satisfied with the prism sectors, and none reported any adaptation difficulty. It should be noted, however, that the study lacked a control group.

11.5.5 Limitations and Remarks of the EP Method

The EP method suffers from two main limitations:

a- binocular rivalry of the image diverted by the prisms induces local suppression that, in turn, decreases the field enlargement pursued by the sectors.

Confusion triggers binocular rivalry so that the binocular rivalry between the image seen through the prismatic sector and the corresponding region of the visual

---

[5]The vertical upward and inward expansion toward the center is given by the formula: $VE = p \times \sin(\beta))$. The reduction in the lateral field expansion is given by the formula: $LE = p \times \cos(\beta))$, where p is the prism power expressed in degrees and β is the tilt of the sector in degrees (Peli *et al.*, 2016).

[6]No visual neglect.

[7]Age: 18–62 years, onset from lesion: 9–48 months.

[8]National Eye Institute 25-Item Visual Functioning Questionnaire (Mangione *et al.*, 2001).

field perceived by the fellow eye is expected. Indeed, in binocular rivalry the weaker stimulus tends to be suppressed; now, the weaker image is the image seen through the prismatic sector (especially the Fresnel press-on), as it is degraded in terms of contrast (Katz, 2004a, 2004b), chromatic aberration, and spatial distortion. It is theorized, therefore, that the binocular predominance of the prism image is reduced, so it is the visual field enlargement.

However, in conditions of static binocular viewing Ross and co-workers (2012) found no binocular rivalry-induced local suppression of the image diverted by the prism in a group of hemianopic patients.

Shen and co-workers (2015) reconsidered the problem and its impact not only in static conditions but also in a real-world dynamic environment. In the presence of a static background, the authors found no differences in the expansion area between the monocular and binocular conditions: this finding is in agreement with what was reported by the group of Ross. On the contrary, the detection rate in the expansion area was significantly lower in binocular conditions over a moving background. These findings suggest that binocular rivalry with the reduced predominance of the image diverted by the prismatic sector is favored by conflicting motion (*i.e.* motion of the scene perceived through the prism *vs.* motion perceived by the fellow eye) in the expanded area. This phenomenon hampers the ameliorative effect of the EP sectors in everyday viewing situations, as theorized.[9]

The results of Shen and associates are in line with what was found the previous year by Haun and Peli (2014), who measured binocular rivalry in simulated right hemianopic conditions with a 40Δ press-on prism fitted on the temporal side of one lens of a pair of spectacles. The prism was placed temporally to the fixation point in the left eye whereas the right part of both lenses was masked to simulate homonymous hemianopia. Targets were red or green squares presented dichoptically to the left of fixation onto a noise-dynamic background. The background drifted in opposite directions in the visual field seen by the eye covered by the prism and in the visual field seen directly by the fellow eye. The subject had to indicate whether a red or a green patch was seen. The authors found that the predominance of the image seen through the Fresnel prism was reduced in binocular conditions but not profoundly disrupted, so the prism remains effective in enlarging the visual field. The same authors argued that the undesirable effect may be less evident in permanent PMMA sectors due to their better optical quality compared to the press-on Fresnel prisms. In addition, they showed that prism images viewed more eccentrically compete in rivalry more effectively than prism images viewed more centrally. Now, EP prisms are fitted more peripherally on the carrier lens compared to the press-on

[9]The authors used static perimetry to estimate detection of stimuli presented over dynamic natural driving scenes in a sample of 9 patients with homonymous hemianopia and no hemineglect. As a comparison, static backgrounds were used as well. Patients wore the 40Δ EP press-on sectors in the oblique configuration (30° tilt) and tests were administered after at least 4 weeks of prism adaptation. The target was a 2 × 2 black-and-white square checkerboard presented for 205 ms in a 6 × 8° zone located in the lower expansion area and in a zone located within the seeing hemifield. The size and contrast of the target were customized for each patient to achieve at least 10% detection in the expansion area and no more than 95% detection in the seeing hemifield.

sectors applied in this experiment: so, the predominance of the peripheral EP, prisms, thereby their effectiveness, is expected to be greater than that found in this experimental condition;

b- total internal reflection of the high-power EP 57Δ prisms limits the advantage of scanning into the affected hemifield.

With the high-power EP 57Δ sectors, the total internal reflection of the prisms limits the advantage of scanning into the affected hemifield (Peli *et al.*, 2016; Jung and Peli, 2014). Indeed, distortion and total internal reflection generally go ignored in prescribing prisms, but with high-power prismatic sectors these effects can consistently hamper the rehabilitative outcome. A 57Δ EP sector produces a slightly magnified image at the apex and severe image compression at the base. In addition, transmittance decreases rapidly toward the base so that total internal reflection takes place beyond 5 degrees of scanning through the prism toward the blind sight. This effect actually neutralizes the further widening of the visual field when looking through the prism toward the blind side expected in ideal no-internal reflection conditions.

Peli considered that:

i- even if, according to Margolis and Suter (2006), the EP sectors require consistent adaptation, most of the treated patients adapted well to the prismatic correction within two to three weeks;
ii- the procedure seems to have no detrimental effect on self-motion, as the optical flow is affected only in peripheral vision, but not centrally;
iii- the method seems not to be effective in patients with abnormal binocular function;
iv- when homonymous hemianopia is associated with non-comitant diplopia (it may occur in case of trauma), the author suggests penalizing the central vision of the eye corresponding to the side of the hemianopia (for example by frosting the central part of the lens with nail polish or with a translucent tape) and fitting the same lens with the prism segment. This way the binocular visual field enlargement is obtained and, at the same time, diplopia is avoided;
v- the method is not suitable with bifocal/progressive lenses;
vi- the method is not suitable for reading or other activities that require a downward gaze. A solution for rapidly switching from far to near position is using a clip-on plano lens with a prismatic sector mounted over it, to be used for far distance and removed where it comes to read or sew;
vii- an after-effect needs to be evaluated, as it could be a problem when switching from far-distance glasses to reading glasses;
viii- detection in the affected side is not fully restored by prisms, due to optical factors and peripheral binocular rivalry (Shen *et al.*, 2015; Haun and Peli, 2014);
ix- the use of press-on prisms is useful to introduce the procedure in patients and assess its usefulness on a subjective basis, but is a temporary solution: the material of the press-on prisms has poor optical quality and tends to

deteriorate with time. To solve this problem and ensure higher optical quality, Peli developed a polymethylmethacrylate Fresnel 57 diopters prism[10] inset embedded into the carrier lens, with conical surfaces and wider extension toward the front side of the carrier for safety reasons.

To improve cosmetics, a dark sunshade clip-on over the glasses can be used: this way, the prismatic sectors are completely invisible (Peli *et al.*, 2020).

11.6 The Multiplexing Prisms of Peli and Jung (2017)

To address the issue of apical scotoma, Peli and Jung devised a new prismatic solution, called *multiplexing prism*, which differs from the conventional Fresnel prisms inasmuch the latter have an array of identical prismatic elements arranged from the base to the apex, whereas in the multiplexing prism the prismatic elements alternate with flat surfaces (Peli and Jung, 2017). The view that passes through the flat elements alternates with the view deviated by the prism so that they are seen simultaneously and should neutralize the effect of the apical scotoma (figure 11.12).

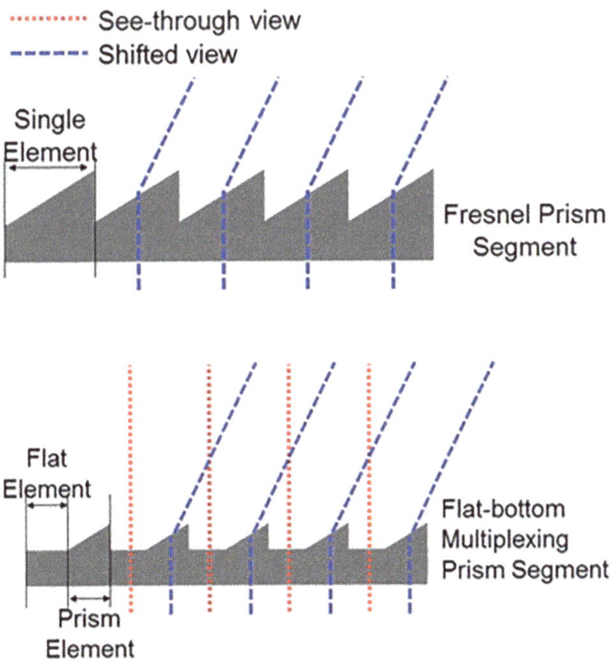

Fig. 11.12 – The multiplexing system of Peli and Jung. From Peli and Jung (2017). With permission of Wolters Kluwer Health.

[10]Height: 8 mm, horizontal extension: 22 mm. The expected visual field enlargement is about 30° (Apfelbaum *et al.*, 2013).

Conclusion

Patients with stroke and visual impairment are not like the others: they are condemned to bear a heavy psychological burden. Loneliness. They feel alone, and abandoned. Indeed, there are no physicians who can care for them after their clinical condition has been stabilized: in fact, neither the neurologist nor the ophthalmologist may help them restore, even in part, their visual field. They feel deeply frustrated for not having answers, for not finding solutions. For this reason and the clinical condition itself, it is easy to imagine the profound deterioration in the quality of life and the risk of developing depression.

The onset of hemianopia is a drama: patients are disoriented, scared by what has just happened and worried about what will become of their daily lives. Hemianopia generates reading and orientation problems: they can no longer drive, and independence and social life are at risk.

Nature in its immense wisdom has shaped the visual brain so that in hemianopia the central visual function is generally preserved: macular sparing helps a lot, as it allows for retaining a good visual acuity. But it is not enough when there are objects all around, when it comes to walking, driving, or reading my favorite book. The scenario is even worse when fate seems to rage and neglect coexists.

We recalled in the introduction of this treatise "The Dogma": "In the brain what is lost is lost". Neurons cannot regenerate so rehabilitation can at best induce axonal sprouting and synaptogenesis, but, beyond this, its boundaries are firmly set. For a long time, indeed, the visual system was thought to have no capacity to recover after occipital damage. Now we can reasonably state this is not the whole story.

Since the article by Eriksson and associates dating back to 1998 that provided evidence of neuronal genesis in the dentate gyrus of the hippocampus in adult human brains, the statement that brain cells cannot regenerate has been challenged. Quoting McMillan and colleagues <<the significance of the Eriksson study is that it may change our conceptualization of what neurorehabilitation can do to the brain in principle, and in the future we may look for a combination of neuropharmacological

and neurorehabilitation treatments that could produce recovery in the everyday function that has been beyond our wildest dreams>> (McMillan *et al.*, 1999, p. 131).

Since the past century, indeed, Research has been challenging the Dogma. Investigations first on animals, and then on humans reveal that systematic and repetitive stimulation of the blind region of the visual field (may) help restore, even if partially, the neuronal function.

Visual restitution is mainly focused on the transition zone. The neuroplasticity of the visual system provides the neurobiological substrate for this strategy. The effective enlargement of the visual field after repetitive stimulation of the region between the seen and the no-seen zone is the most debated topic. The results reported after visual restitution, indeed, have been undermined by the biasing effect of fixation instability or unnoticed ocular movements and by the failure in replicating the visual field enlargement reported at "high resolution" non-conventional perimetry when a conventional visual field analyzer is used. Even if controversial, visual restitution seems to be effective, but the training is time-consuming and results are limited in terms of visual field expansion. Sabel and Kastel recommend using visual restitution only in patients with some residual function, with two sessions a day for at least 6 months. They warn against treating subjects with photosensitive epilepsy and conclude that <<[...] although complete restitution seems unlikely at present, significant visual field enlargement can be accomplished, and patients with visual field defects such as scotoma or hemianopia benefit from it>>. They conclude that for these patients it should become the standard therapy (Sabel and Kasten, 2000). Contrary to this statement, Hämäläinen and Julkunen wrote in their review that <<It seems evident that many patients with visual field defects benefit from training, but certainly not all of them. Currently, it is nearly impossible to select those patients who would benefit from visual field treatment. At least in chronic stages, a sufficiently long and intense period of treatment (almost daily for months) will be needed to gain benefit. On the other hand, if the treatment is easy to access and use and is not costly, there should be no objection to trying it out>> (Hämäläinen and Julkunen, 2004, p. 17).

Pharmacological supplementation (like amphetamine) may help reduce the time of treatment and improve the outcome but further research is needed to understand the potential of this approach and the benefit-risk ratio. Overall, modulation of the treatment and improvement of the procedures are expected to yield better results in the future.

Even if visual restitution is mainly focused on the transition zone, this does not preclude the possibility of training the inner regions of the hemiscotoma as well, with the aim to enhance the function of the extrastriate pathway responsible for blindsight.

It is well known that man is a highly adaptive being: it is not surprising, therefore, that hemianopes learn by themselves new oculomotor strategies to overcome their hemifield loss. In this respect, visual compensation training is found to improve the capacity to explore the lost part of the visual world. Even if visual compensation adds nothing in terms of visual field expansion, it seems more effective than visual restitution in rehabilitating patients in daily life activities, and rehabilitation time is consistently shorter. Again, rehabilitative protocols that associate visual restitution and visual compensation are worth to be investigated. Indeed, visual restitution and visual compensation can have a synergistic effect, as explained by Nelles and colleagues (2009). As the visual field loss contributes to saccadic abnormality, a combined treatment strategy should be considered with visual restitution therapy administered before visual compensation.

Finally, the intact region of vision can make up for the defective area when appropriate optic devices are developed and applied. The use of a mirror is aesthetically unacceptable, and the reverse image makes adaptation troublesome. Prisms seem to be a more suitable solution.

Monocular prismatic sectors have been designed to supply the loss of function in the hemianopic region with the spared visual hemifield. Sectors determine enlargement of the field of view by creating a region of visual confusion when part of the image that falls onto the blind hemifield is diverted towards the intact region. Expansion can be intermittent, when the half-prism is placed to the side of the loss, and takes place only when the gaze intercepts the system, or constant, occurring in any direction of gaze, when the EP prisms are applied in the superior and inferior part of the lens.

According to Lawton Smith and colleagues, the best candidates for visual substitution are hemianopic patients whose visual field defect is their main complaint, but we are obtaining encouraging results also in subjects for whom the main problem is motor.[1]

Whatever the type of treatment adopted, the co-occurrence of neglect is a detrimental factor for rehabilitation. The outcome will be poor in the presence of neglect: so, rehabilitation of heminattention should precede any visual treatment, be it restoration, compensation, or substitution. Yoked full-field prisms can be of avail, as shown in several studies, and in the short term this is probably the research stream that should be developed.

But that's not all.

If, on the one hand, the investigation of the potential for visual restitution, substitution, and compensation is in progress, parallel research directions are evolving. Considering the positive results in motor rehabilitation, recently a strand of research has been probing the effect of transcranial current stimulation on the visual function of hemianopes. Noninvasive current stimulation, indeed, is found to enhance neuronal excitability (see Raffin *et al.*, 2020 for a discussion), thereby it increases the likelihood of neuronal firing in the affected cortical region. This way, it could help functional recovery, especially if associated with visual restoration training. In transcranial direct current stimulation (tDCS), subthreshold current is applied through saline-soaked sponge electrodes placed along the midline of the scalp, over the Oz (anode electrode) and the Cz position. The pursued effect is a change in neuronal membrane polarization that, in turn, translates into increased cortical

[1]Data not yet published at the time of the publication of this treatise.

excitability. When used in conjunction with VRT, a visual field enlargement at the transition zone of 4° has been reported in a single-case study (Halko *et al.*, 2011) and in a sample of 10 patients (Plow *et al.*, 2012) after 3 months of combined treatment. However, the subjective improvement and the effect on the recovery of function in activities of daily living remain controversial. Combined administration of tDCT and blindsight training is reported to improve functional, clinical, and ecological tests more than blindsight training alone (Matteo *et al.*, 2017). In transcranial random noise stimulation (tRNS), frequencies of alternating current are applied with electrodes placed bilaterally over the visual cortex. In a pilot study on 11 patients who underwent tRNS coupled with training at the transition zone, improvement in visual performance was recorded after 10 days of treatment, and the effect persisted for 6 months (Herpich *et al.*, 2019). Finally, repetitive transorbital alternating current stimulation (rtACS) focuses on the orbital region to stimulate the functional activity of the visual pathways and visual cortex. After 10 days of treatment, increased contrast sensitivity was reported in one patient (Sabel *et al.*, 2020). Taken together, these results make electric cerebral stimulation an interesting add-on approach for the rehabilitation of hemianopia; however, at the moment only a few clinical studies are available, and the real potential must be clarified.

Finally, there is the postural approach: the direction of gaze, that is orbital eye position, seems to yield a modulatory effect on the scotoma: turning the head toward the blind field to shift the gaze ipsilesionally (toward the spared hemifield) is found to normalize the scotoma, as reported by Nadeau and Heilman (1991) in a patient with left upper quadrantanopia following right temporo-occipital lesion, and by Kerkhoff in a subject with right upper quadrantanopia due to left posterior cerebral artery infarction (Kerkhoff, 1999). In both cases the improvement did not depend on a visual field shift, was transient, and disappeared as the head and, consequently, the gaze returned to the primary position. Maybe eccentric gaze, proprioceptive neck afferents, or both, modulate the neuronal activity of the damaged cortex, and this modulation is interesting for rehabilitative purposes.

It is somehow reassuring that cerebral lesions do not annihilate the whole pattern of visual information: visual processing is overlapping and complementary so that shape, for example, can be derived from contour, contrast, or relative motion. It follows that patients can rely on the preserved aspects of their visual perception for initiating a recovery strategy. Future rehabilitation procedures may exploit the overlapping pattern to enhance the overall visual processing of hemianopes (Anderson, 2003).

Last but not least, visual function in hemianopia seems to be somehow degraded even in the intact field. As recalled by Kerkhoff, the "useful field of view" (UFOV) is the visual area in which information can be acquired at a glance, *i.e.* during a single fixation. The difference with the conventional visual field is that in perimetry the task is detecting an isolated target presented against a uniform background, whereas in the UFOV examination a stimulus is presented in a cluttered visual background with many distractors, and the task consists of peripheral localization (Kerkhoff, 2000). This experimental condition, indeed, reproduces the visual daily experience better than the conventional perimetric examination.

It is weird and worrying that the UFOV is defective not only in the affected hemifield, as expected, but also in the contralateral, spared region. In a study on 12 patients with unilateral lesions of the striate area, Rizzo and Robin (1996) found that the UFOV was reduced by 30%–57%. The reduction, indeed, was not detected at standard perimetry. UFOV reduction in the "surviving" region could contribute to the perceptual difficulties complained about by patients in real life, especially in tasks like driving or reading. Now, what is of interest from a translational perspective is that the UFOV seems responsive to visual training in hemianopics (Kerkhoff *et al.*, 1994).

Visual restitution, compensation, substitution.... pharmacological treatment, current stimulation, postural rehabilitation. Training of the overlapping visual pattern. UFOV enhancement.... There is room for thought. And for hope.

A lot of work has been done, important results have been achieved.

Yet, far more needs to be done; it is worth going on, unfortunate people are waiting.

In the end, their partial eclipse of the sight will be defeated. And their Moon will not be doomed to have a dark side forever.

Research is my faith.

And I am a believer.

Appendix. Pure Alexia

Pure alexia is an acquired reading disorder that affects subjects suffering from a lesion to the left occipitotemporal cortex. In pure alexia "[...] patients appear to have lost the ability to process letters as whole word recognition units" (Warrington and Langdon, 1994, p. 211). In other terms, the "mapping of the visual structure of the whole world onto its neutrally encoded representation in the long-term memory store (lexicon) of familiar words is impaired" (Leff *et al.*, 2001b, p. 511): thereby, words cannot be recognized whereas individual letters do.[2] It follows that pure alexics, contrary to normal readers, adopt a serial rather than parallel decoding strategy (Behrmann *et al.*, 2001): they read a letter at a time and, after completing the sequence, name the word. Letter-by-letter reading makes the lexical process remarkably slow albeit quite accurate,[3] and it is revealed by the so-called *word length effect* [WLE]. WLE is an abnormally large increase in naming latency as a function of the number of letters in the string[4] (Behrmann *et al.*, 2001). The WLE, at least for words made of 3–6 letters, is absent in normal subjects (Lavidor and Ellis, 2002; Weekes, 1997) and in hemianopic subjects or, when present, it is far less pronounced than in pure alexics (Leff *et al.*, 2001b, 2006; Behrmann *et al.*, 2001).[5]

The pathophysiology of letter-by-letter reading in pure alexics remains a matter of debate. A line of research states the WLE depends on a defective deployment of spatial attention across the word that induces the reader to allocate attention sequentially (serially) to each letter rather than in parallel, as it occurs in normal readers (Rapp and Caramazza, 1991). This perspective is supported by the correlation reported by Rapp and Caramazza in their alexic patient between the visual

[2]Contrary to pure alexia, global alexia is characterized by failure to recognize individual letters. Patients who, immediately after the cerebral accident, suffer from global alexia, may "recover" over days or weeks to a condition of pure alexia (Leff *et al.*, 2001b).

[3]The use of this strategy is confirmed by the fact that the tachistoscopic presentation of words (that forces to process words in parallel, *i.e.* as a whole rather than letter-by-letter) is profoundly impaired in pure alexics (Warrington and Langdon, 1994).

[4]The WLE is generated by an increase in viewing time and fixation frequency per additional letter (Pflugshaupt *et al.*, 2009).

[5]In hemianopia, reading is not as impaired as in pure alexia. Reading speed (silent reading) of texts has been estimated to be 66%–68% slower in pure alexics compared to right-sided hemianopic alexics (Pflugshaupt *et al.*, 2009; Leff *et al.*, 2001b, 2006).

search time of a target embedded in an array of distractors and the number of distractors. From a different perspective, Johnson and Rayner argued that the WLE reflects a defect at a low level of visual processing of the text, namely during the extraction of visual information performed by a particular region of the brain called the *visual word form area* (Johnson and Rayner, 2007).

A.1 Etiology of Pure Alexia and the VWFA

Pure alexia is supposed to depend on the damage or disconnection from a specific region of the cortex devoted to the lexical task at a presemantic stage: the so-called *Visual Word Form Area (VWFA)*.

The VWFA is an area in the posterior region of the left temporal cortex activated by visual words. For this reason, it is argued to be specialized in word recognition.[6] With an fMRI and electrophysiological study, Gaillard and colleagues provided direct evidence of the specialization of the VWFA in reading. They measured the reading function in a patient before and after surgical remotion of a small part of the left occipitotemporal cortex corresponding to the VWFA. Reading was profoundly impaired after surgery, whereas recognition of categories of objects other than words remained intact. This comes out in favor of the selective lexical activation of the VWFA (Gaillard *et al.*, 2006).

The VWFA is sensitive to the abstract form of the words, that is to say to the abstract representation of groups of letters integrated into a perceptual unit, irrespective of font, case, or size. In other terms, the VWFA recognizes holistically words as lexical objects and not by processing serially the letters they are made up of. The holistic recognition of words is made possible as the VWFA contains neurons tuned to their invariant stimulus properties, even if it is responsive also to faces and objects (McCandliss *et al.*, 2003).[7] The parallel processing of words performed by this area accounts for the lack of the so-called "word length effect" in normal readers, in which the recognition time of words does not increase as a function of the number of letters.

---

[6]Despite a consistent number of studies indicating the VWFA is a specialized region devoted to word identification (*e.g.* Gaillard *et al.*, 2006), this statement is not completely accepted. According to Price and Devlin, for example, neuroimaging and neuropsychological data are not consistent with a cortical region specialized to visual word form representation. In fact, the authors reported evidence that the so-called VWFA is not specific for words, but extends to tasks that do not engage visual word form processing, like naming pictures or colors (Price and Devlin, 2003).

[7]An intriguing question deals with the origin of the VWFA: the VWFA is a region that seems specialized to process stimuli like words that never existed before the relatively recent invention of alphabetic writing. According to McCandliss and colleagues "the functional property of the VWFA is a special case of "perceptual expertise", in which extensive visual experience with a class of stimuli drives enhancement of perceptual mechanisms and changes in the supporting functional architecture in the left fusiform gyrus [...]" (McCandliss *et al.*, 2003, p. 296). This theory is supported by the evidence that perceptual expertise can stem from the visual experience in a particular domain of objects like cars or birds (in these cases the right (and not the left) fusiform gyrus is activated: Gauthier *et al.*, 2000). The fact that patients with pure alexia are also impaired at object identification, *e.g.* pictures, supports the theory that the VWFA is not strictly devoted to processing orthographic symbols (Behrman *et al.*, 1998).

The VWFA is insensitive to size, fonts, letter cases, and position in the visual field.[8] Its activation is elicitable also in conditions of unawareness (Dehaene *et al.*, 2001).

The VWFA is localized in the left fusiform gyrus (Brodmann's area 37), more precisely between the posterior fusiform gyrus and inferior temporal gyrus at the left occipitotemporal junction (Leff *et al.*, 2001b, 2006; McCandliss *et al.*, 2003; Dehaene *et al.*, 2002; Polk *et al.*, 2002; Menard *et al.*, 1996; Henderson *et al.*, 1985). It receives projections from the occipital area. In turn, it projects to the left angular gyrus, which is considered more responsive than the VWFA to real words (the left angular gyrus would be the "repository to visual images of words", as recalled by Cohen *et al.* (2003)). When the word is presented in the right hemifield (thereby it is projected onto the left occipital hemisphere) the signal transits directly to the left occipitotemporal junction, where the VWFA is located. When the word is presented in the left hemifield (it is projected onto the right occipital hemisphere) the signal is conveyed by the interhemispheric fibers of the splenium of the corpus callosum to the left occipitotemporal junction (Molko *et al.*, 2002; Cohen *et al.*, 2000; Binder and Mohr, 1992; Henderson *et al.*, 1985) (figure A1).

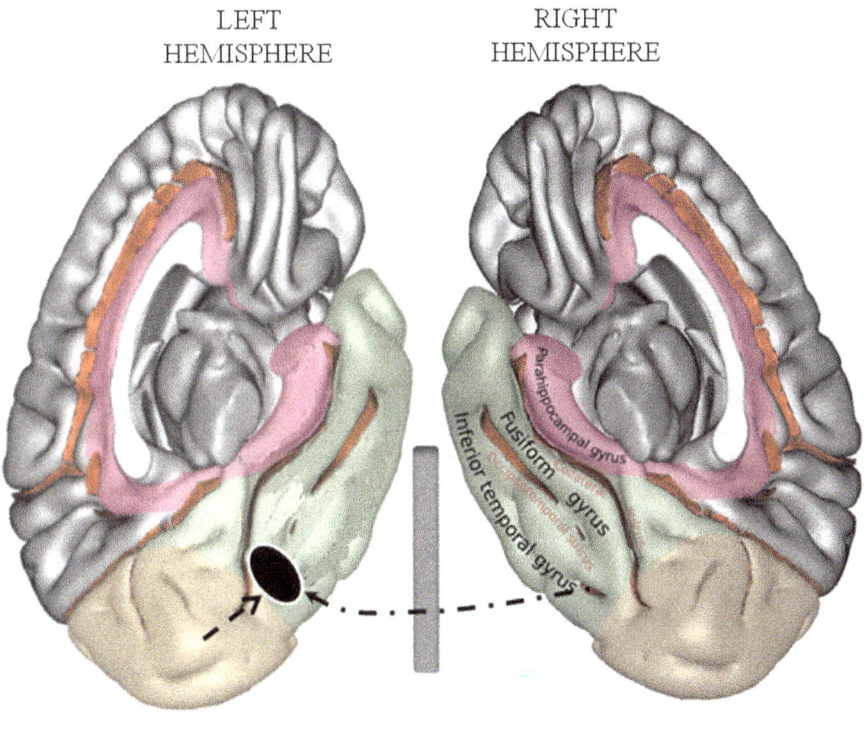

FIG. A1 – The VWFA (black region). See text for explanation.

So, words presented in the left and the right hemi-visual field are equally readable since the VWFA activation is expected to be the same irrespective of the left/right

[8]Even if the latency is slightly longer for stimuli presented to the left hemifield (Brown *et al.*, 1998).

stimulation. However, due to the callosal right-left signal transfer, the left hemifield stimulation shows a delay of about 10–15 ms (Brown *et al.*, 1998).

The VWFA has some peculiar characteristics:

- it responds selectively to letters, syllables, or words, even if neurons sensitive to other complex visual tasks such as faces or objects are intermingled in this region (Puce *et al.*, 1996);
- it is insensitive to upper- and lowercase letters as well as to fonts and size (Polk and Farah, 2002);
- its activation is the same irrespective of the position of the word in the visual field (Cohen *et al.*, 2000);
- it responds better to words and pseudo-words than to random consonant strings (Cohen *et al.*, 2002; Dehaene *et al.*, 2002). In this respect it is worth considering the study by Nobre and colleagues, who recorded the cortical event-related potentials (ERP) in 27 subjects who were stimulated with a variety of visual stimuli, including words, letter strings, faces, and checkerboard stimuli (Nobre *et al.*, 1994). The authors reported large potentials with peak latencies of about 200 ms in the posterior fusiform gyrus. The response was elicited by strings of letters but not by the other types of stimuli. In turn, a potential with a peak at 400 ms was recorded in the anterior fusiform gyrus when words with semantic content were presented but not in the presence of the other types of stimuli, non-words included. The study suggests that the VWFA is made up of two distinct regions: the posterior sector, responsive to strings of letters (pre-lexical processing), and an anterior part, sensitive to the semantic content of words;
- neurons in the VWFA are topographically tuned from its posterior to the anterior side to progressively larger (more invariant) lexical units: simple graphemes, then syllables, then familiar clusters of letters, and finally entire words[9] (Cohen and Dehaene, 2004; McCandliss *et al.*, 2003).

The presence of a strong word-length effect in children aged 6–7 years that fades gradually up to 11–12 years of age (Aghababian and Nazir, 2000) suggests that the normal development of the VWFA is complete at that time and is not the natural course of a developmental process but depends on the maturation of the reading skill.

A bulk of research suggests that pure alexics suffer from damage or deafferentiation of the VWFA so that the automatic activation of the abstract visual representation of the word is prevented (Johnson and Rayner, 2007).

---

[9]According to Pelli and associates, the hypothesis of neurons tuned for complex stimuli (*i.e.* words and not features of letters or whole letters) is not supported by the fact that "[...] rather than directly recognizing complex familiar objects, such as words, our visual system detects smaller components-letters or perhaps features of letters and only then recognizes the object specified by these components. Nothing is seen unless its components are detected" (Pelli *et al.*, 2003, p. 753). In line with this statement, the authors consider unlikely the existence of high-order neurons that integrate over complex receptive fields matching entire words. On the contrary, they suggest that word identification follows necessarily independent detection of letters or, more probably, of features of letters.

The involvement of the VWFA in pure alexia is the consequence of an infarction of the left posterior cerebral artery that affects the left occipitotemporal junction and includes, to a variable extent, the left occipital cortex. This is the reason why a right homonymous hemianopia is generally present in pure alexia (in 91.5% of the cases according to Leff *et al.*, 2001b). However, reading disability in pure alexics is not related to perimetric deprivation (Leff *et al.*, 2006): on the one hand, reading in pure alexics is hampered also when the whole word is placed within the boundary of the spared hemifield (Behrmann *et al.*, 2001), on the other hand, damage restricted to the occipitotemporal junction with no involvement of the occipital cortex[10] produces reading disability without hemianopia.

It should be noted in this respect that the prevalence of pure alexia is lower compared to hemianopic alexia. The explanation is anatomical: of the four branches of the posterior cerebral artery (anterior and posterior temporal artery, parieto-occipital artery, and calcarine artery), the anterior and the posterior temporal artery originate from the posterior cerebral artery at almost 90° angle and feed the fusiform gyrus. The abrupt deviation of the circulatory flow at this level reduces the probability for emboli to enter the temporal branches causing infarction of the VWFA; on the contrary, it is more probable they continue along the parieto-occipital and calcarine artery, reaching the striate cortex (Leff *et al.*, 2006). It remains, however, that, as highlighted by Leff and associates, <<[...,] pure alexia and hemianopic alexia form a continuum, and patients with aspects of both syndromes will have an intermediate lesion profile [...]>> (Leff *et al.*, 2006, p. 1007).

Interestingly, the callosal fibers connecting the right occipitotemporal junction (ROTJ: *i.e.* the correspondent region of the VWFA in the right hemifield that Cohen and colleagues (2003) call R-VWFA) to the left occipitotemporal junction may compensate for the defective function of the VWFA, preventing or reducing the severity of pure alexia (Cohen *et al.*, 2003; Leff *et al.*, 2001b). For this reason, the syndrome is more common in the presence of white matter destruction, especially of the splenium. In other terms, if the VWFA is damaged but the white matter is only partially involved, symptoms may be less severe as the R-VWFA in the ROTJ may mitigate the reading disability (Bartolomeo *et al.*, 1998). The letter-by-letter reading strategy of pure alexics, indeed, may be driven by the R-VWFA in the ROTJ that acts as a letter identification center (Cohen *et al.*, 2003).

In general, any cortical damage that blocks access to the VWFA from both hemispheres may generate pure alexia (Patterson and Kay, 1982). Cohen and associates (2004) reported the case of a patient with letter-by-letter reading following surgical removal of left occipitotemporal regions that spared the VWFA. Evidently, the deafferentiation of the left fusiform gyrus, where the VWFA is located, was the factor responsible for the reading disability.

The lexical "information processing" model described by Coslett (2000) clarifies the possible reading strategies used by normal and pure alexic subjects (figure A.2). In normal conditions the lexical route, which implies parallel processing of words

[10]A rare occurrence: see Benito-León *et al.*, 1997; Iragui and Kritchevsky, 1991; Caffarra, 1987; Henderson *et al.*, 1985; Greenblatt, 1973, 1976.

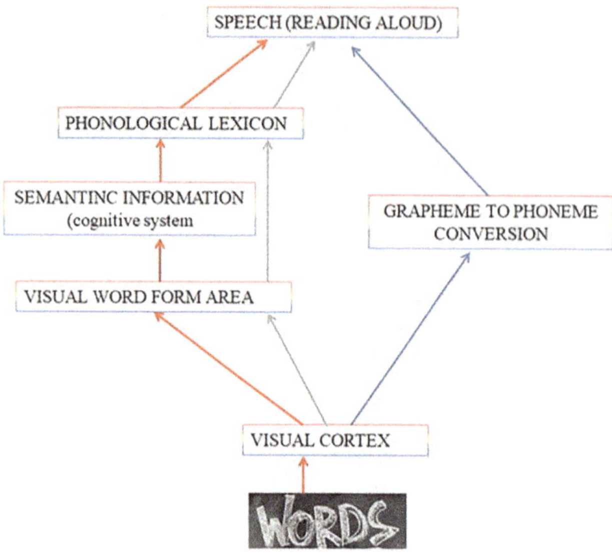

FIG. A2 – The information processing model for oral reading. Based on Coslett (2000, p. 421, fig. 1). Red: normal reading (lexical route); blue: letter-by-letter reading (sublexical route); gray: lexical route with no semantic information ("direct reading route"). Subjects who use the direct reading route can read aloud words that they are not able to comprehend.

and activation of the VWFA, is used. In the case of letter-by-letter reading, there is direct grapheme–to–phoneme conversion.

In pure alexia, the deficit takes place at an early stage of the lexical processing, precisely when visual information is extracted from the text and processed by the VWFA, and not at the higher level of activation of semantic representations (top-down processing). The impaired bottom-up information is suggested by the word-length effect and by the frequent substitution of letters. In support of this hypothesis, low-pass filtered text (early degradation of the lexical content) is read by normal subjects as if they were pure alexics, with increased letter confusability and word length effect (Fiset *et al.*, 2006). According to Johnson and Rayner, the reading characteristics of pure alexics can be clarified by the Interactive Activation Model (IAM: Behrmann *et al.*, 1998) which assumes that reading is the result of the integration of bottom-up and top-down processing. Quoting Johnson and Rayner: "The reader extracts low-level perceptual conformation about the visual letter features which provide bottom-up information about the stimulus. At the same time, processing occurs at higher levels, thereby providing top-down information" (Johnson and Rayner, 2007, p. 2248). Top-down information, which includes word frequency, facilitates low-level processing. In pure alexia bottom-up processing related to the VWFA is impaired, as revealed by the word length effect and frequent letter confusability. On the contrary, higher-order processing is intact, as demonstrated by the shorter fixation duration and the few number of fixations on high-frequency words compared to low-frequency words: short fixation duration and their reduced number are signs that high-frequency words are read more easily. This indicates that patients rely heavily on top-down processing (Johnson and Rayner, 2007; Behrmann *et al.*, 2001). In their study on a patient suffering from pure alexia, Johnson and Rayner reported that this frequency effect was even greater than in normal control readers. Behrmann and colleagues quantified the frequency effect of pure alexics as 2.4 times greater than that of normal readers. The same applies to word predictability (Johnson and Rayner, 2007).

In sum, the abnormal word length effect in the presence of normal or super-normal sensitivity to word frequency reveals that bottom-up and top-down levels of text processing interact and that in pure alexics the defective bottom-up effect tends to be compensated by the strong reliance on higher order lexical processing (Johnson and Rayner, 2007; Behrmann *et al.*, 2001). If the low level-impairment of pure alexics is believed to be localized in the VWFA, the cerebral regions supposedly in charge of the top-down compensatory effect are in more frontal regions: these areas, in fact, would be related to word frequency effects according to Fiebach and Friederici (fMRI study: Fiebach and Friederici, 2002).

The variability of the word length effect among word-by-word readers is characteristic (see for example Leff *et al.*, 2001b; Behrmann *et al.*, 1998). It depends on the fact that the high-order lexical representations intervene to support bottom-up information in each subject to a different extent. This is explained by Behrmann *et al.* (1998b) in terms of different reliance on higher-order processing. In the most severe cases, profoundly weakened bottom-up information makes the engagement of the top-down processing scarce; likewise, in milder cases, the top-down support is largely unnecessary as the bottom-up information is effective enough. Instead, pure alexics in the middle range of severity are those who most of all benefit from the higher-order activation.

Yet, a stream of research argued against the selective damage to the VWFA and posits that the reading disability of pure alexics is a specific manifestation of a generalized defect in object processing (Behrmann *et al.*, 1998; Sekuler and Behrmann, 1996; Farah, 1992; Farah and Wallace, 1991; Friedman and Alexander, 1984; Kinsbourne and Warrington, 1962). In effect, even if pure alexics do not suffer from evident visual agnosia, they are found to perform worse than controls in object recognition (Behrmann *et al.*, 1998). Within this visuoperceptive impairment, the selective reading deficit is explained by the particular difficulty (thereby the increased susceptibility to damage) of the lexical function.

According to Friedman and Alexander (1984), the global perceptual impairment of pure alexics refers specifically to the rapid identification of the visual input: rapid visual identification, indeed, is crucial in reading and less important in object recognition. So, a generalized reduced speed in visual identification would be the factor responsible for defective object identification, and, even more, for the reading difficulty of pure alexics.

A.2 Classifications of Pure Alexias

Based on the type of errors, Patterson and Kay (1982) classified letter-by-letter reading into two types:

- in type I, patients suffer solely from a letter processing deficit: patients of this class generally do not make errors when reading a word after they have read correctly each letter ("classical letter-by-letter readers").
- in type II, patients suffer not only from a letter processing deficit but also from a deficit at the lexical level. These patients tend to make word recognition errors also if they have identified all the letters of the word: as a consequence, type II patients generally read slower than type I. The presence of these subtypes accounts for the large variability in reading speed among pure alexics. However, the reason for this distinction is not yet clear. Hanley and Kay (1996) examined two type I and type II alexic patients to assess if the faster reading rate of type I depends on residual (even if inefficient) parallel word processing,[11] on better letter recognition[12], or, finally, on a different speed of reading identification. They ruled out the parallel processing and did not produce evidence that the faster reading speed of type I alexics depends on better letter recognition. The authors concluded that type II reading is slower than type I because type II process individual letters at a lower speed, and make word recognition errors despite correctly identifying the letters of the word. These findings suggest that in type II the involvement of the visual word form area is more severe than in type I.

Damasio and Damasio (1983) provided an anatomo-functional classification of pure alexia:

- type I is characterized by an impairment of the anterior and ventral occipitotemporal cortex including the VWFA and interhemispheric connections. This type corresponds to the case of global alexia described by Cohen *et al.* (2003);
- type II follows a lesion of the left calcarine cortex and deafferentiation of the VWFA (pure alexia with right-sided hemianopia);
- type III is due to small lesions to the left ventral occipitotemporal cortex with partial or complete sparing of the visual field.

In addition, selective destruction of the splenium that interrupts the connection between the VWFA and the right occipital area determines a form of pure alexia limited to the left visual hemifield (so-called "callosal alexia": Cohen *et al.*, 2000; Abe *et al.*, 1986; Levine and Calvanio, 1980): in fact, the efference from the left occipital area (right hemifield) to the VWFA is preserved, while the efference from the right occipital area (left hemifield) is disrupted. Cohen and associates reported an fMRI study of two patients with damage to the posterior part of their corpus callosum who were unable to read tachistoscopic words presented in their left hemifield but performed like controls for words displayed in the right hemifield (Cohen *et al.*, 2000). Interestingly, non-words in the left hemifield were read correctly, suggesting the right hemisphere may have a role in the recognition of non-words (see further; see Cohen *et al.*, 2000 for details).

[11]Residual parallel letter processing takes place in pure alexics, but is largely inefficient as it is hampered by a level of background noise that prevents the identification of the word (Arguin *et al.*, 2002; Howard, 1991).

[12]The more accurate is letter recognition, the faster is word recognition (Shallice, 1988).

Finally, in 1986 Horner and Massey described a case, they defined as "dynamic spelling alexia", in a subject who suffered a left posterior temporal stroke with right superior quadrantanopia. He developed a dynamic form of pure alexia as he was unable to read static words, but could read letter-by-letter words presented dynamically (1 letter per second). Right hemineglect, disorganized left-to-right scanning, and visuospatial misperception leading to copying deficits were associated. The authors interpreted this clinical condition as a particular form of "impaired recognition of statically-presented stimuli with relatively preserved recognition of dynamically-presented stimuli" (Horner and Massey, 1986). The authors pinpointed that the lesion of their patient was larger than those generally responsible for typical pure alexia.

A.3 Differential Diagnosis with Hemianopic Alexia

Disentangling pure alexia from hemianopic alexia is not easy as most pure alexics show right-sided hemianopic defects. The differential diagnosis relies on:

- the word length effect, absent or far less evident in hemianopes[13]: an arbitrary cut-off to differentiate pure alexics from hemianopic alexics is 100 ms per additional letter when reading single words (Leff *et al.*, 2006) and 50 ms per additional letter when reading a text (Pflugshaupt *et al.*, 2009). The main limitation in the use of this parameter is the variability of the magnitude of the WLE;
- lesion analysis with imaging showing a lesion to the VWFA. The involvement of the cerebral region corresponding to the VWFA, indeed, is highly indicative of pure alexia (Pflugshaupt *et al.*, 2009; Leff *et al.*, 2006; Henry *et al.*, 2005; Cohen *et al.*, 2003). Yet, it is worth recalling that in rare cases letter-by-letter reading has been reported in patients with intact VWFA and left thalamic hemorrhage (Hanley and Kay, 1996) or even after right-sided cortical lesion (Tsapkini *et al.*, 2005; Leśniak *et al.*, 2014);
- the oculomotor pattern: pure alexics show a consistent positive correlation between the number of fixations per word and word length, contrary to left- and right-sided hemianopic patients (Pflugshaupt *et al.*, 2009; Behrmann *et al.*, 2001). So, when present, the homonymous visual field defects in pure alexics are not causally related to their characteristic letter-by-letter reading.

A.4 The Oculomotor Pattern of Pure Alexics

Pure alexics do not show a primary impairment of the ocular movements that accounts for their reading disability, as demonstrated by a normal visual search performance (Behrmann *et al.*, 2001). However, ocular movements during reading differ greatly from normal readers, and are characterized by more fixations per word, longer fixation time, smaller amplitude of forward saccades, and more backward

[13]When present, the slight WLE in right-sided hemianopia is inversely related to the macular sparing (Pflugshaupt *et al.*, 2009).

saccades (Pflugshaupt *et al.*, 2009; Behrmann *et al.*, 2001). In addition, a positive correlation between the number of fixations per word and word length reveals WLE (Pflugshaupt *et al.*, 2009; Behrmann *et al.*, 2001: figure A4).

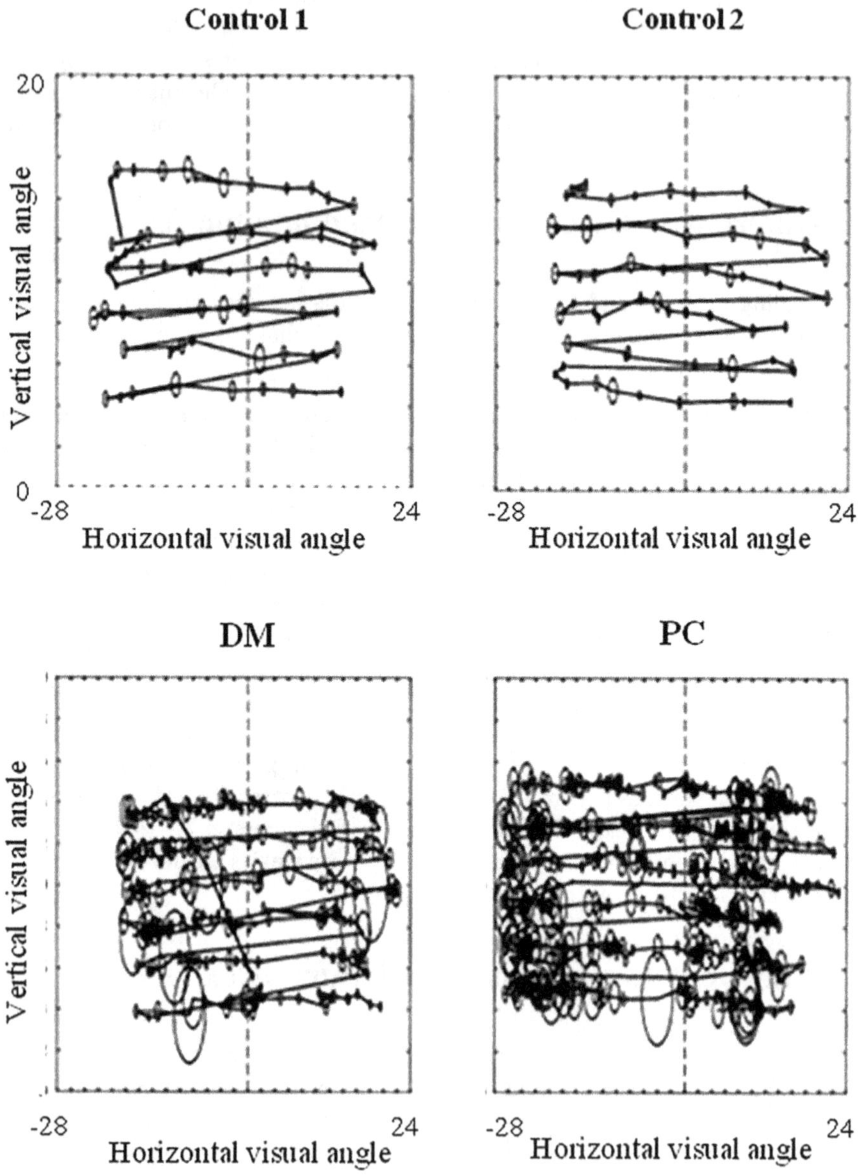

FIG. A4 – The oculomotor pattern (number and duration of fixations) in the two pure alexics examined by Behrmann and colleagues. From Behrmann *et al.* (2001). With permission of Elsevier.

Rayner and Johnson (2005) compared the oculomotor pattern of a pure alexic patient with that of six normal subjects forced to read in a letter-by-letter fashion by applying the moving-window paradigm (see Rayner and Bertera, 1979; McConkie and Rayner, 1975). The moving window was calibrated so that only one letter at a time or three letters at a time could be read. Reading time, number of fixations, fixation durations, and saccade length of the normal readers were similar to that of the pure alexic patient in the one-letter-at-a-time simulated condition. This finding confirms that pure alexics are letter-by-letter readers, and their oculomotor pattern is the consequence of this lexical strategy.

A.5 The Residual Reading Ability of Pure Alexics

The residual reading ability of pure alexics may depend on a residual function of the VWFA, as suggested by Behrmann and colleagues (1998), or on the activation of the right hemisphere. As recalled by Coslett and his group, indeed, there is evidence that the right hemisphere, traditionally considered “illiterate”, has the capacity to read to some extent, therefore could be responsible for the residual lexical function in patients (*e.g.* Coslett, 2000; Coslett and Monsul, 1994; Coslett and Saffran, 1989). This is shown by the case described by Patterson and colleagues: N.I. was a girl with Rasmussen’s encephalitis who underwent a left hemispherectomy for intractable epilepsy. After the operation, she could read about one-third of single words (Patterson *et al.*, 1989). Another example is the case of a pure alexic subject who had partially recovered the lexical function. The recovery was disrupted by transcranial magnetic stimulation of the right hemisphere [See Coslett, 2000 for a more exhaustive explanation].

It remains that higher-order lexical factors in terms of activation of semantic or lexical representation are intact in alexic patients and are maximally exploited to overcome their lexical problems (Johnson and Rayner, 2007).

References

Abe T., Nakamura N., Sugishita M., Kato Y., Iwata M. (1986) Partial disconnection syndrome following penetrating stab wound of the brain, *Eur. Neurol.* **25**, 233–239.

Adair J.C., Williamson D.J., Jacobs D.H., Heilman K.M. (1995) Neglect of radial and vertical space: Importance of the retinotopic reference frame, *J. Neurol. Neurosurg. Psychiatry* **58**, 724–728.

Aghababian V., Nazir T.A. (2000) Developing normal reading skills: Aspects of the visual processes underlying word recognition, *J. Exp. Child Psychol.* **76**, 123–150.

Ahissar M., Hochstein S. (1997) Task difficulty and the specificity of perceptual learning, *Nature* **387**, 401–406.

Albert M.L. (1973) A simple test of visual neglect, *Neurology* **23**, 658–664.

Aleci C. (2021) *Measuring the soul-psychophysics for non-psychophysicists.* EDP Sciences Publisher, Les Ulis, France.

Aleci C., Pira F. (2018) Bidimensional spatial distortion in quadrantanopia depends on the cortical damage and not on the deprived region in the visual field, *Ophthalmol. Res.: Int. J.* **9**(3), 1–11.

Ali M., Hazelton C., Lyden P., Pollock A., Brady M. (2013) Recovery from poststroke visual impairment: Evidence from a clinical trials resource, *Neurorehabil. Neural Repair* **27**(2), 133–141.

Allegri R.F. (2000) Attention and neglect: Neurological basis, assessment and disorders, *Rev. Neurol.* **30**(5), 491–494.

Anderson S.W. (2003) Neuropsychologic rehabilitation for visuoperceptual impairments, *Neurol. Clin.* **21**, 729–740.

Anderson S.W., Rizzo M. (1994) Hallucinations following occipital lobe damage: The pathological activation of visual representations, *J. Clin. Exp. Neuropsychol.* **16**, 651–663.

Angeli V., Benassi M.G., Làdavas E. (2004) Recovery of oculo-motor bias in neglect patients after prism adaptation, *Neuropsychologia* **42**, 1223–1234.

Antonucci G., Judica A., Menghini G., Pizzamiglio L. (1992) Optokinetic stimulation in the rehabilitation of visual neglect [Abstract], *J. Clin. Exp. Neuropsychol.* **14**, 387.

Apfelbaum H.L., Ross N.C., Bowers A.R., Peli E. (2013) Considering apical scotomas, confusion, and diplopia when prescribing prisms for homonymous hemianopia, *Transl. Vision Sci. Technol.* **2** (4), 2. https://doi.org/10.1167/tvst.2.4.2.

Arguin M., Fiset S., Bub D. (2002) Sequential and parallel letter processing in letter-by-letter dyslexia, *Cognit. Neuropsychol.* **19**, 535–555.

Bach-y-Rita P. (1983) Controlling variables eliminates hemianopia rehabilitation results, *Behav. Brain Sci.* **6**(3), 488.

Bailey I. (1978) Mirrors for visual field defects, *Optom. Mon.* **69**, 1073–1078.

Bailey I. (2007) The optometric examination of the older adult, *Rosenbloom and Morgan's vision and aging* (A.A.J. Rosenbloom, Ed.). Butterworth-Heinemann, St. Louis, USA, pp. 133–162.

Balliet R., Blood K., Bach-y-Rita P. (1985) Visual field rehabilitation in the cortically blind? *J. Neurol. Neurosurg. Psychiatry* **48**(11), 1113–1124.

Barbieri C., De Renzi E. (1989) Patterns of neglect dissociation, *Behav. Neurol.* **2**(1), 13–24.

Barbur J.L., Harlow A.J., Weiskrantz L. (1994) Spatial and temporal response properties of residual vision in a case of hemianopia, *Philos. Trans. R. Soc. Lond. B: Biol. Sci.* **343**, 157–166.

Barbur J.L., Ruddock K.H., Waterfield V.A. (1980) Human visual responses in the absence of the geniculo-calcarine projection, *Brain* **103**, 905–928.

Barbur J.L., Watson J.D., Frackowiak R.S., Zeki S. (1993) Conscious visual perception without V1, *Brain* **116**, 1293–1302.

Bartolomeo P., Bachoud-Levi A.C., Degos J.D., Boller F. (1998) Disruption of residual reading capacity in a pure alexic patient after a mirror-image right-hemispheric lesion, *Neurology* **50**, 286–288.

Barton J.J., Behrmann M., Black S. (1998) Ocular search during line bisection. The effects of hemi-neglect and hemianopia, *Brain* **121**, 1117–1131.

Barton J.J., Black S.E. (1998) Line bisection in hemianopia, *J. Neurol. Neurosurg. Psychiatry* **64**, 660–662.

Barton J.J.S., Behrmann M., Black S.E., *et al.* (1997) Eye movements during line bisection in left hemi-neglect and left hemianopia, *Neurology* **48**(suppl), A197.

Baumann T.P., Spear P.D. (1977) Role of the lateral suprasylvian visual area in behavioral recovery from effects of visual cortex damage in cats, *Brain Res.* **138**, 445–468.

Behrmann M., Black S.E., McKeeff T.J., Barton J.J.S. (2002) Oculographic analysis of word reading in hemispatial neglect, *Physiol. Behav.* **77**, 613–619.

Behrmann M., Moscovitch M., Black S.E., Mozer M. (1990) Perceptual and conceptual mechanisms in neglect dyslexia, *Brain* **113**, 1163–1183.

Behrmann M., Nelson J., Sekuler E.B. (1998) Visual complexity in letter-by-letter reading: 'Pure' alexia is not so pure, *Neuropsychologia* **36**, 1115–1132.

Behrmann M., Plaut D.C., Nelson J. (1998b) A literature review and new data supporting an interactive account of letter-by-letter reading, *Cognit. Neuropsychol.* **15**, 7–51.

Behrmann M., Shomstein S.S., Black S.E., Barton J.J.S. (2001) The eye movements of pure alexic patients during reading and nonreading tasks, *Neuropsychologia* **9**, 983–1002.

Behrmann M., Watt S., Black S.E., Barton J.J.S. (1997) Impaired visual search in patients with unilateral neglect: An oculographic analysis, *Neuropsychologia* **35**, 1445–1458.

Belliveau J.W., Kennedy D.N., McKinstry R.C., Buchbinder B.R., Weisskoff R.M., Cohen M.S., Vevea J.M., Brady T.J., Rosen B.R. (1991) Functional mapping of the human visual cortex by magnetic resonance imaging, *Science* **254**, 716–719.

Bender M.B., Strauss I. (1937) Defects in visual field of one eye only in patients with a lesion of one optic radiation, *Arch. Ophthalmol.* **17**, 765–787.

Benito-León J., Sánchez-Suarez C., Díaz-Guzmán J., Martinez-Salio A. (1997) Pure alexia could not be a disconnection syndrome, *Neurology* **49**, 305–306.

Benton S., Levy I., Swash M. (1980) Vision in the temporal crescent in occipital infarction, *Brain* **103**, 83–97.

Berberovic N., Pisella L., Morris A.P., Mattingley J.B. (2004) Prismatic adaptation reduces biased temporal order judgements in spatial neglect, *Neuroreport* **15**, 1199–1204.

Bergsma D.P., van der Wildt G. (2010) Visual training of cerebral blindness patients gradually enlarges the visual field, *Br. J. Ophthalmol.* **94**, 88–96.

Bertini C., Leo F., Làdavas E. (2008) Temporonasal asymmetry in multisensory integration mediated by the Superior Colliculus, *Brain Res.* **1242**, 37–44.

Binder J.R., Mohr J.P. (1992) The topography of callosal reading pathways. A case-control analysis, *Brain* **115**, 1807–1826.

Bischoff P., Lang J., Huber A. (1995) Macular sparing as a perimetric artifact, *Am. J. Ophthalmol.* **119**, 72–80.

Bisiach E. (1991) Extinction and neglect: Same or different? *Brain and space* (J. Paillard, Ed.). Oxford University Press, Oxford, UK, pp. 251–257.

Bisiach E., Capitani E., Porta E. (1985) Two basic properties of space representation in the brain, *J. Neurol. Neurosurg. Psychiatry* **48**, 141–144.

Bisiach E., Meregalli S., Berti A. (1990) Mechanisms of production control and belief fixation in human visuospatial processing: Clinical evidence from hemispatial neglect and misrepresentation, *Quantitative analyses of behavior. Computational and clinical approaches to pattern recognition and concept formation*, vol. IX (M.L. Commons, R.J. Herrnstein, S.M. Kosslyn and D.B. Mumford, Eds). Lawrence Erlbaum, Hillsdale, NJ, pp. 3–21.

Bisiach E., Vallar G., Perani D., Papagno C., Berti A. (1986) Unawareness of disease following lesions of the right hemisphere: Anosognosia for hemiplegia and anosognosia for hemianopia, *Neuropsychologia* **24**, 471–482.

Blanchard H.E., Pollatsek A., Rayner K. (1989) The acquisition of parafoveal word information in reading, *Percept. Psychophys.* **46**, 85–94.

Bodis-Wollner I., Diamond S.P. (1976) The measurements of spatial contrast sensitivity in cases of blurred vision associated with cerebral lesions, *Brain* **99**, 695–710.

Bogousslavsky J., Miklossy J., Regli F., Deruaz J.P., Assal G., Delaloye B. (1988) Subcortical neglect: Neuropsychological, SPECT, and neuropathological correlations with anterior choroidal artery territory infarction, *Ann. Neurol.* **23**, 448–452.

Bolognini N., Frassinetti F., Làdavas E. (2005b) Acoustical vision of below threshold stimuli: Interaction among spatially converging stimuli, *Exp. Brain Res.* **160**, 273–282.

Bolognini N., Rasi F., Coccia M., Làdavas E. (2005a) Visual search improvement in hemianopic patients after audio-visual stimulation, *Brain* **128**, 2830–2842.

Bosley T.M., Dann R., Silver F.L., Alavi A., Kushner M., Chawluk J.B., Savino P.J., Sergott R.C., Schatz N.J., Reivich M. (1987) Recovery of vision after ischemic lesions: Positron emission tomography, *Ann. Neurol.* **21**(5), 444–450.

Bosley T.M., Rosenquist A.C., Kushner M., Burke A., Stein A., Dann R. (1985) Ischemic lesions of the occipital cortex and optic radiations: Positron emission tomography, *Neurology* **35**, 470–484.

Bowers A.R., Keeney K., Peli E. (2008) Community-based trial of a peripheral prism visual field expansion device for hemianopia, *Arch. Ophthalmol.* **126**, 657–664.

Bowers A.R., Keeney K., Peli E. (2014) Randomized crossover clinical trial of real and sham peripheral prism glasses for hemianopia, *JAMA Ophthalmol.* **132**, 214–222.

Bowers A.R., Tant M., Peli E. (2012) A pilot evaluation of on-road detection performance by drivers with hemianopia using oblique peripheral prisms, *Stroke Res. Treat.* **2012**, 176806. https://doi.org/10.1155/2012/176806.

Boyer J.L., Harrison S., Ro T. (2005) Unconscious processing of orientation and color without primary visual cortex, *Proc. Natl. Acad. Sci. USA* **102**(46), 16875–16879.

Brandt T., Thie A., Caplan L.R., Hacke W. (1995) Infarcts in the brain areas supplied by the posterior cerebral artery. Clinical aspects, pathogenesis and prognosis, *Nervenarzt* **66**(4), 267–274.

Braun C., Weber J., Schiefer U., Skalej M., Dietrich T. (2001) Hyperexcitatory activity in visual cortex in homonymous hemianopia after stroke, *Clin. Neurophysiol.* **112**, 336–343.

Braun J.J., Meyer P.P., Meyer D.R. (1966) Sparing of a brightness habit in rats following visual decortication, *J. Comp. Physiol. Psychol.* **61**, 79–82.

Bridge H., Thomas O., Jbabdi S., Cowey A. (2008) Changes in connectivity after visual cortical brain damage underlie altered visual function, *Brain* **131**, 1433–1444.

Brown W.S., Bierke M.D., Galbraith G.C. (1998) Interhemispheric transfer in normals and acallosals: Latency adjusted evoked potential averaging, *Cortex* **34**, 677–692.

Bruce C.J., Goldberg M.E. (1985) Primate frontal eye fields. I. Single neurons discharging before saccades, *J. Neurophysiol.* **53**, 603–635.

Brunn J.L., Farah M.J. (1981) The relation between spatial attention and reading: Evidence from the neglect syndrome, *Cognit. Neuropsychol.* **8**, 59–75.

Buchkremer-Ratzmann I., Witte O.W. (1997) Extended brain disinhibition following small photothrombotic lesions in rat frontal cortex, *NeuroReport* **8**, 519–522.

Bulens C., Meerwaldt J.D., Van Der Wildt G.J., Keemink C.J. (1989) Spatial contrast sensitivity in unilateral cerebral ischaemic lesions involving the posterior visual pathway, *Brain* **112**, 507–520.

Bullier J., Kennedy H. (1983) Projection of the lateral geniculate nucleus onto cortical area V2 in the macaque monkey, *Exp. Brain Res.* **53**, 168–172.

Bunt A.H., Minckler D.S. (1977) Foveal sparing: New anatomical evidence for bilateral representation of the central retina, *Arch. Ophthalmol.* **95**, 1445–1447.

Bunt A.H., Minckler D.S., Johanson G.W. (1977) Demonstration of bilateral projections of the central retina of the monkey with horseradish peroxidase neuronography, *J. Comp. Neurol.* **171**, 619–630.

Caffarra P. (1987) Alexia without agraphia or hemianopia, *Eur. Neurol.* **27**, 65–71. https://doi.org/10.1159/000116133.

Campion J., Latto R., Smith Y.M. (1983) Is blindsight an effect of scattered light, spared cortex, and near-threshold vision? *Behav. Brain Sci.* **6**, 423–486.

Cantoni C., Piccirilli M. (1997) Dissociation in the recovery from neglect dyslexia and visuo-spatial unilateral neglect: A case report, *Ital. J. Neurol. Sci.* **18**, 41–43.

Cappelletti M., Freeman E.D., Cipolotti L. (2007) The middle house or the middle floor: Bisecting horizontal and vertical mental number lines in neglect, *Neuropsychologia* **45**, 2989–3000.

Cassidy T.P., Bruce D.W., Lewis S., Gray C.S. (1999) The association of visual field deficits and visuo-spatial neglect in acute right-hemisphere stroke patients, *Age Ageing* **28**(3), 257–260.

Çelebisoy M., Çelebisoy N., Bayam E., Köse T. (2011) Recovery of visual-field defects after occipital lobe infarction: A perimetric study, *J. Neurol. Neurosurg. Psychiatry* **82**(6), 695–702.

Celesia G.G., Brigell M.G., Vaphiades M.S. (1997) Hemianopic anosognosia, *Neurology* **49**, 88–97.

Celesia G.G., Bushnell D., Toleikis S.C., Brigell M.G. (1991) Cortical blindness and residual vision: Is the second visual system in humans capable of more than rudimentary visual perception? *Neurology* **41**, 862–869.

Chatterjee A. (1994) Picturing unilateral spatial neglect: Viewer versus object centred reference frames, *J. Neurol. Neurosurg. Psychiatry* **57**, 1236–1240.

Chédru F., Leblanc M., Lhermitte F. (1973) Visual searching in normal and brain-damaged subjects (contribution to the study of unilateral inattention), *Cortex* **9**, 94–111.

Cherney L.R., Halper A.S., Kwasnica C.M., Harvey R.L., Zhang M. (2001) Recovery of functional status after right hemisphere stroke: Relationship with unilateral neglect, *Arch. Phys. Med. Rehabil.* **82**(3), 322–328.

Chokron S., Imbert M. (1995) Variations of the egocentric reference among normal subjects and a patient with unilateral neglect, *Neuropsychologia* **35**, 703–711.

Clisby C. (1995) Visual assessment of patients with cerebrovascular accident on the elderly care wards, *Br. Orthopt. J.* **52**, 38–40.

Clower D.M., Hoffman J.M., Votaw J.R., Faber T.L., Woods R.P., Alexander G.E. (1996) Role of posterior parietal cortex in the recalibration of visually guided reaching, *Nature* **383**, 618–621.

Cohen J.M., Wass B. (1996) Visual field remediation, *Remediation and management of low vision* (R.G. Cole and B.P. Rosenthal, Eds). Mosby, St. Louis, USA, pp. 1–24.

Cohen L., Dehaene S. (2004) Specialization within the ventral stream: The case for the visual word form area, *NeuroImage* **22**(1), 466–476.

Cohen L., Dehaene S., Naccache L., Lehéricy S., Dehaene-Lambertz G., Hénaff M.A., Michel F. (2000) The visual word form area: Spatial and temporal characterization of an initial stage of reading in normal subjects and posterior split-brain patients, *Brain* **123**, 291–307.

Cohen L., Henry C., Dehaene S., Martinaud O., Lehericy S., Lemer C., Ferrieux S. (2004) The pathophysiology of letter-by-letter reading, *Neuropsychologia* **42**, 1768–1780.

Cohen L., Lehéricy S., Chochon F., Lemer C., Rivaud S., Dehahene S. (2002) Language-specific tuning of visual cortex? Functional properties of the visual word form area, *Brain* **125**(5), 1054–1069.

Cohen L., Martinaud O., Lemer C., Lehéricy S., Samson Y., Obadia M., Slachevsky A., Dehaene S. (2003) Visual word recognition in the left and right hemispheres: Anatomical and functional correlates of peripheral alexias, *Cereb. Cortex* **13**, 1313–1333.

Corbetta M. (1998) Frontoparietal cortical networks for directing attention and the eye to visual locations: Identical, independent, or overlapping neural systems? *Proc. Natl. Acad. Sci.* **95**, 831–838.

Coslett H.B. (2000) Acquired dyslexias, *Semin. Neurol.* **20**(4), 419–426.

Coslett H.B., Monsul N. (1994) Reading and the right hemisphere: Evidence from transcranial magnetic stimulation, *Brain Lang.* **46**, 198–211.

Coslett H.B., Saffran E.M. (1989) Evidence for preserved reading in pure alexia, *Brain* **112**, 327–359.

Costello A.D., Warrington E.K. (1987) The dissociation of visuospatial neglect and neglect dyslexia, *J. Neurol. Neurosurg. Psychiatry* **50**, 1110–1116.

Cowey A. (1967) Perimetric study of field defects in monkeys after cortical and retinal ablations, *Q. J. Exp. Psychol.* **19**, 232–245.

Cowey A., Rolls E.T. (1974) Human cortical magnification factor and its relation to visual acuity, *Exp. Brain Res.* **21**, 447–454.

Cubelli R., Nichelli P., Bonito V., De Tanti A., Inzaghi M.G. (1991) Different patterns of dissociation in unilateral spatial neglect, *Brain Cognit.* **15**, 139–159.

Damasio A.R., Damasio H. (1983) The anatomic basis of pure alexia, *Neurology* **33**, 1573–1583.

Darian-Smith C., Gilbert C.D. (1994) Axonal sprouting accompanies functional reorganization in adult cat striate cortex, *Nature* **368**, 737–740.

Darian-Smith C., Gilbert C.D. (1995) Topographic reorganization in the striate cortex of the adult cat and monkey is cortically mediated, *J. Neurosci.* **15**, 1631–1647.

Das A. (1997) Plasticity in adult sensory cortex: A review, *Netw.: Comput. Neural Syst.* **8**, R33–R76.

Das A., Gilbert C.D. (1995) Receptive field expansion in adult visual cortex is linked to dynamic changes in strength of cortical connections, *J. Neurophysiol.* **74**, 779–792.

De Luca M., Spinelli D., Zoccolotti P. (1996) Eye movement patterns in reading as a function of visual field defects and contrast sensitivity loss, *Cortex* **32**, 491–502.

Dehaene S., Le Clec H.G., Poline J.B., Le Bihan D., Cohen L. (2002) The visual word form area: A prelexical representation of visual words in the fusiform gyrus, *Neuroreport* **13**, 321–325.

Dehaene S., Naccache L., Cohen L., Le Bihan D., Mangin J.F., Poline J.B., Rivière D. (2001) Cerebral mechanisms of word masking and unconscious repetition priming, *Nat. Neurosci.* **4**, 752–758.

Denes G., Semenza C., Stoppa E., Lis A. (1982) Unilateral spatial neglect and recovery from hemiplegia: A follow-up study, *Brain* **105**, 543–552.

di Pellegrino G., Ladavas E., Galletti C. (2001) Lexical processes and eye movements in neglect dyslexia, *Behav. Neurol.* 2001–2002 **13**, 61–74.

Dilks D.D., Serences J.T., Rosenau B.J., Yantis S., McCloskey M. (2007) Human adult cortical reorganization and consequent visual distortion, *J. Neurosci.* **27**(36), 9585–9594. https://doi.org/10.1523/JNEUROSCI.2650-07.2007.

Dombovy M.L., Aggarwal U. (2000) Stroke rehabilitation, *Physical medicine and rehabilitation: The complete approach* (M. Grabois, S.J. Garrison, K.A. Hart, *et al.*, Eds). Blackwell Scientific Publications, Malden, Mass.

Donaldson I.M.L., Long A.C. (1980) Interactions between extraocular proprioceptive and visual signals in the superior colliculus of the cat, *J. Physiol. (Lond.)* **298**, 85–110.

Driver J., Baylis G.C., Goodrich S.J., Rafal R.D. (1994) Axis-based neglect of visual shapes, *Neuropsychologia* **11**, 1353–1365.

Driver J., Halligan P.W. (1991) Can visual neglect operate in object-centered coordinates: An affirmative single case study, *Cognit. Neuropsychol.* **8**, 475–496.

Duszynski L.R. (1955) Hemianopsia dichroic mirror device, *Am. J. Ophthalmol.* **39**, 876–878.

Ellis A.W., Flude B.M., Young A.W. (1987) Neglect dyslexia and the early visual processing of letters in words and nonwords, *Cognit. Neuropsychol.* **4**, 439–464.

Eriksson P.S., Perfilieva E., Bjork-Eriksson T., Alborn A.M., Nordbord C., Peterson D.A., Gage F. H. (1998) Neurogenesis in the adult human hippocampus, *Nat. Med.* **4**, 1313–1317.

Eysel U., Schmidt-Kastner R. (1991) Neuronal dysfunction at the border of focal cortical lesions in cat visual cortex, *Neurosci. Lett.* **131**, 45–48.

Eysel U.T., Eyding D., Schweigart G. (1998) Repetitive optical stimulation elicits fast receptive field changes in mature visual cortex, *NeuroReport* **9**(5), 949–954.

Eysel U.T., Schweigart G. (1999) Increased receptive field size in the surround of chronic lesions in the adult cat visual cortex, *Cereb. Cortex* **9**, 101–109.

Eysel U.T., Schweigart G., Mittmann T., Eyding D., Arckens L., Qu Y., Vandesande F., Orban G. (1999) Reorganization in the visual cortex after retinal and cortical damage, *Restor. Neurol. Neurosci.* **15**, 153–164.

Farah M.J. (1992) Is an object an object? Cognitive and neuropsychological investigations of domain specificity in visual object recognition, *Curr. Dir. Psychol. Sci.* **1**(5), 164–169.

Farah M.J., Monheit M.A., Wallace M.A. (1991) Unconscious perception of 'extinguished' visual stimuli: Reassessing the evidence, *Neuropsychologia* **29**, 949–958.

Farah M.J., Wallace M. (1991) Pure alexia as a visual impairment: A reconsideration, *Cognit. Neuropsychol.* **8**, 1–19.

Farnè A., Rossetti Y., Toniolo S., Làdavas E. (2002) Ameliorating neglect with prism adaptation: Visuo-manual and visuo-verbal measures, *Neuropsychologia* **40**(7), 718–729.

Fendrich R., Wessinger C.M., Gazzaniga M.S. (1992) Residual vision in a scotoma: Implications for blindsight, *Science* **258**, 1489–1491.

Ferber S., Karnath H.O. (1999) Parietal and occipital lobe contribution to perception of straight ahead orientation, *J. Neurol. Neurosurg. Psychiatry* **67**, 572–578.

Fiebach C.J., Friederici A.D. (2002) fMRI evidence for dual routes to the mental lexicon in visual word recognition, *J. Cognit. Neurosci.* **14**, 11–23.

Findlay J.M. (1982) Global visual processing for saccadic eye movements, *Vision Res.* **22**, 1033–1045.

Fischer B. (1987) The preparation of visually guided saccades, *Rev. Physiol. Biochem. Pharmacol.* **106**, 1–35.

Fischer B., Breitmeyer B. (1987) Mechanisms of visual attention revealed by saccadic eye movements, *Neuropsychologia* **25**, 73–83.

Fischman M.W., Meikle T.H. Jr. (1965) Visual intensity discrimination in cats after serial tectal and cortical lesions, *J. Comp. Physiol. Psychol.* **59**, 193–201.

Fiset S., Arguin M., Fiset D. (2006) An attempt to simulate letter-by-letter dyslexia in normal readers, *Brain Lang.* **98**, 251–263.

Fowler M.S., Wade D.T., Richardson A.J., Stein J.F. (1996) Squints and diplopia seen after brain damage, *J. Neurol.* **243**(1), 86–90. https://doi.org/10.1007/BF00878537.

Fox P.T., Fox J.M., Raichle M.E., Burde R.M. (1985) The role of cerebral cortex in the generation of voluntary saccades: A positron emission tomographic study, *J. Neurophysiol.* **54**, 348–369.

Fox P.T., Miezin F.M., Allman J.M., Van Essen D.C., Raichle M.E. (1987) Retinotopic organization of human visual cortex mapped with positron emission tomography, *J. Neurosci.* **7**, 913–922.

Foxe J.J., Simpson G.V. (2002) Flow of activation from V1 to frontal cortex in humans. A framework for defining "early" visual processing, *Exp. Brain Res.* **142**, 139–150.

Frassinetti F., Angeli V., Meneghello F., Avanzi S., Làdavas E. (2002a) Long-lasting amelioration of visuospatial neglect by prism adaptation, *Brain* **125**, 608–623.

Frassinetti F., Bolognini N., Bottari D., Bonora A., Làdavas E. (2005) Audiovisual integration in patients with visual deficit, *J. Cognit. Neurosci.* **17**, 1442–1452.

Frassinetti F., Bolognini N., Làdavas E. (2002b) Enhancement of visual perception by crossmodal visual-auditory interaction, *Exp. Brain Res.* **147**, 332–343.

Freeman C.F., Rudge N.B. (1988) Cerebrovascular accident and the orthoptist, *Br. Orthopt. J.* **45**, 8–18.

Friedman R.B., Alexander M.P. (1984) Picture, images, and pure alexia, *Cognit. Neuropsychol.* **1**, 9–23.

Fries W. (1981) The projection from the lateral geniculate nucleus to the prestriate cortex of the macaque monkey, *Proc. R. Soc. Lond. B: Biol. Sci.* **213**, 73–86.

Fruhmann-Berger M., Karnath H.-O. (2005) Spontaneous eye and head position in patients with spatial neglect, *J. Neurol.* **252**, 1194–2000.

Fujino T., Kigazawa K., Yamada R. (1986) Homonymous hemianopia. A retrospective review of 140 cases, *Neuro-Ophthalmol.* **6**, 17–21.

Gaillard R., Naccache L., Pinel P., Clémenceau S., Volle E., Hasboun D., Dupont S., Baulac M., Dehaene S., Adam C., Cohen L. (2006) Direct intracranial, fMRI, and lesion evidence for the causal role of left inferotemporal cortex in reading, *Neuron* **50**(2), 191–204. https://doi.org/10.1016/j.neuron.2006.03.031.

Gall C., Franke G.H., Sabel B.A. (2010) Vision-related quality of life in first stroke patients with homonymous visual field defects, *Health Quality Life Outcomes* **8**, 33. http://www.hqlo.com/content/8/1/33.

Gall C., Lucklum J., Sabel B.A., Franke G.H. (2009) Vision- and health-related quality of life in subjects with visual field loss after postchiasmatic lesions, *Invest. Ophthalmol. Visual Sci.* **50**, 2765–2776.

Gall C., Mueller I., Kaufmann C., Sabel B.A. (2006) Effects of long-term use of Vision Restoration Therapy (VRT) and stability of visual field improvements $>$ 3 years. 67th AAPM&R Annual Assembly; Nov, 9–12.

Gall C., Sabel B.A. (2012) Reading performance after vision rehabilitation of subjects with homonymous visual field defects, *PM&R* **4**(12), 928–935.

Gauthier I., Skudlarski P., Gore J.C., Anderson A.W. (2000) Expertise for cars and birds recruits brain areas involved in face recognition, *Nat. Neurosci.* **3**, 191–197.

Gaymard B., Ploner C.J., Rivaud S., Vermersch A.I., Pierrot-Deseilligny C. (1998) Cortical control of saccades, *Exp. Eye Res.* **123**, 159–163.

Gaymard B., Rivaud S., Cassarini J.F., Dubard T., Rancurel G., Agid Y., Pierrot-Deseilligny C. (1998b) Effects of anterior cingulate cortex lesions on ocular saccades in humans, *Exp. Brain Res.* **120**, 173–183.

Giard M.H., Peronnet F. (1999) Auditory-visual integration during multimodal object recognition in humans: A behavioral and electrophysiological study, *J. Cognit. Neurosci.* **11**(5), 473–490. https://doi.org/10.1162/089892999563544.

Gilbert C.D. (1998) Adult cortical dynamics, *Physiol. Rev.* **78**, 467–485.

Gilbert C.D., Das A., Ito M., Kapadia M., Westheimer G. (1996) Spatial integration and cortical dynamics, *Proc. Natl. Acad. Sci. USA* **93**, 615–622.

Gilbert C.D., Wiesel T.N. (1992) Receptive field dynamics in adult primary visual cortex, *Nature* **356**, 150–152.

Giorgi R.G., Woods R.L., Peli E. (2009) Clinical and laboratory evaluation of peripheral prism glasses for hemianopia, *Optom. Visual Sci.* **86**, 492–502.

Girotti F., Casazza M., Musicco M., Avanzini G. (1983) Oculomotor disorders in cortical lesions in man: The role of unilateral neglect, *Neuropsychologia* **21**(5), 543–553. https://doi.org/10.1016/0028-3932(83)90010-6.

Gottlieb D.D. (1988) *Method of using a prism in lens for the treatment of visual field loss.* U.S. Patent 4,779,972.

Gottlieb D.D., Freeman P., Williams M. (1992) Clinical research and statistical analysis of a visual field awareness system, *J. Am. Optom. Assoc.* **63**, 581–588.

Gottlieb D.D., Fuhr A., Hatch W.V., Wright K.D. (1998) Neuro-optometric facilitation of vision recovery after acquired brain injury, *NeuroRehabilitation* **11**(3), 175–199.

Gray C.S., French J.M., Bates D., Cartlidge N.E., Venavles G.S., James O.F. (1989) Recovery of visual fields in acute stroke: Homonymous hemianopia with adverse prognosis, *Age Aging* **18**(6), 419–421.

Greenblatt S.H. (1973) Alexia without agraphia or hemianopsia. Anatomical analysis of an autopsied case, *Brain* **96**, 307–316.

Greenblatt S.H. (1976) Subangular alexia without agraphia or hemianopsia, *Brain Lang.* **3**, 229–245.

Habekost T., Starrfelt R. (2006) Alexia and quadrant-amblyopia: Reading disability after a minor visual field deficit, *Neuropsychologia* **44**, 2465–2476.

Hadidi N., Treat-Jacobson D.J., Lindquist R. (2009) Poststroke depression and functional outcome: A critical review of literature, *Heart Lung* **38**, 151–162.

Halko M., Datta A., Plow E.B., Scaturro J., Bikson M., Merabet L.B. (2011) Neuroplastic changes following rehabilitative training correlate with regional electrical field induced with tDCS, *Neuroimage* **57**, 885–891.

Halligan P.W. (1999) Hemianopia and visual neglect: A question of balance? *J. Neurol. Neurosurg. Psychiatry* **67**, 565–566.

Halligan P.W., Marshall J.C. (1991) Spatial compression and visual neglect, *Cortex* **27**, 623–629.

Halligan P.W., Marshall J.C., Wade D.T. (1990) Do visual field deficits exacerbate visuo-spatial neglect? *J. Neurol. Neurosurg. Psychiatry* **53**, 487–491.

Hämäläinen H.A., Julkunen L.A. (2004) Treatment of visual field defects after stroke, *Adv. Clin. Neurosci. Rehabil.* **3**(6), 17–18.

Hanley J.R., Kay J. (1996) Reading speed in pure alexia, *Neuropsychologia* **34**, 1165–1174.

Hari R., Salmelin R. (1997) Human cortical oscillations: A neuromagnetic view through the skull, *Trends Neurosci.* **20**, 44–49.

Haun A.M., Peli E. (2014) Binocular rivalry with peripheral prisms used for hemianopia rehabilitation, *Ophthalmic Physiol. Opt.* **34**, 573–579.

Haywood M., Coltheart M. (2000) Neglect dyslexia and the early stages of visual word recognition, *Neurocase* **6**, 33–44.

He H.Y., Hodos W., Quinlan E.M. (2006) Visual deprivation reactivates rapid ocular dominance plasticity in adult visual cortex, *J. Neurosci.* **26**, 2951–2955.

Heide W., Kömpf D. (1998) Combined deficits of saccades and visuo-spatial orientation after cortical lesions, *Exp. Brain Res.* **23**, 164–171.

Heilman K.M., Bowers D., Watson R.M. (1983) Performance on hemispatial pointing task by patients with neglect syndrome, *Neurology* **33**, 663–664.

Henderson V.W., Friedman R.B., Teng E.L., Weiner J.M. (1985) Left hemisphere pathways in reading: Inferences from pure alexia without hemianopia, *Neurology* **35**(7), 962–968. https://doi.org/10.1212/wnl.35.7.962.

Henriksson L., Raninen A.N., Näsänen R., Hyvarinen L., Vanni S. (2007) Training-induced cortical representation of a hemianopic hemifield, *J. Neurol. Neurosurg. Psychiatry* (1), 74–81.

Henry C., Gaillard R., Volle E., Chiras J., Ferrieux S., Dehaene S., Cohen L. (2005) Brain activations during letter-by-letter reading: A follow-up study, *Neuropsychologia* **43**, 1983–1989.

Herman P. (1975) The Behr pupil revisited. Anisocoria following cerebrovascular accidents, *Stroke* **6**(6), 697–702.

Herpich F., Melnick M.D., Agosta S., Huxlin K.R., Tadin D., Battelli L. (2019) Boosting learning efficacy with noninvasive brain stimulation in intact and brain-damaged humans, *J. Neurosci.* **39** (28), 5551–5561.

Hillis A.E., Caramazza A. (1995) A framework for interpreting distinctive patterns of hemispatial neglect, *Neurocase* **1**, 189–207.

Hillis A.E., Newhart M., Heidler J., Barker P.B., Herskovits E.H., Degaonkar M. (2005) Anatomy of spatial attention: Insights from perfusion imaging and hemispatial neglect in acute stroke, *J. Neurosci.* **25**, 3161–3167.

Hillis A.E., Rapp B., Benzing L., Caramazza A. (1998) Dissociable coordinate frames of unilateral spatial neglect: "Viewer-centered" neglect, *Brain Cognit.* **37**, 491–526.

Hirsch J., Gilbert C.D. (1993) Long-term changes in synaptic strength along specific intrinsic pathways in the cat's visual cortex, *J. Physiol. (Lond.)* **461**, 247–262.

Hochstein S., Ahissar M. (2002) View from the top: Hierarchies and reverse hierarchies in the visual system, *Neuron* **36**, 791–804.

Holmes G. (1918) Disturbances of vision by cerebral lesions, *Br. J. Ophthalmol.* **2**(7), 353–384.

Holmes G. (1945) The organization of the visual cortex in man, *Proc. R. Soc. Lond. B Biol. Sci.* **132**, 348–361.

Hornak J. (1992) Ocular exploration in the dark by patients with visual neglect, *Neuropsychologia* **30**, 547–552.

Horner J., Massey W. (1986) Dynamic spelling alexia, *J. Neurol. Neurosurg. Psychiatry* **49**, 455–457.

Horton J.C. (2005a) Disappointing results from Nova Vision's visual restoration therapy, *Br. J. Ophthalmol.* **89**, 1–2.

Horton J.C. (2005b) Vision restoration therapy: Confounded by eye movements, *Br. J. Ophthalmol.* **89**, 792–794.

Horton J.C., Dagi L.R., McCrane E.P., de Monasterio F.M. (1990) Arrangement of ocular dominance columns in human visual cortex, *Arch. Ophthalmol.* **108**, 1025–1031.

Horton J.C., Hoyt W.F. (1991) The representation of the visual field in human striate cortex: A revision of the classic Holmes map, *Arch. Ophthalmol.* **109**, 816–824.

Howard D. (1991) Letter-by-letter readers: Evidence for parallel processing, *Basic processes in reading: Visual word recognition* (D. Besner and G.W. Humphreys, Eds). Lawrence Erlbaum Associates Inc., Hillsdale, NJ, pp. 34–76.

Huber A. (1962) Homonymous hemianopia after occipital lobectomy, *Am. J. Ophthalmol.* **54**, 623–629.

Huber A. (1992) Homonymous hemianopia, *Neuro-Ophthalmol.* **12**, 351–366.

Husain M., Mannan S., Hodgson T., Wojciulik E., Driver J., Kennard C. (2001) Impaired spatial working memory across saccades contributes to abnormal search in parietal neglect, *Brain* **124**(5), 941–952.

Huxlin K.R., Riley M.E., Martin T., Kelly K.N., Friedman D.I., Burgin W.S., Hayhoe M. (2009) Perceptual relearning of complex visual motion after V1 damage in humans, *J. Neurosci.* **29**, 3981–3991.

Hyvärinen L., Raninen A.N., Näsänen R.E. (2002) Vision rehabilitation in homonymous hemianopia, *Neuro-Ophthalmol.* **27**, 97–102.

Ikeda M., Saida S. (1978) Span of recognition in reading, *Vision Res.* **18**, 83–88.

Iragui V.J., Kritchevsky M. (1991) Alexia without agraphia or hemianopia in parietal infarction, *J. Neurol. Neurosurg. Psychiatry* **54**, 841–842.

Ishiai S., Furukawa T., Tsukagoshi H. (1987) Eye-fixation patterns in homonymous hemianopia and unilateral spatial neglect, *Neuropsychologia* **25**, 675–679.

Ishiai S., Furukawa T., Tsukagoshi H. (1989) Visuospatial processes of line bisection and the mechanisms underlying unilateral spatial neglect, *Brain* **112**, 1485–1502.

Ishiai S., Sugushita M., Mitani K., Ishizawa M. (1992) Leftward search in left unilateral spatial neglect, *J. Neurol. Neurosurg. Psychiatry* **55**(1), 40–44.

Jamara R.J., Van De Velde F., Peli E. (2003) Scanning eye movements in homonymous hemianopia documented by scanning laser ophthalmoscope retinal perimetry, *Optom. Vision Sci.* **80**, 495–504.

Jeannerod M., Rossetti Y. (1993) Visuonotor coordination as a dissociable visual function: Experimental and clinical evidence, *Baillière's Clin. Neurol.* **2**(2), 439–460.

Jobke S., Kasten E., Sabel B.A. (2009) Visual restoration through extrastriate stimulation in patients with visual field defects: A double-blind and randomized experimental study, *Neural Rehabil. Neural Repair* **23**, 246–255.

Johnson C.W., Diller L. (1986) Exploratory eye movements and visual hemi-neglect, *J. Clin. Exp. Neuropsychol.* **8**, 93–101.

Johnson R.L., Rayner K. (2007) Top-down and bottom-up effects in pure alexia: Evidence from eye movements, *Neuropsychologia* **45**, 2246–2257.

Juan C.H., Walsh V. (2003) Feedback to V1: A reverse hierarchy in vision, *Exp. Brain Res.* **150**, 259–263.

Julkunen L., Tenovuo O., Jääskeläinen S., Hämäläinen H. (2003) Rehabilitation of chronic post-stroke visual field defect with computer-assisted training: A clinical and neurophysiological study, *Restor. Neurol. Neurosci.* **21**, 19–28.

Julkunen L., Tenovuo O., Vorobyev V., Hiltunen J., Teräs M., Jääskeläinen S.K., Hämäläinen H. (2006) Functional brain imaging, clinical and neurophysiological outcome of visual rehabilitation in a chronic stroke patient, *Restor. Neurol. Neurosci.* **24**, 123–132.

Jung J.H., Peli E. (2014) Impact of high power and angle of incidence on prism corrections for visual field loss, *Opt. Eng.* **53**(6), 061707.

Jung J.H., Peli E. (2018) No useful field expansion with full-field prisms, *Optom. Vision Sci.* **95**, 805–813.

Kaas J.H., Krubitzer L.A., Chino Y.M., Langston A.L., Polley E.H., Blair N. (1990) Reorganization of retinotopic cortical maps in adult mammals after lesions of the retina, *Science* **248**, 229–231.

Karmarka U.R., Dan Y. (2006) Experience-dependent plasticity in adult visual cortex, *Neuron* **52** (4), 577–585.

Karnath H.O. (1996) Optokinetic stimulation influences the disturbed perception of body orientation in spatial neglect, *J. Neurol. Neurosurg. Psychiatry* **60**, 217–220.

Karnath H.O., Ferber S., Himmelbach M. (2001) Spatial awareness is a function of the temporal not the posterior parietal lobe, *Nature* **411**, 950–953.

Karnath H.O., Fruhmann Berger M., Kuker W., Rorden C. (2004) The anatomy of spatial neglect based on voxelwise statistical analysis: A study of 140 patients, *Cereb. Cortex* **14**, 1164–1172.

Karnath H.O., Huber W. (1992) Abnormal eye movement behavior during text reading in neglect syndrome: A case study, *Neuropsychologia* **30**, 593–598.

Karnath H.O., Niemeier M., Dichgans J. (1998) Space exploration in neglect, *Brain* **121**, 2357–2367.

Karnath H.O., Schenkel P., Fischer B. (1997) Trunk orientation as the determining factor of the "contralateral" deficit in the neglect syndrome and as the physical anchor of the internal representation of body orientation in space, *Brain* **114**, 1997–2014.

Kasneci E., Sippel K., Aehling K., Heister M., Rosenstiel W., Schiefer U., Papageorgiou E. (2014, Feb 11) Driving with binocular visual field loss? A study on a supervised on-road parcours with simultaneous eye and head tracking. *PLoS One* **9**(2), e87470. https://doi.org/10.1371/journal.pone.0087470. eCollection 2014.

Kasten E., Bunzenthal U., Sabel B.A. (2006) Visual field recovery after vision restoration therapy (VRT) is independent of eye movements: An eye tracker study, *Behav. Brain Res.* **175**, 18–26.

Kasten E., Müller-Oehring E., Sabel B.A. (2001) Stability of visual field enlargement following computer-based restitution training in patients with cerebral damage – Results of a follow-up study, *J. Clin. Exp. Neuropsychol.* **23**, 297–305.

Kasten E., Poggel D.A., Muller-Oehring E., Gothe J., Schulte T., Sabel B.A. (1999) Restoration of vision II: Residual functions and training-induced visual field enlargement in brain-damaged patients, *Restor. Neurol. Neurosci.* **15**, 273–287.

Kasten E., Poggel D.A., Sabel B.A. (2000) Computer-based training of stimulus detection improves color and simple pattern recognition in the defective field of hemianopic subjects, *J. Cognit. Neurosci.* **12**, 1001–1012.

Kasten E., Strasburger H., Sabel B.A. (1997) Programs for diagnosis and therapy of visual field deficits in vision rehabilitation, *Spat. Vision* **10**, 499–503.

Kasten E., Wuest S., Sabel B.A. (1998b) Residual vision in transition zones in patients with cerebral blindness, *J. Clin. Exp. Neuropsychol.* **20**, 581–598.

Kasten E., Wüst S., Behrens-Baumann W., Sabel B.A. (1998a) Computer-based training for the treatment of partial blindness, *Nat. Med.* **4**, 1083–1087.

Katz M. (2004a) Visual acuity through Fresnel, refractive, and hybrid refractive/diffractive prisms, *Optometry* **75**(8), 503–508.

Katz M. (2004b) Contrast sensitivity through hybrid diffractive, Fresnel, and refractive prisms, *Optometry* **75**(8), 509–516.

Katz N.A., Hartman-Maeir A.H., Ring H., Soroker N. (1999) Functional disability and rehabilitation outcome in right hemisphere damaged patients with and without unilateral spatial neglect, *Arch. Phys. Med. Rehabil.* **80**(4), 379–384. https://doi.org/10.1016/s0003-9993(99)90273-3.

Kaul S.N., Boulay G.H.D., Kendall B.E., Russell R.W.R. (1974) Relationship between visual field defect and arterial occlusion in the posterior cerebral circulation, *J. Neurol. Neurosurg. Psychiatry* **37**, 1022–1030.

Kennedy A., Brooks R., Flynn L.-A., Prophet C. (2003) The reader's spatial code, *The mind's eye: Cognitive and applied aspects of eye movement research* (J. Hyönä, R. Radach and H. Deubel, Eds). Elsevier, Oxford, pp. 193–212.

Kentridge R.W., Heywood C.A., Weiskrantz L. (1997) Residual vision in multiple retinal locations within a scotoma: Implications for blindsight, *J. Cognit. Neurosci.* **9**, 191–202.

Kerkhoff G. (1993) Displacement of the egocentric visual midline in altitudinal postchiasmatic scotomata, *Neuropsychologia* **31**(3), 261–265.

Kerkhoff G. (1999) Restorative and compensatory therapy approaches in cerebral blindness – A review, *Restor. Neurol. Neurosci.* **15**, 255–271.

Kerkhoff G. (2000) Neurovisual rehabilitation: Recent developments and future directions, *J. Neurol. Neurosurg. Psychiatry* **68**, 691–706.

Kerkhoff G., Bucher L. (2008) Line bisection as an early method to assess homonymous hemianopia, *Cortex* **44**(2), 200–205.

Kerkhoff G., Münßinger G., Eberle-Strauss G., Stögerer E. (1992a) Rehabilitation of hemianopic alexia in patients with postgeniculate visual field disorders, *Neuropsychol. Rehabil.* **2**, 21–42.

Kerkhoff G., Münßinger G., Haaf E., Eberle-Strauss G., Stögerer E. (1992b) Rehabilitation of homonymous scotomata in patients with postgeniculate damage of the visual system: Saccadic compensation training, *Restor. Neurol. Neurosci.* **4**, 245–254.

Kerkhoff G., Keller I., Ritter V., Marquardt C. (2006) Repetitive optokinetic stimulation induces lasting recovery from visual neglect, *Restor. Neurol. Neurosci.* **24**, 357–369.

Kerkhoff G., Münßinger G., Meier E.K. (1994) Neurovisual rehabilitation in cerebral blindness, *Arch. Neurol.* **51**, 474–481.

Kerkhoff G., Schindler I., Keller I., Marquarot C. (1999) Visual background motion reduces size distortion in spatial neglect, *Neuroreport* **10**, 319–323.

Kinsbourne M. (1970) A model for the mechanism of unilateral neglect of space, *Trans. Am. Neurol. Soc.* **95**, 143–146.

Kinsbourne M. (1987) Mechanisms of unilateral neglect, *Neurophysiological and neuropsychological aspects of spatial neglect* (M. Jeannerod, Ed.). Advances in psychology. No. 45. North-Holland, Amsterdam.

Kinsbourne M. (1993) Orientational bias model of unilateral neglect: Evidence from attentional gradients within hemispace, *Unilateral neglect: Clinical and experimental studies* (I.H. Robertson and J.C. Marshall, Eds). Lawrence Erlbaum Associates, Hillsdale, NJ, pp. 63–86.

Kinsbourne M., Warrington E.K. (1962) A disorder of simultaneous form perception, *Brain* **85**, 461–486.

Kinsbourne M., Warrington E.K. (1962b) A variety of reading disability associated with right hemisphere lesions, *J. Neurol. Neurosurg. Psychiatry* **25**, 339–344.

Koehler P.J., Endtz L.J., Te Velde J., Hekster R.E.M. (1986) Aware or non-aware: On the significance of awareness for the localization of the lesion responsible for homonymous hemianopia, *J. Neurol. Sci.* **75**, 255–262.

Kölmel H.W. (1985) Complex visual hallucinations in the hemianopic field, *J. Neurol. Neurosurg. Psychiatry* **48**(1), 29–38. https://doi.org/10.1136/jnnp.48.1.29.

Kooistra C.A., Heilman K.M. (1989) Hemispatial visual inattention masquerading as hemianopia, *Neurology* **39**, 1125–1127.

Kowler E., Anton S. (1987) Reading twisted text: Implications for the role of saccades, *Vision Res.* **27**, 45–60.

Kurtzberg D., Vaughan H.G. (1977) Electrophysiological observations on the visuomotor system and visual neurosensorium, *Visual evoked potentials in man: New developments* (J.E. Desmedt, Ed.). Clarendon Press, Oxford, pp. 314–331.

Ladavas E. (1987) Is the hemispatial deficit produced by right parietal damage associated with retinal or gravitational coordinates? *Brain* **110**, 167–180.

Ladavas E., Petronio A., Umiltà C. (1990) The deployment of visual attention in the intact field of hemineglect patients, *Cortex* **26**, 307–317.

Lance J.W. (1976) Simple formed hallucinations confined to the area of a specific visual field defect, *Brain* **99**(4), 719–734. https://doi.org/10.1093/brain/99.4.719.

Landau K., Wichmann W., Valavanis A.T. (1995) The missing temporal crescent, *Am. J. Ophthalmol.* **119**(3), 345–349. https://doi.org/10.1016/S0002-9394(14)71178-X.

Lashley K. (1939) The mechanisms of vision XVI. The function of small remnants of the visual cortex, *J. Comp. Neurol.* **70**, 45–67.

Lavidor M., Ellis A.W. (2002) Word length and orthographic neighborhood size effects in the left and right cerebral hemispheres, *Brain Lang.* **80**, 45–62.

Lavidor M., Walsh V. (2004) The nature of foveal representation, *Nat. Rev.* **5**, 729–735.

Lawton Smith J., Weiner I.G., Lucero A.J. (1982) Hemianopic Fresnel prisms, *J. Clin. Neuro-Ophthalmol.* **2**, 19–22.

Lee A.G., Perez A.M. (1999) Improving awareness of peripheral visual field using sectorial prisms, *J. Am. Optom. Assoc.* **70**, 624–628.

Lee B.H., Suh M.K., Kim E.J., Seo S.W., Choi K.-M., Kim G.M., Chung C.S., Heilman K.M., Na D.L. (2009) Neglect dyslexia: Frequency, association with other hemispatial neglects, and lesion localization, *Neuropsychologia* **47**, 704–710.

Leff A.P. (2004) A historical review of the representation of the visual field in primary visual cortex with special reference to the neural mechanisms underlying macular sparing, *Brain Lang.* **88**, 268–278.

Leff A.P., Behrmann M. (2008) Treatment of reading impairment after stroke, *Curr. Opin. Neurol.* **21**, 1–5.

Leff A.P., Crewes H., Plant G.T., Scott S.K., Kennard C., Wise R.J. (2001b) The functional anatomy of single-word reading in patients with hemianopic and pure alexia, *Brain* **124**, 510–521.

Leff A.P., Scott S.K., Crewes H., Hodgson T.L., Cowey A., Howard D., Wise R.J. (2000) Impaired reading in patients with right hemianopia, *Ann. Neurol.* **47**, 171–178.

Leff A.P., Scott S.K., Rothwell J.C., Wise R.J.S. (2001a) The planning and guiding of reading saccades: A repetitive transcranial magnetic stimulation study, *Cereb. Cortex* **11**, 918–923.

Leff A.P., Spitzyna G.A., Plant G.T., Wise R.J.S. (2006) Structural anatomy of pure and hemianopic alexia, *J. Neurol. Neurosurg. Psychiatry* **77**, 1004–1007.

Legge G.E., Mansfield J.S., Chung S.T. (2001) Psychophysics of reading. XX. Linking letter recognition to reading speed in central and peripheral vision, *Vision Res.* **41**, 725–743.

Legge G.E., Rubin G.S., Lubker A. (1987) Psychophysics of reading V. The role of contrast in normal vision, *Vision Res.* **27**, 1165–1177.

Legge G.E., Rubin G.S., Pelli D.G., Schleske M.M. (1985) Psychophysics of reading – II. Low vision, *Vision Res.* **25**, 253–266.

Leo F., Bertini C., di Pellegrino G., Làdavas E. (2008) Multisensory integration for orienting responses in humans requires the activation of the superior colliculus, *Exp. Brain Res.* **186**(1), 67–77.

Lepore F.E. (2001) The preserved temporal crescent: The clinical implications of an "endangered" finding, *Neurology* **57**, 1918–1921.

Leśniak M., Soluch P., Stępień U., Czepiel W., Seniów J. (2014) Pure alexia after damage to the right fusiform gyrus in a right-handed male, *Neurol. Neurochir. Pol.* **48**, 373–377.

Levine D.N., Calvanio R. (1980) Visual discrimination after lesion of the posterior corpus callosum, *Neurology* **30**, 21–30.

Lindegger D.J., Pless M. (2019) The discovery of visual field representation in the brain, *J. Ophthalmol. Sci.* **1**(1), 6–12.

Lovie-Kitchin J., Mainstone J.M., Robinson J., Brown B. (1990) What areas of the visual field are important for mobility in low vision patients, *Clin. Vision Sci.* **5**, 249–263.

Lutzemberger L., Marzi C.A., Tassinari G. (1985) On inferring blindsight from normal vision, *Behav. Brain Sci.* **8**(4), 754–755.

Lynch J.C., McLaren J.W. (1989) Deficits of visual attention and saccadic eye movements after lesions of parieto-occipital cortex in monkeys, *J. Neurophysiol.* **61**, 74–90.

Machner B., Sprenger A., Sander T., Heide W., Kimmig H., Helmchen C., Kömpf D. (2009) Visual search disorders in acute and chronic homonymous hemianopia: Lesion effects and adaptive strategies, *Ann. N. Y. Acad. Sci.* **1164**, 419–426.

MacIntosh C. (2003) Stroke re-visited: Visual problems following stroke and their effect on rehabilitation, *Br. Orthopt. J.* **60**, 10–14.

Mackensen G. (1962) Examining the ability to read as clinical functional analysis [German], *Fortschr. Augenheilk.* **12**, 344–379.

Mangione C.M., Lee P.P., Gutierrez P.R., Spritzer K., Berry S., Hays R.D. (2001) Development of the 25-item national eye institute visual function questionnaire, *Arch. Ophthalmol.* **119**(7), 1050–1058. https://doi.org/10.1001/archopht.119.7.1050.

Mannan S.K., Pambakian A.L., Kennard C. (2010) Compensatory strategies following visual search training in patients with homonymous hemianopia: An eye movement study, *J. Neurol.* **257** (11), 1812–1821.

Margolis N.W., Suter P.S. (2006) Visual field defects & unilateral spatial inattention: Diagnosis and treatment, *J. Behav. Optom.* **17**, 31–37.

Marshall R.S., Ferrera J.J., Barnes A., Zhang X., O'Brian K.A., Chmayssani M., Hirsch J., Lazar R.M. (2008) Brain activity associated with stimulation therapy of the visual borderzone in hemianopic stroke patients, *Neurorehabil. Neural Repair* **22**(2), 136–144. https://doi.org/10.1177/1545968307305522.

Martin T., Riley M.E., Kelly K.N., Haynoe M., Huxlin K.R. (2007) Visually-guided behavior of homonymous hemianopes in a naturalistic task, *Vision Res.* **47**, 3434–3446.

Marzi C.A., Smania N., Martini M.C., Gambina G., Tomelleri G., Palamara A., Alessandrini F., Prior M. (1996) Implicit redundant-targets effect in visual extinction, *Neuropsychologia* **34**, 9–22.

Marzi C.A., Tassinari G., Aglioti S., Lutzemberger L. (1986) Spatial summation across the vertical meridian in hemianopics: A test of blindsight, *Neuropsychologia* **24**(6), 749–758. https://doi.org/10.1016/0028-3932(86)90074-6.

Matteo B.M., Viganò B., Cerri C.G., Meroni R., Cornaggia C.M., Perin C. (2017) Transcranial direct current stimulation (tDCS) combined with blindsight rehabilitation for the treatment of homonymous hemianopia: A report of two-cases, *J. Phys. Ther. Sci.* **29**(9), 1700–1705.

Mauthner L. (1881) *Gehirn und Auge (brain and eye)*. Bergmann, Wiesbaden, Germany.

McAuley D.L., Russell R. (1979) Correlation of CAT scan and visual field defects in vascular lesions of the posterior visual pathways, *J. Neurol. Neurosurg. Psychiatry* **42**, 298–311.

McCandliss B.D., Cohen L., Dehaene S. (2003) The visual word form area: Expertise for reading in the fusiform gyrus, *Trends Cognit. Sci.* **7**, 293–299.

McConkie G.W., Kerr P.W., Reddix M.D., Zola D. (1988) Eye movement control during reading: I. The location of initial eye fixations on words, *Vision Res.* **28**, 1107–1118.

McConkie G.W., Kerr P.W., Reddlx M.D., Zola D., Jacobs A.M. (1989) Eye movement control during reading: II. Frequency of refixating a word, *Percept. Psychophys.* **46**, 245–253.

McConkie G.W., Rayner K. (1975) The span of the effective stimulus during a fixation in reading, *Percept. Psychophys.* **17**, 578–586.

McConkie G.W., Rayner K. (1976) Asymmetry of the perceptual span in reading, *Bull. Psychon. Soc.* **8**, 365–368.

McConkie G.W., Zola D. (1989) Some characteristics in readers' eyes movements, *Brain and reading* (C. von Euler, I. Lundberg and G. Lennerstrand, Eds). Macmillian Press, London.

McDonald S.A., Spitzyna G., Shillcock R., Wise R.J.S., Leff A.P. (2006) Patients with hemianopic alexia adopt an inefficient eye movement strategy when reading text, *Brain* **129**, 158–167.

McFadzean R., Brosnahan D., Hadley D., Mutlukan E. (1994) Representation of the visual field in the occipital striate cortex, *Br. J. Ophthalmol.* **78**, 185–190.

McIntosh R.D., Rossetti Y., Milner A.D. (2002) Prism adaptation improves chronic visual and haptic neglect, *Cortex* **38**, 309–320.

McMillan T.M., Robertson I.H., Wilson B.A. (1999) Neurogenesis after brain injury: Implications for neurorehabilitation, *Neuropsychol. Rehabil.* **9**, 129–133.

Meienberg O. (1988) Eye movement patterns in homonymous hemianopia and visual hemineglect, *Klin Monbl Augenheilkd* **192**(2), 108–112. https://doi.org/10.1055/s-2008-1050084.

Meienberg O., Harrer M., Wehren C. (1986) Oculographic diagnosis of hemineglect in patients with homonymous hemianopia, *J. Neurol.* **233**, 97–101.

Meienberg O., Zangemeister W.H., Rosenberg M., Hoyt W.F., Stark L. (1981) Saccadic eye movement strategies in patients with homonymous hemianopia, *Ann. Neurol.* **9**, 537–544.

Menard M.T., Kosslyn S.M., Thompson W.L., Alpert N.M., Rauch S.L. (1996) Encoding words and pictures: A positron emission tomography study, *Neuropsychologia* **34**(3), 185–194.

Meredith M.A., Stein B.E. (1986) Spatial factors determine the activity of multisensory neurons in cat superior colliculus, *Brain Res.* **369**, 350–354.

Messing B., Ganshirt H. (1987) Follow-up of visual field defects with vascular damage of the geniculostriate visual pathway, *Neuro-Ophthalmol.* **7**, 231–242.

Milner A.D., Harvey M. (1995) Distortion of size perception in visuospatial neglect, *Curr. Biol.* **5** (1), 85–89. https://doi.org/10.1016/s0960-9822(95)00020-0.

Mintz M.J. (1979) A mirror for hemianopia, *Am. J. Ophthalmol.* **88**(4), 768. https://doi.org/10.1016/0002-9394(79)90681-0.

Mohler C.W., Wurtz R.H. (1977) Role of striate cortex and superior colliculus in visual guidance of saccadic eye movements in monkeys, *J. Neurophysiol.* **40**, 74–94.

Molko N., Cohen L., Mangin J.F., Chochon F., Lehéricy S., Le Bihan D., Dehaene S. (2002) Visualizing the neural bases of a disconnection syndrome with diffusion tensor imaging, *J. Cognit. Neurosci.* **14**, 629–636.

Morgan M.W. (1963) Distortions of ophthalmic prisms, *Am. J. Ophthalmol.* **40**, 111.

Mort D.J., Kennard C. (2003) Visual search and its disorders, *Curr. Opin. Neurol.* **16**(1), 51–57.

Mort D.J., Malhotra P., Mannan S.K., Rorden C., Pambakian A., Kennard C., Husain M. (2003) The anatomy of visual neglect, *Brain* **126**, 1986–1997.

Moss A.M., Harrison A.R., Lee M.S. (2014) Patients with homonymous hemianopia become visually qualified to drive using monocular sector prisms, *J. Neuro-Ophthalmol.* **34**, 53–56.

Mueller I., Gall C., Kasten E., Sabel B.A. (2008) Long-term learning of visual functions in patients after brain damage, *Behav. Brain Res.* **191**, 32–42.

Mueller I., Mast H., Sabel B.A. (2007) Recovery of visual field defects: A large clinical observational study using vision restoration therapy, *Restor. Neurol. Neurosci.* **25**, 563–572.

Mueller I., Poggel D.A., Kenkel S., Kasten E., Sabel B.A. (2003) Vision restoration therapy after brain damage: Subjective improvements of activities of daily life and their relationship to visual field enlargements, *Vision Impairment Res.* **5**, 157–178.

Müller-Oehring E.M., Kasten E., Poggel D.A., Schulte T., Strasburger H., Sabel B.A. (2003) Neglect and hemianopia superimposed, *J. Clin. Exp. Neuropsychol.* **25**(8), 1154–1168.

Müri R.M., Cazzoli D., Nyffeler T., Pflugshaupt T. (2009) Visual exploration pattern in hemineglect, *Psychol. Res.* **73**(2), 147–157.

Müri R.M., Vermersch A.I., Rivaud S., Gaymard B., Pierrot-Deseilligny C. (1996) Effects of single-pulse transcranial magnetic stimulation over the prefrontal and posterior parietal cortices during memory-guided saccades in humans, *J. Neurophysiol.* **76**, 2102–2106.

Nadeau S.F., Heilman K.M. (1991) Gaze-dependant hemianopia without hemispatial neglect, *Neurology* **41**, 1244–1250.

Nazir T.A., Heller D., Sussmann C. (1992) Letter visibility and word recognition. The optimal viewing position in printed words, *Percept. Psychophys.* **52**(3), 315–328.

Nelles G., De Greiff A., Pscherer A., Forsting M., Gerhard H., Esser J., Diener H.C. (2007b) Cortical activation in hemianopia after stroke, *Neurosci. Lett.* **426**, 34–38.

Nelles G., De Greiff A., Pscherer A., Stude P., Forsting M., Hufnagel A., Gerhard H., Esser J., Diener H.C. (2007) Saccade induced cortical activation in patients with post-stroke visual field defects, *J. Neurol.* **254**, 1432–1459.

Nelles G., Esser J., Eckstein A., Tiede A., Horst G., Diener H.C. (2001) Compensatory visual field training for patients with hemianopia after stroke, *Neurosci. Lett.* **306**, 189–192.

Nelles G., Pscherer A., de Greiff A., Forsting M., Gerhard H., Esser J., Diener H.C. (2009) Eye-movement training-induced plasticity in patients with post-stroke hemianopia, *J. Neurol.* **256**, 726–733.

Nelles G., Widman G., de Greiff A., Meistrowitz A., Dimitrova A., Weber J., Forsting M., Esser J., Diener H.C. (2002) Brain representation of hemifield stimulation in poststroke visual field defects, *Stroke* **33**(5), 1286–1293. https://doi.org/10.1161/01.str.0000013685.76973.67.

Nerenberg B. (1980) A new mirror design for hemianopia, *Am. J. Optom. Physiol. Opt.* **53**, 464–467.

Newman S.A., Miller N.R. (1983) Optic tract syndrome. Neuro-ophthalmologic considerations, *Arch. Ophthalmol.* **101**(8), 1241–1250. https://doi.org/10.1001/archopht.1983.01040020243018.

Nichelli P., Rinaldi M., Cubelli R. (1989) Selective spatial attention and length representation in normal subjects and in patients with unilateral spatial neglect, *Brain Cognit.* **9**(1), 57–70.

Nobre A.C., Allison C., McCarthy G. (1994) Word recognition in the human inferior temporal lobe, *Nature* **372**(6503), 260–263.

Nooney T. (1986) Partial visual rehabilitation of hemianopic patients, *Am. J. Optom. Physiol. Opt.* **63**(5), 382–386.

Ogren M.P., Mateer C.A., Wyler A.R. (1984) Alterations in visually related eye movements following left pulvinar damage in man, *Neuropsychologia* **22**, 187–196.

O'Neill E.C., Connell P.P., O'Connor J.C., Brady J., Reid I., Logan P. (2011) Prism therapy and visual rehabilitation in homonymous visual field loss, *Optom. Vision Sci.* **88**, 263–268.

Ong Y.H., Brown M.M., Robinson P., Plant G.T., Husain M., Leff A.P. (2012) Read-right: A "web app" that improves reading speeds in patients with hemianopia, *J. Neurol.* **259**(12), 2611–2615.

O'Regan J.K. (1990) Eye movements and reading, *Eye movements and their role in visual and cognitive processes* (E. Kowler, Ed.). Elsevier, Amsterdam, Holland.

Ownsworth T., Clare L. (2006) The association between awareness deficits and rehabilitation outcome following acquired brain injury, *Clin. Psychol. Rev.* **26**, 783–795.

Palomar-Mascaró F.J., Palomar-Mascaró M.V., De Miguel Simó P.V. (2018) Rehabilitation of hemianopic patients with Palomar Prisms, *Ophthalmol. Clin. Res.* **1**(2), 28–34.

Pambakian A.L., Currie J., Kennard C. (2005) Rehabilitation strategies for patients with homonymous visual field defects, *J. Neuro-Ophthalmol.* **25**(2), 136–142.

Pambakian A.L., Kennard C. (1997) Can visual function be restored in patients with homonymous hemianopia? *Br. J. Ophthalmol.* **81**, 324–328.

Pambakian A.L.M., Mannan S.K., Hodgson T.L., Kennard C. (2004) Saccadic visual search training: A treatment for patients with homonymous hemianopia, *J. Neurol. Neurosurg. Psychiatry* **75**, 1443–1448.

Pambakian A.L.M., Wooding D.S., Patel N., Morland A.B., Kennard C., Mannan S.K. (2000) Scanning the visual world: A study of patients with homonymous hemianopia, *J. Neurol. Neurosurg. Psychiatry* **69**, 751–759.

Papageorgiou E., Hardiess G., Schaeffel F., Wiethoelter H., Karnath H.-O., Mallot H., Schoenfisch B., Sciefer U. (2007) Assessment of vision-related quality of life in patients with homonymous visual field defects, *Graefe's Arch. Clin. Exp. Ophthalmol.* **245**, 1749–1758.

Passamonti C., Bertini C., Làdavas E. (2009) Audiovisual stimulation improves oculomotor patterns in patients with hemianopia, *Neuropsychologia* **47**, 546–555.

Patterson K., Kay J. (1982) Letter-by-letter reading: Psychological descriptions of a neurological syndrome, *Q. J. Exp. Psychol. A* **34**, 411–441.

Patterson K., Vargha-Khadem F., Polkey C.F. (1989) Reading with one hemisphere, *Brain* **112**, 39–63.

Patterson K.E., Wilson B. (1990) A ROSE is a ROSE or a NOSE: A deficit in initial letter identification, *Cognit. Neuropsychol.* **7**, 447–477.

Paus T. (1996) Location and function of the human frontal eye field: A selective review, *Neuropsychologia* **734**, 475–483.

Peli E. (2000) Field expansion for homonymous hemianopia by optically induced peripheral exotropia, *Optom. Vision Sci.* **77**, 453–464.

Peli E. (2020) Peripheral prisms for visual field expansion: A translational journey, *Optom. Vision Sci.* **97**(10), 833–846.

Peli E., Bowers A.R., Keeney K., Jung J.H. (2016) High-power prismatic devices for oblique peripheral prisms, *Optom. Vision Sci.* **93**, 521–533.

Peli E., Jung J.H. (2017) Multiplexing prisms for field expansion, *Optom. Vision Sci.* **94**, 817–829.

Pelli D.G., Farell B., Moore D.C. (2003) The remarkable inefficiency of word recognition, *Nature* **423**, 752–756.

Perenin M.T. (1991) Discrimination of motion direction in perimetrically blind fields, *NeuroReport* **2**, 397–400.

Pessin M.S., Lathi E.S., Cohen M.B., Kwan E.S., Hedges T.R. 3rd, Caplan L.R. (1987) Clinical features and mechanism of occipital infarction, *Ann. Neurol.* **21**, 290–299.

Petter M.W., Gilbert C.D. (1992) Dynamic changes in receptive-field size in cat primary visual cortex, *Proc. Natl. Acad. Sci. USA* **89**, 8366–8370.

Pflugshaupt T., Gutbrod K., Wurtz P., von Wartburg R., Nyffeler T., de Haan B., Karnath H.O., Mueri R.M. (2009) About the role of visual field defects in pure alexia, *Brain* **132**, 1907–1917.

Pierrot-Deseilligny C. (1994) Saccade and smooth-pursuit impairment after cerebral hemispheric lesions, *Eur. Neurol.* **34**, 121–134.

Pierrot-Deseilligny C., Rivaud S., Gaymard B., Agid Y. (1991a) Cortical control of reflexive visually-guided saccades, *Brain* **114**, 1473–1485.

Pierrot-Deseilligny C., Rivaud S., Gaymard B., Agid Y. (1991b) Cortical control of memory-guided saccades in man, *Exp. Brain Res.* **83**, 607–617.

Pierrot-Deseilligny C., Rivaud S., Gaymard B., Müri R., Vermersch A.I. (1995) Cortical control of saccades, *Ann. Neurol.* **37**, 557–567.

Pisella L., Rode G., Farnè A., Boisson D., Rossetti Y. (2002) Dissociated long lasting improvements of straight-ahead pointing and line bisection tasks in two hemineglect patients, *Neuropsychologia* **40**, 327–334.

Pizzamiglio L., Frasca R., Guariglia C., Incoccia C., Antonucci C. (1990) Effect of optokinetic stimulation in patients with visual neglect, *Cortex* **26**, 535–540.

Plant G.T. (2005) A work out for hemianopia, *Br. J. Ophthalmol.* **89**, 2.

Pleger B., Foerster A.F., Widdig W., Henschel M., Nicolas V., Jansen A., Frank A., Knecht S., Schwenkreis P., Tegenthoff M. (2003) Functional magnetic resonance imaging mirrors recovery of visual perception after repetitive tachistoscopic stimulation in patients with partial cortical blindness, *Neurosci. Lett.* **335**, 192–196.

Plow E.B., Maguire S., Obretenova S., Pascual-Leone A., Merabet L.B. (2009) Approaches to rehabilitation for visual field defects following brain lesions, *Exp. Rev. Med. Dev.* **6**(3), 291–305.

Plow E.B., Obretenova S.N., Fregni F., Pascual-Leone A., Merabet L.B. (2012) Comparison of visual field training for hemianopia with active versus sham transcranial direct cortical stimulation, *Neurorehabil. Neural Repair* **26**(6), 616–626.

Poggel D.A., Kasten E., Müller-Oehring E.M., Sabel B.A., Brandt S.A. (2001) Unusual spontaneous and training induced visual field recovery in a patient with a gunshot lesion, *J. Neurol. Neurosurg. Psychiatry* **70**, 236–239.

Poggel D.A., Kasten E., Sabel B.A. (2004) Attentional cueing improves vision restoration therapy in patients with visual field defects, *Neurology* **63**(11), 2069–2076.

Poggel D.A., Mueller I., Kasten E., Bunzenthal U., Sabel B.A. (2010) Subjective and objective outcome measures of computer-based vision restoration training, *NeuroRehabilitation* **27**, 173–187.

Poggel D.A., Mueller I., Kasten E., Sabel B.A. (2008a) Multifactorial predictors and outcome variables of vision restoration training in patients with postgeniculate visual field loss, *Restor. Neurol. Neurosci.* **26**, 321–339.

Poggel D.A., Mueller-Oehring E.M., Kasten E., Buzenthal U., Sabel B.A. (2008b) The topography of training-induced visual recovery: Perimetric maps and subjective representations, *Visual Cognit.* **16**, 1059–1077.

Poggel D.A., Müller-Oehring E.M., Gothe J., Kenkel S., Kasten E., Sabel B.A. (2007) Visual hallucinations during spontaneous and training-induced visual field recovery, *Neuropsychologia* **45** (11), 2598–2607. https://doi.org/10.1016/j.neuropsychologia.2007.03.005.

Polk T.A., Farah M.J. (2002) Functional MRI evidence for an abstract, not perceptual, word-form area, *J. Exp. Psychol.: Gen.* **131**, 65–72.

Polk T.A., Stallcup M., Aguirre G.K., Alsop D.C., D'Esposito M., Detre J.A., Farah M.J. (2002) Neural specialization for letter recognition, *J. Cognit. Neurosci.* **14**, 145–159.

Pollatsek A., Bolozky S., Well A.D., Rayner K. (1981) Asymmetries in the perceptual span for Israeli readers, *Brain Lang.* **14**, 174–180.

Pommerenke K., Markowitsch H.J. (1989) Rehabilitation training of homonymous visual field defects in patients with postgeniculate damage of the visual system, *Restor. Neurol. Neurosci.* **1**, 47–63.

Potthoff R.D. (1995) Regeneration of specific nerve cells in lesioned visual cortex of the human brain: An indirect evidence after constant stimulation with different spots of light, *J. Neurosci. Res.* **15**, 787–796.

Price C.J., Devlin J.T. (2003) The myth of the visual word form area, *Neuroimage* **19**, 473–481.

Ptak R., Schnider A., Golay L., Müri R.M. (2007) A non-spatial bias favouring fixated stimuli revealed in patients with spatial neglect, *Brain* **130**, 3211–3222.

Ptito A., Lepore F., Ptito M., Lassonde M. (1991) Target detection and movement discrimination in the blind field of hemispherectomized patients, *Brain* **114**, 497–512.

Puce A., Allison T., Asgari M., Gore J.C., McCarthy G. (1996) Differential sensitivity of human visual cortex to faces, letter strings, and textures: A functional magnetic resonance imaging study, *J. Neurosci.* **16**, 5205–5215.

Rafal R.D. (1994) Neglect, *Curr. Opin. Neurobiol.* **4**, 2312–2316.

Raffin E., Salamanca-Giron R.F., Hummel F.C. (2020, Jan) Perspectives: Hemianopia-toward novel treatment options based on oscillatory activity? *Neurorehabil. Neural Repair* **34**(1), 13–25.

Raninen A., Vanni S., Hyvärinen L., Näsänen R. (2007) Temporal sensitivity in a hemianopic visual field can be improved by long-term training using flicker stimulation, *J. Neurol. Neurosurg. Psychiatry* **78**, 66–73.

Rapcsak S.Z., Cimino C.R., Heilman K.M. (1988) Altitudinal neglect, *Neurology* **38**, 277–281.

Rapp B., Caramazza A. (1991) Spatially determined deficits in letter and word processing, *Cognit. Neuropsychol.* **8**(3/4), 275–311.

Rayner K. (1975) The perceptual span and peripheral cues in reading, *Cognit. Psychol.* **7**, 65–81.

Rayner K. (1978) Eye movements in reading and information processing, *Psychol. Bull.* **85**, 618–660.

Rayner K. (1979) Eye guidance in reading: Fixation localization within words, *Perception* **8**, 21–30.

Rayner K. (1998) Eye movements in reading and information processing: 20 years of research, *Psychol. Bull.* **124**, 372–422.

Rayner K., Bertera J.H. (1979) Reading without a fovea, *Science* **206**, 468–469.

Rayner K., Inhoff A.W., Morrison R.E., Sowiaczek M.L., Bertera J.H. (1981) Masking of foveal and parafoveal vision during eye fixations in reading, *J. Exp. Psychol.: Hum. Percept. Perform.* **7**, 167–179.

Rayner K., Johnson R.L. (2005) Letter-by-letter acquired dyslexia is due to the serial encoding of letters, *Psychol. Sci.* **16**, 530–534.

Rayner K., Pollatsek A. (1987) Eye movements in reading: A tutorial review, *Attention and performance XII: The psychology of reading* (M. Coltheart, Ed.). Erlbaum, London.

Rayner K., Pollatsek A. (1989) *The psychology of reading.* Lawrence Erlbaum, Hillsdale.

Rayner K., Well A.D., Pollatsek A. (1980) Asymmetry of the effective visual field in reading, *Percept. Psychophys.* **27**, 537–544.

Rayner K., Well A.D., Pollatsek A., Bertera J.H. (1982) The availability of useful information to the right of fixation in reading, *Percept. Psychophys.* **31**, 537–550.

Redding G.M., Wallace B. (2006) Prism adaptation and unilateral neglect: Review and analysis, *Neuropsychologia* **44**, 1–20.

Reding M., Potes E. (1988) Rehabilitation outcome following initial unilateral hemispheric stroke. Life table analysis approach, *Stroke* **19**, 1354–1358.

Reinhard J., Schreiber A., Schiefer U., Kasten E., Sabel B.A., Kenkel S., Vonthein R., Trauzettel-Klosinski S. (2005) Does visual restitution training change absolute homonymous visual field defects? A fundus controlled study, *Br. J. Ophthalmol.* **89**, 30–35.

Reinhard J., Trauzettel-Klosinski S. (2003) Nasotemporal overlap of retinal ganglion cells in humans: A functional study, *Invest. Ophthalmol. Visual Sci.* **44**, 1568–1572.

Rivaud S., Müri R.M., Gaymard B., Vermesch A.I., Pierrot-Deseilligny C. (1994) Eye movement disorders after frontal eye field lesions in humans, *Exp. Brain Res.* **102**, 110–120.

Rizzo M., Robin D.A. (1996) Bilateral effects of unilateral visual cortex lesions in human, *Brain* **119**, 951–963.

Ro T., Shelton D., Lee O.L., Chang E. (2004) Extrageniculate mediation of unconscious vision is transcranial magnetic stimulation-induced blindsight, *PNAS* **101**(26), 9933–9935.

Robertson I.H., Halligan P.W. (1999) *Spatial neglect: A clinical handbook for diagnosis and treatment.* Psychol Press Ltd. Ed, East Sussex, U.K.

Rode G., Rossetti Y., Li L., Boisson D. (1998/1999) Improvement of mental imagery after prism exposure in neglect: A case study, *Behav. Neurol.* **11**, 251–258.

Romano J.G., Schulz P., Kenkel S., Todd D.P. (2008) Visual field changes after a rehabilitation intervention: Vision restoration therapy, *J. Neurol. Sci.* **273**(1–2), 70–74. https://doi.org/10.1016/j.jns.2008.06.026.

Ross N.C., Bowers A.R., Peli E. (2012) Peripheral prism glasses: Effects of dominance, suppression, and background, *Optom. Vision Sci.* **89**, 1343–1352.

Rossetti Y., Rode G., Pisella L., Farnè A., Li L., Boisson D., Perenin M.T. (1998) Prism adaptation to a rightward optical deviation rehabilitates left-hemispatial neglect, *Nature* **395**(6698), 166–169.

Rossi O.W., Kheyfets S., Reding M.J. (1990) Fresnel prisms improve visual perception in stroke patients with homonymous hemianopia or unilateral visual neglect, *Neurology* **40**, 1597–1599.

Roth T., Sokolov A.N., Messias A., Roth P., Weller M., Trauzettel-Klosinski S. (2009) Comparing explorative saccade and flicker training in hemianopia: A randomized controlled study, *Neurology* **72**, 324–331.

Rousseaux M., Bernati T., Saj A., Kozlowski O. (2006) Ineffectiveness of prism adaptation on spatial neglect signs, *Stroke* **37**, 542–543.

Rowe F., Brand D., Jackson C.A., Price A., Walker L., Harrison S., Eccleston C., Scott C., Akerman N., Dodridge C., Howard C., Shipman T., Sperring U., MacDiarmid S., Freeman C. (2009) Visual impairment following stroke: Do stroke patients require vision assessment? *Age Aging* **38**, 188–193.

Rowe F., VIS Group UK. (2009) Visual perceptual consequences of stroke, *Strabismus* **17**, 24–28.

Rowe F., Wright D., Brand D., Jackson C., Price A., Walker L., Harrison S., Eccleston C., Maan T., Scott C., Vogwell L., Peel S., Robson L., Akerman N., Dodridge C., Howard C., Shipman T., Sperring U., Yarde S., Macdarmid S., Freeman C. (2011) Reading difficulty after stroke: Ocular and non ocular causes, *Int. J. Stroke* **6**, 404–411. World Stroke Organization. https://doi.org/10.1111/j.1747-4949.2011.00583.x.

Sabel B.A. (1997) Unrecognized potential of surviving neurons: Within systems plasticity, recovery of function, and the hypothesis of minimal residual structure, *Neuroscientist* **3**, 366–370.

Sabel B.A. (1999) Restoration of vision: I. Neurobiological mechanisms of visual restitution and plasticity after brain damage—A review, *Restor. Neurol. Neurosci.* **15**, 177–200.

Sabel B.A. (2006) Vision restoration therapy and raising red flags too early, *Br. J. Ophthalmol.* **90**, 659–660.

Sabel B.A., Hamid A.I.A., Borrmann C., Speck O., Antal A. (2020) Transorbital alternating current stimulation modifies BOLD activity in healthy subjects and in a stroke patient with hemianopia: A 7 Tesla fMRI feasibility study, *Int. J. Psychophysiol.* **154**, 80–92.

Sabel B.A., Kasten E. (2000) Restoration of vision by training of residual functions, *Curr. Opin. Ophthalmol.* **11**, 430–436.

Sabel B.A., Kenkel S., Kasten E. (2004) Vision restoration therapy (VRT) efficacy as assessed by comparative perimetric analysis and subjective questionnaires, *Restor. Neurol. Neurosci.* **22**, 399–420.

Sabel B.A., Trauzettel-Klosinski S. (2005) Improving vision in a patient with homonymous hemianopia, *J. Neuro-Ophthalmol.* **25**(2), 143–149.

Sahraie A., Trevethan C.T., MacLeod M.J., Murray A.D., Olson J.A., Weiskrantz L. (2006) Increased sensitivity after repeated stimulation of residual spatial channels in blindsight, *Proc. Natl. Acad. Sci. USA* **103**(40), 14971–14976.

Sahraie A., Trevethan C.T., Weiskrantz L., Olson J., MacLeod M.J., Murray A.D., Dijkhuizen R.S., Counsell C., Coleman R. (2003) Spatial channels of visual processing in cortical blindness, *Eur. J. Neurosci.* **18**, 1189–1196.

Saslow M.G. (1967) Effects of components of displacement-step stimuli upon latency for saccadic eye movement, *J. Opt. Soc. Am.* **57**, 1024–1029.

Savino P.J., Paris M., Schatz N.J., Orr L.S., Corbett J.J. (1978) Optic tract syndrome: A review of 21 patients, *Arch. Ophthalmol.* **96**, 656–663.

Schenkenberg T., Bradford D.C., Ajax E.T. (1980) Line bisection and unilateral visual neglect in patients with neurologic impairment, *Neurology* **30**, 509–517.

Schlag J., Schlag-Rey M. (1987) Evidence for a supplementary eye field, *J. Neurophysiol.* **57**, 179–200.

Schmid M., Mrowka S., Turchi J., Saunders R., Wilke M., Peters A., Ye F., Leopold D. (2010) Blindsight depends on the lateral geniculate nucleus, *Nature* **466**, 373–377.

Schmielau F., Wong E.K. (2007) Recovery of visual fields in brain-lesioned patients by reaction perimetry treatment, *J. Neuroeng. Rehabil.* **4**, 31. https://doi.org/10.1186/1743-0003-4-31.

Schoenfeld M.A., Heinze H.J., Woldorff M.G. (2002a) Unmasking motion-processing activity in human brain area V5/MT + mediated by pathways that bypass primary visual cortex, *Neuroimage* **17**, 769–779.

Schoenfeld M.A., Noesselt T., Poggel D., *et al.* (2002b) Analysis of pathways mediating preserved vision after striate cortex lesions, *Ann. Neurol.* **52**, 814–824.

Schoepf D., Zangemeister W.H. (1993) Correlation of ocular motor reading strategies to the status of adaptation in patients with hemianopic visual field defects, *Ann. N. Y. Acad. Sci.* **682**, 404–408.

Schreiber A., Vonthein R., Reinhard J., Trauzettel-Klosinski S., Connert C., Schiefer U. (2006) Effect of visual restitution training on absolute homonymous scotomas, *Neurology* **67**, 143–145.

Schuett S. (2009) The rehabilitation of hemianopic dyslexia, *Nat. Rev. Neurol.* **5**(8), 427–437. https://doi.org/10.1038/nrneurol.2009.97.

Schuett S., Heywood C.A., Kentridge R.W., Zihl J. (2008a) The significance of visual information processing in reading: Insights from hemianopic dyslexia, *Neuropsychologia* **46**, 2445–2462.

Schuett S., Heywood C.A., Kentridge R.W., Zihl J. (2008b) Rehabilitation of hemianopic dyslexia: Are words necessary for re-learning oculomotor control? *Brain* **131**, 3156–3168.

Schuett S., Kentridge R.W., Zihl J., Heywood C.A. (2009a) Are hemianopic reading and visual exploration impairments visually elicited? New insights from eye movements in simulated hemianopia, *Neuropsychologia* **47**, 733–746.

Schuett S., Kentridge R.W., Zihl J., Heywood C.A. (2009b) Adaptation of eye movements to simulated hemianopia in reading and visual exploration: Transfer or specificity? *Neuropsychologia* **47**, 1712–1720.

Schulte T., Strasburger H., Müller-Oehring E.M., Kasten E., Sabel B.A. (1999) Automobile driving performance of brain-injured patients with visual field defects, *Am. J. Phys. Med. Rehabil.* **78**(2), 136–142. https://doi.org/10.1097/00002060-199903000-00010.

Sekuler E.B., Behrmann M. (1996) Perceptual cues in pure alexia, *Cognit. Neuropsychol.* **13**, 941–974.

Sereno M.I., Dale A.M., Reppas J.B., Kwong K.K., Belliveau J.W., Brady T.J., Rosen B.R., Tootell R.B.H. (1995) Borders of visual areas in humans revealed by functional magnetic resonance imaging, *Science* **268**(5212), 889–893. https://doi.org/10.1126/science.7754376.

Shallice T. (1988) *From neuropsychology to mental structure.* Cambridge University Press, Cambridge.

Shen J., Peli E., Bowers A.R. (2015) Peripheral prism glasses: Effects of moving and stationary backgrounds, *Optom. Vision Sci.* **92**, 412–420.

Sincich L.C., Park K.F., Wohlgemuth M.J., Horton J.C. (2004) Bypassing V1: A direct geniculate input to area MT, *Nat. Neurosci.* **7**(10), 1123–1128. https://doi.org/10.1038/nn1318.

Smith C.G., Richardson W.F.G. (1966) The course and distribution of the arteries supplying the visual (striate) cortex, *Am. J. Ophthalmol.* **61**, 1391–1396.

Solomon J.A., Pelli D.G. (1994) The visual filter mediating letter identification, *Nature* **369**, 395–397.

Sommer M.A., Tehovnik E.J. (1997) Reversible inactivation of macaque frontal eye field, *Exp. Brain Res.* **116**, 229–249.

Sparks D.L. (1986) Translation of sensory signals into commands for control of saccadic eye movements: Role of primate superior colliculus, *Physiol. Rev.* **66**, 118–171.

Spear P.D., Barbas H. (1975) Recovery of pattern discrimination ability in rats receiving serial or one-stage visual cortex lesions, *Brain Res.* **94**, 337–346.

Spitzyna G.A., Wise R.J., McDonald S.A., Plant G.T., Kidd D., Crewes H., Leff A.P. (2007) Optokinetic therapy improves text reading in patients with hemianopic alexia: A controlled trial, *Neurology* **68**, 1922–1930.

Sprague J.M. (1966) Interaction of cortex and superior colliculus in mediation of visually guided behavior in the cat, *Science* **153**, 1544–1547.

Stein B.E. (1998) Neural mechanisms for synthesizing sensory information and producing adaptive behaviors, *Exp. Brain Res.* **123**(1–2), 124–135. https://doi.org/10.1007/s002210050553.

Stein B.E., London N., Wilkinson L.K., Price D.D. (1996) Enhancement of perceived visual intensity by auditory stimuli: A psychophysical analysis, *J. Cognit. Neurosci.* **8**, 497–506.

Stein B.E., Meredith M.A. (1993) *Merging of the senses.* MIT Press, Cambridge, Mass.

Stein J.F. (1989) Representation of egocentric space in the posterior parietal cortex, *Q. J. Exp. Physiol.* **74**, 583–606.

Stein J.F. (1992) The representation of egocentric space in the posterior parietal cortex, *Behav. Brain Sci.* **4**, 691–700. https://doi.org/10.1017/S0140525X00072605.

Stoerig P., Cowey A. (1989) Wavelength sensitivity in blindsight, *Nature* **342**(6252), 916–918. https://doi.org/10.1038/342916a0.

Stoerig P., Cowey A. (1992) Wavelength discrimination in blindsight, *Brain* **115**, 425–444.

Stoerig P., Kleinschmidt A., Frahm J. (1998) No visual responses in denervated V1: High-resolution functional magnetic resonance imaging of a blindsight patient, *NeuroReport* **9**, 21–25.

Stone J. (1966) The naso-temporal division of the cat's retina, *J. Comp. Neurol.* **136**, 585–600.

Stone J., Leicester J., Sherman S.M. (1973) The nasotemporal division of the monkey's retina, *J. Comp. Neurol.* **150**, 333–348.

Stone S.P., Halligan P.W., Greenwood R.J. (1993) The incidence of neglect phenomena and related disorders in patients with an acute right or left hemisphere stroke, *Age Aging* **22**, 46–52.

Stone S.P., Patel P., Greenwood R.J., Halligan P.W. (1992) Measuring visual neglect in acute stroke and predicting its recovery: The visual neglect recovery index, *J. Neurol. Neurosurg. Psychiatry* **55**(6), 431–436. https://doi.org/10.1136/jnnp.55.6.431.

Sturm W., Thimm W., Küst J., Karbe H., Fink G.R. (2006) Alertness-training in neglect: Behavioral and imaging results, *Restor. Neurol. Neurosci.* **24**(4–6), 371–384.

Suchoff I.B., Ciuffreda K.J. (2004) A primer for the optometric management of unilateral spatial inattention, *J. Am. Optom. Assoc.* **75**, 305–319.

Suchoff I.B., Kapoor N., Ciuffreda K.J., Rutner D., Han E., Craig S. (2008) The frequency of occurrence, types, and characteristics of visual field defects in acquired brain injury: A retrospective analysis, *Optometry* **79**, 259–265.

Sugita Y. (1996) Global plasticity in adult visual cortex following reversal of visual input, *Nature* **380**, 523–526.

Sunderland A., Wade D.T., Langton Hewer R. (1987) The natural history of visual neglect after stroke. Indications from two methods of assessment, *Int. Disabil. Stud.* **9**, 55–59.

Suzuki Y., Kiyosawa M., Oda K., Ishiwara K., Ishii K. (2016) Improvement of glucose metabolism in the visual cortex accompanies visual field recovery in a patient with hemianopia, *J. Exp. Med.* **238**(4), 267–271. https://doi.org/10.1620/tjem.238.267.

Szlyk J.P., Brigell M., Seiple W. (1993) Effects of age and hemianopic visual field loss on driving, *Optom. Vision Sci.* **70**, 1031–1037.

Szlyk J.P., Seiple W., Stelmack J., McMahon T. (2005) Use of prisms for navigation and driving in hemianopic patients, *Ophthalmic Physiol. Opt.* **25**, 128–135.

Tant M.L.M., Cornelissen F.W., Kooijman A.C., Brouwer W.H. (2002) Hemianopic visual field defects elicit hemianopic scanning, *Vision Res.* **42**, 1339–1348.

Tardif E., Clarke S. (2002) Commissural connections of human superior colliculus, *Neuroscience* **111**, 363–372.

Terao N., Inatomi A., Maeda T. (1982) Anatomical evidence for the overlapped distribution of ipsilaterally and contralaterally projecting ganglion cells to the lateral geniculate nucleus in the cat retina: A morphologic study with fluorescent tracers, *Invest. Ophthalmol. Visual Sci.* **23**, 796–798.

Tiel K., Kolmel H.W. (1991) Patterns of recovery from homonymous hemianopia subsequent to infarction in the distribution of posterior cerebral artery, *Neuro-Ophthalmol.* **11**, 33–39.

Tipper S.P., Behrmann M. (1996) Object-centered not scene-based visual neglect, *J. Exp. Psychol.: Hum. Percept. Perform.* **22**, 1261–1278.

Tootell R.B., Mendola J.D., Hadjikhani N.K., Liu A.K., Dale A.M. (1998) The representation of the ipsilateral visual field in human cerebral cortex, *Proc. Natl. Acad. Sci. USA* **95**, 818–824.

Trauzettel-Klosinski S. (1997) Eccentric fixation with hemianopic field defects: A valuable strategy to improve reading ability and an indication of cortical plasticity, *Neuro-Ophthalmol.* **18**(3), 117–131. https://doi.org/10.3109/01658109709044129.

Trauzettel-Klosinski S., Brendler K. (1998) Eye movements in reading with hemianopic field defects: The significance of clinical parameters, *Graefe's Arch. Clin. Exp. Ophthalmol.* **236**, 91–102.

Trauzettel-Klosinski S., Reinhard J. (1998) The vertical field border in hemianopia and its significance for fixation and reading, *Invest. Ophthalmol. Visual Sci.* **39**, 2177–2186.

Trobe J.D., Lorber M.L., Schlezinger N.S. (1973) Isolated homonymous hemianopia: A review of 104 cases, *Arch. Ophthalmol.* **89**, 373–381.

Tsapkini K., Dimos O., Katsarou Z. (2005) Pure alexia without agraphia after a lesion at the right hemisphere: A case study, *Brain Lang.* **95**, 239–240.

Ungerleider L.G., Christensen C.A. (1977) Pulvinar lesions in monkeys produce abnormal eye movements during visual discrimination training, *Brain Res.* **136**, 189–196.

Ungerleider L.G., Christensen C.A. (1979) Pulvinar lesions in monkeys produce abnormal scanning of a complex visual array, *Neuropsychologia* **17**, 493–501.

Urbaitis J.C., Meikle T.H. Jr. (1968) Relearning a dark-light discrimination by cats after cortical and cullicular lesions, *Exp. Neurol.* **20**, 295–311.

Vallar G., Burani C., Arduio L.S. (2010) Neglect dyslexia: A review of the neuropsychological literature, *Exp. Brain Res.* **206**, 219–235.

Vallar G., Lobel E., Galati G., Berthoz A., Pizzamiglio L., Le Bihan D. (1999) A fronto-parietal system for computing the egocentric spatial frame of reference in humans, *Exp. Brain Res.* **124**, 281–286.

Vallar G., Perani D. (1986) The anatomy of unilateral neglect after right-hemisphere stroke lesions. A clinical/CT-scan correlation study in man, *Neuropsychologia* **24**, 609–622.

Vallar G., Ronchi R. (2006) Anosognosia for motor and sensory deficits after unilateral brain damage: A review, *Restor. Neurol. Neurosci.* **24**, 247–257.

Van der Wildt G.J., Bergsma D.P. (1998) Visual field enlargement by neuropsychological training of a hemianopsia patient, *Doc. Ophthalmol.* **93**, 277–292.

Vaphiades M.S., Celesia G.G., Brigell M.G. (1996) Positive spontaneous visual phenomena limited to the hemianopic field in lesions of the central visual pathways, *Neurology* **47**(2), 408–417.

Vuilleumier P.O., Rafal R.D. (2000) A systematic study of visual extinction. Between- and within-field deficits of attention in hemispatial neglect, *Brain* **123**, 1263–1279.

Walker R., Deubel H., Schneider W.X., Findlay J.M. (1997) Effect of remote distractors on saccade programming: Evidence for an extended fixation zone, *J. Neurophysiol.* **78**, 1108–1119.

Walker R., Findlay J.M. (1996) Saccadic eye movement programming in unilateral neglect, *Neuropsychologia* **34**, 493–508.

Walker R., Findlay J.M., Young A.W., Welch J. (1991) Disentangling neglect and hemianopia, *Neuropsychologia* **29**, 1019–1027.

Walker R., Kentridge R.W., Findlay J.M. (1995) Independent contributions of the orienting of attention, fixation offset and bilateral stimulation on human saccadic latencies, *Exp. Brain Res.* **103**, 294–310.

Wall M., Kutzko K.E., Chauan B.C. (2002) The relationship of visual threshold and reaction time to visual field eccentricity with conventional automated perimetry, *Vision Res.* **42**, 781–787.

Wallace M.T., Meredith M.A., Stein B.E. (1992) Integration of multiple sensory modalities in cat cortex, *Exp. Brain Res.* **91**, 484–488.

Wang M.K. (2003) Reading with a right homonymous hemianopia, *Lancet* **361**, 1138. https://doi.org/10.1016/s0140-6736(03)12885-1.

Warrington E.K., Langdon D. (1994) Spelling dyslexia: A deficit of the visual word-form, *J. Neurol. Neurosurg. Psychiatry* **57**, 211–216.

Weekes B.S. (1997) Differential effects of number of letters on word and non-word naming latency, *Q. J. Exp. Psychol.* **50A**, 439–456.

Weiskrantz L. (1980) Varieties of residual experience, *Q. J. Exp. Psychol.* **32**, 365–386.

Weiskrantz L. (1986) *Blindsight: A case study and implications.* Clarendon Press, Oxford.

Weiskrantz L. (1987) Residual vision in a scotoma. A follow-up study of 'form' discrimination, *Brain* **110**, 77–92. https://doi.org/10.1093/brain/110.1.77.

Weiskrantz L. (1998) *Introduction to the new paperback edition of blindsight. Blindsight: A case study and implications.* Clarendon Press, Oxford.

Weiskrantz L., Warrington E.K., Sanders M.D., Marshall J. (1974) Visual capacity in the hemianopic field following a restricted occipital ablation, *Brain* **97**, 709–728.

Weiss N.J. (1969) Management of the low vision patient with peripheral field loss, *J. Am. Optom. Assoc.* **40**, 830–832.

Wellings P.C. (1989) Detection and recognition of visual field defects resulting from lesions involving the visual pathways, *Aust. N. Z. J. Ophthalmol.* **17**, 331–335.

Wessinger C.M., Fendrich R., Gazzaniga M.S. (1997) Islands of residual vision in hemianopic patients, *J. Cognit. Neurosci.* **9**, 203–221.

Wessinger C.M., Fendrich R., Gazzaniga M.S. (1999) Variability of residual vision in hemianopic subjects, *Restor. Neurol. Neurosci.* **15**, 243–253.

Widdig W., Pleger B., Rommel O., Malin J.P., Tegenthoff M. (2003) Repetitive visual stimulation: A neuropsychological approach to the treatment of cortical blindness, *NeuroRehabilitation* **18**, 227–237.

Wong A.M.F., Sharpe J.A. (1999) Representation of the visual field in the human occipital cortex. A magnetic resonance imaging and perimetric correlation, *Arch. Ophthalmol.* **117**, 208–217.

Wood J.M., McGwin G. Jr., Elgin J., Vaphiades M.S., Braswell R.A., DeCarlo D.K., Kline L.B., Owsley C. (2011) Hemianopic and quadrantanopic field loss, eye and head movements, and driving, *Invest. Ophthalmol. Visual Sci.* **52**(3), 1220–1225.

Yoshida M., Ida M., Nguyen T.H., Iba-Zizen M.T., Bellinger L., Stievenart J.J., Nagao T., Kikuchi S., Hara T., Shiba T., Kitahara K., Cabanis E.A. (2006) Resolution of homonymous visual field loss documented with functional magnetic resonance and diffusion tensor imaging, *J. Neuro-Ophthalol.* **26**(1), 11–17. https://doi.org/10.1097/01.wno.0000205620.60510.01.

Young A.W., Newcombe F., Ellis A.W. (1991) Different impairments contribute to neglect dyslexia, *Cognit. Neuropsychol.* **8**, 177–191.

Yukie M., Iwai E. (1981) Direct projection from the dorsal lateral geniculate nucleus to the prestriate cortex in macaque monkeys, *J. Comp. Neurol.* **201**, 81–97.

Zangemeister W.H., Meienberg O., Stark L., Hoyt W.F. (1982) Eye-head coordination in homonymous hemianopia, *J. Neurol.* **226**, 243–254.

Zangemeister W.H., Oechsner U., Freska C. (1995) Short-term adaptation of eye movements in patients with visual hemifield defects indicates high level control of human scanpath, *Optom. Vision Sci.* **72**(7), 467–477.

Zangemeister W.H., Utz P. (2002) An increase in a virtual hemianopic field defect enhances the efficiency of secondary adaptive gaze strategies, *Curr. Psychol. Cognit.* **21**, 281–303.

Zeki S. (2015) Area V5-A microcosm of the visual brain, *Front. Integr. Neurosci.* **9**, 21. https://doi.org/10.3389/fnint.2015.00021.

Zeki S., Shipp S. (1988) The functional logic of cortical connections, *Nature* **335**, 311–316.

Zepeda A., Vaca L., Arias C., Sengpiel F. (2003) Reorganization of visual cortical maps after focal ischemic lesions, *J. Cereb. Blood Flow Metab.* **23**, 811–820.

Zhang X., Kedar S., Lynn M.J., Newman N.J., Biousse V. (2006a) Natural history of homonymous hemianopia, *Neurology* **66**, 901–905.

Zhang X., Kedar S., Lynn M.J., Newman N.J., Biousse V. (2006b) Homonymous hemianopias: Clinical-anatomic correlations in 904 cases, *Neurology* **66**, 906–910.

Zihl J. (1980) "Blindsight": Improvement of visually guided eye movements by systematic practice in patients with cerebral blindness, *Neuropsychologia* **18**(1), 71–78. https://doi.org/10.1016/0028-3932(80)90085-8.

Zihl J. (1981) Recovery of visual functions in patients with cerebral blindness. Effects of specific practice with saccadic localization, *Exp. Brain Res.* **44**, 159–169.

Zihl J. (1989) Cerebral disturbances of elementary visual functions, *Neuropsychology of visual perception* (J.W. Brown, Ed.). Lawrence Erlbaum Associates Inc., Hillsdale, NJ.

Zihl J. (1994) Rehabilitation of visual impairments in patients with brain damage, *Low vision: Research and new development in rehabilitation* (A.C. Kooijman, P.L. Looijestijn, J.A. Welling and G.J. van der Wildt, Eds). IOS Press, Amsterdam, pp. 287–295.

Zihl J. (1995a) Eye movement patterns in hemianopic dyslexia, *Brain* **118**, 891–912.

Zihl J. (1995b) Visual scanning behavior in patients with homonymous hemianopia, *Neuropsychologia* **33**, 287–303.

Zihl J. (2000) *Rehabilitation of visual disorders after brain injury.* Psychology Press, Hove, UK.

Zihl J. (2009) Oculomotor scanning performance in subjects with homonymous visual field disorders, *Visual Impairment Res.* **1**, 23–31.

Zihl J., Hebel N. (1997) Patterns of oculomotor scanning in patients with unilateral posterior parietal or frontal lobe damage, *Neuropsychologia* **35**, 893–906.

Zihl J., von Cramon D. (1979) Restitution of visual function in patients with cerebral blindness, *J. Neurol. Neurosurg. Psychiatry* **42**, 312–322.

Zihl J., von Cramon D. (1982) Restitution of visual field in patients with damage to the geniculostriate visual pathway, *Hum. Neurobiol.* **181**, 5–8.

Zihl J., von Cramon D. (1985) Visual field recovery from scotoma in patients with postgeniculate damage. A review of 55 cases, *Brain* **108**, 335–365.

Zihl J., von Cramon D. (1986) *Zerebrale Sehstörungen.* Kohlhammer, Stuttgart, Germany, pp. 87–101.

www.ingramcontent.com/pod-product-compliance
Lightning Source LLC
Chambersburg PA
CBHW071436230926
51846CB00001B/251